2024

Changes | An Insider's View

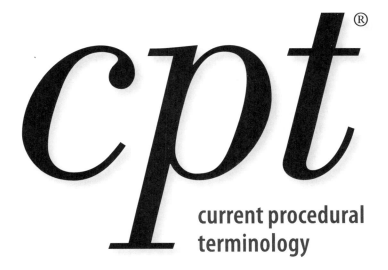

cpt®

current procedural
terminology

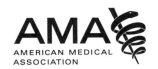

AMA
AMERICAN MEDICAL
ASSOCIATION

Contents

Foreword vii

Using This Book viii

The Symbols viii

The Rationale viii

Reading the Clinical Examples ix

Summary of Additions, Deletions, and Revisions and Indexes ix

CPT Codebook Conventions and Styles ix

Introduction 1

Instructions for Use of the
CPT Codebook 1

▶Audio-Video (Appendix P) and Audio-Only (Appendix T) Telemedicine Services Criteria◀ . . . 2

Unlisted Procedure or Service 3

Time 4

Evaluation and Management 5

Summary of Additions, Deletions, and Revisions 5

Evaluation and Management (E/M) Services Guidelines 7

Classification of Evaluation and Management (E/M) Services 7

Initial and Subsequent Services 7

▶Split or Shared Visits◀ 7

▶Multiple Evaluation and Management Services on the Same Date◀ 8

Levels of E/M Services 9

Guidelines for Selecting Level of Service Based on Medical Decision Making 9

Number and Complexity of Problems Addressed at the Encounter 12

Risk of Complications and/or Morbidity or Mortality of Patient Management 12

Guidelines for Selecting Level of Service Based on Time 13

Office or Other Outpatient Services 15

New Patient 15

Established Patient 15

Hospital Inpatient and Observation Care Services 16

Initial Hospital Inpatient or Observation Care 16

Hospital Inpatient or Observation Care Services (Including Admission and
Discharge Services) 17

Hospital Inpatient or Observation Discharge Services 18

Nursing Facility Services 18

Initial Nursing Facility Care 18

Subsequent Nursing Facility Care 19

Prolonged Services 19

▶Prolonged Service Without Direct Patient Contact on Date Other Than the
Face-to-Face Evaluation and Management Service◀ 19

Prolonged Service With or Without Direct Patient Contact on the Date of an
Evaluation and Management Service 20

Preventive Medicine Services 21

Non-Face-to-Face Services 22

Digitally Stored Data Services/Remote Physiologic Monitoring 22

Contents

Special Evaluation and Management Services 22

    Work Related or Medical Disability Evaluation Services 22

Other Evaluation and Management Services. 22

Surgery 23

Summary of Additions, Deletions, and Revisions 23

Musculoskeletal System. 25

    Spine (Vertebral Column) 25

    Pelvis and Hip Joint 29

    Foot and Toes 30

Respiratory System. 31

    Nose 31

    Accessory Sinuses 31

    Lungs and Pleura. 32

Cardiovascular System. 32

    Heart and Pericardium 32

Digestive System 39

    Stomach 39

Urinary System 39

    Bladder 39

Female Genital System. 41

    Corpus Uteri 41

    Oviduct/Ovary 42

Nervous System 42

    Skull, Meninges, and Brain 42

    Spine and Spinal Cord 44

    Extracranial Nerves, Peripheral Nerves, and Autonomic Nervous System. 45

Eye and Ocular Adnexa. 48

    Ocular Adnexa. 48

Auditory System 49

    Middle Ear. 49

Radiology 51

Summary of Additions, Deletions, and Revisions 51

Diagnostic Radiology (Diagnostic Imaging) 52

    Gynecological and Obstetrical 52

    Heart 52

    Other Procedures 53

Diagnostic Ultrasound 53

    Ultrasonic Guidance Procedures. 53

    Other Procedures 53

Radiation Oncology. 56

    Hyperthermia 56

Pathology and Laboratory **57**

Summary of Additions, Deletions, and Revisions 57

Urinalysis 63

Molecular Pathology. 63

Tier 1 Molecular Pathology Procedures 63

Tier 2 Molecular Pathology Procedures 64

Genomic Sequencing Procedures and Other Molecular Multianalyte Assays 76

Multianalyte Assays with Algorithmic Analyses. 81

Chemistry 82

Hematology and Coagulation 83

Immunology. 84

Transfusion Medicine 86

Microbiology. 86

Anatomic Pathology 87

Postmortem Examination 87

Cytopathology. 87

Cytogenetic Studies 90

Surgical Pathology 90

In Vivo (eg, Transcutaneous) Laboratory Procedures 94

Other Procedures 94

Reproductive Medicine Procedures 94

Proprietary Laboratory Analyses. 94

Medicine. **109**

Summary of Additions, Deletions, and Revisions 109

Immune Globulins, Serum or Recombinant Products. 112

Immunization Administration for Vaccines/Toxoids 113

Vaccines, Toxoids 121

Psychiatry 128

Psychiatric Diagnostic Procedures 128

Gastroenterology 128

Other Procedures 128

Special Otorhinolaryngologic Services. 128

Evaluative and Therapeutic Services 128

Cardiovascular 130

Therapeutic Services and Procedures 130

Cardiography. 133

▶Phrenic Nerve Stimulation System◀ 133

Cardiac Catheterization 135

Intracardiac Electrophysiological Procedures/Studies. 140

Neurology and Neuromuscular Procedures 140

Sleep Medicine Testing 140

Electromyography 141

Nerve Conduction Tests 141

Contents

Hydration, Therapeutic, Prophylactic, Diagnostic Injections and Infusions, and Chemotherapy and Other Highly Complex Drug or Highly Complex Biologic Agent Administration 141

Therapeutic, Prophylactic, and Diagnostic Injections and Infusions (Excludes Chemotherapy and Other Highly Complex Drug or Highly Complex Biologic Agent Administration). 141

Chemotherapy and Other Highly Complex Drug or Highly Complex Biologic Agent Administration 142

Special Dermatological Procedures 143

Physical Medicine and Rehabilitation 144

Modalities. 144

Therapeutic Procedures 144

Category II Codes **149**

Category III Codes. **151**

Summary of Additions, Deletions, and Revisions 151

Appendix K. **201**

Summary of Additions, Deletions, and Revisions 201

Product Pending FDA Approval. 202

Appendix O. **203**

Summary of Additions, Deletions, and Revisions 203

Multianalyte Assays with Algorithmic Analyses and Proprietary Laboratory Analyses. 208

Appendix P. **257**

▶CPT Codes That May Be Used for Synchronous Real-Time Interactive Audio-Video Telemedicine Services◀ 257

Appendix Q. **259**

Severe Acute Respiratory Syndrome Coronavirus 2 (SARS-CoV-2) (coronavirus disease [COVID-19]) Vaccines. 259

Appendix S. **265**

Artificial Intelligence Taxonomy for Medical Services and Procedures 265

Appendix T. **267**

CPT Codes That May Be Used for Synchronous Real-Time Interactive Audio-Only Telemedicine Services. 267

Index **269**

Foreword

The American Medical Association (AMA) is pleased to offer *CPT® Changes 2024: An Insider's View (CPT Changes)*. Since this book was first published in 2000, it has served as the definitive text on additions, revisions, and deletions to the CPT code set.

In developing this book, our intention was to provide CPT users with a glimpse of the logic, rationale, and proposed function of the changes in the CPT code set that resulted from the decisions of the CPT Editorial Panel and the yearly update process. The AMA staff members have the unique perspective of being both participants in the CPT editorial process and users of the CPT code set.

CPT Changes is intended to bridge understanding between clinical decisions made by the CPT Editorial Panel regarding appropriate service or procedure descriptions with functional interpretations of coding guidelines, code intent, and code combinations, which are necessary for users of the CPT code set. A new edition of this book, like the codebook, is published annually.

To assist CPT users in applying the new and revised CPT codes, this book includes clinical examples that describe the typical patient who might undergo the procedure and detailed descriptions of the procedure. Both of these are required as a part of the CPT code change proposal process, which are used by the CPT Editorial Panel in crafting language, guidelines, and parenthetical notes associated with the new or revised codes. In addition, many of the clinical examples and descriptions of the procedures are used in the AMA/Specialty Society Relative Value Scale (RVS) Update (RUC) process to conduct surveys on physician work and to develop work relative value recommendations to the Centers for Medicare & Medicaid Services (CMS) as part of the Medicare physician fee schedule (MPFS).

We are confident that the information provided in *CPT Changes* will prove to be a valuable resource to CPT users, not only as they apply changes for the year of publication, but also as a resource for frequent reference as they continue their education in CPT coding. The AMA makes every effort to be a voice of clarity and consistency in an otherwise confusing system of health care claims and payment, and *CPT Changes 2024: An Insider's View* demonstrates our continued commitment to assist users of the CPT code set.

Using This Book

This book is designed to serve as a reference guide to understanding the changes contained in the Current Procedural Terminology (CPT®) 2024 code set and is not intended to replace the CPT codebook. Every effort is made to ensure accuracy; however, if differences exist, you should always defer to the information in the *CPT® 2024* codebook

The Symbols

This book uses the same coding conventions as those used in the CPT nomenclature.

● Indicates a new procedure number was added to the CPT nomenclature

▲ Indicates a code revision has resulted in a substantially altered procedure descriptor

✛ Indicates a CPT add-on code

⊘ Indicates a code that is exempt from the use of modifier 51 but is not designated as a CPT add-on procedure or service

►◄ Indicates revised guidelines, cross-references, and/or explanatory text

⭢ Indicates a code for a vaccine that is pending FDA approval

\# Indicates a resequenced code. Note that rather than deleting and renumbering, resequencing allows existing codes to be relocated to an appropriate location for the code concept, regardless of the numeric sequence. Numerically placed references (ie, Code is out of numerical sequence. See...) are used as navigational alerts in the CPT codebook to direct the user to the location of an out-of-sequence code. Therefore, remember to refer to the CPT codebook for these references.

★ Indicates a telemedicine code

⌘ Indicates a duplicate PLA test

⇅ Indicates a Category I PLA

◀ Indicates Audio-only Telemedicine Services

Whenever possible, complete segments of text from the CPT codebook are provided; however, in some instances, only pertinent text is included.

The Rationale

After listing each change or series of changes from the CPT codebook, a rationale is provided. The rationale is intended to provide a brief clarification and explanation of the changes. Nevertheless, it is important to note that they may not address every question that may arise as a result of the changes.

Reading the Clinical Examples

The clinical examples and their procedural descriptions, which reflect typical clinical situations found in the healthcare setting, are included in this text with many of the codes to provide practical situations for which the new and/or revised codes in the CPT 2024 code set would be appropriately reported. It is important to note that these examples do not suggest limiting the use of a code; instead, they are meant to represent the typical patient and service or procedure, as previously stated. In addition, they do not describe the universe of patients for whom the service or procedure would be appropriate. It is important also to note that third-party payer reporting policies may differ.

Summary of Additions, Deletions, and Revisions and Indexes

A **summary of additions, deletions, and revisions** for the section is presented in a tabular format at the beginning of each section. This table provides readers with the ability to quickly search and have an overview of all of the new, revised, and deleted codes for 2024. In addition to the tabular review of changes, the coding index individually lists all of the new, revised, and deleted codes with each code's status (new, revised, deleted) in parentheses. For more information about these indexes, please read the Instructions for the **Use of the Changes Indexes** on page 269.

CPT Codebook Conventions and Styles

Similar to the CPT codebook, the guidelines and revised and new CPT code descriptors and parenthetical notes in *CPT Changes 2024* are set in green type. Any revised text, guidelines, and/or headings are indicated with the ▶◀ symbols. To match the style used in the codebook, the revised or new text symbol is placed at the beginning and end of a paragraph or section that contains revisions, and the use of green text visually indicates new and/or revised content. Similarly, each section's and subsections' (Surgery) complete code range is listed in the tabs, regardless of whether these codes are discussed in this book. In addition, all of the different level of headings in the codebook are also picked up, as appropriate, and set in the same style and color. Besides matching the convention and style used in the CPT codebook, the Rationales are placed within a shaded box to distinguish them from the rest of the content for quick and easy reference.

Introduction

Current Procedural Terminology (CPT®), Fourth Edition, is a set of codes, descriptions, and guidelines intended to describe procedures and services performed by physicians and other qualified health care professionals, or entities. Each procedure or service is identified with a five-digit code. The use of CPT codes simplifies the reporting of procedures and services. In the CPT code set, the term "procedure" is used to describe services, including diagnostic tests.

Inclusion of a descriptor and its associated five-digit code number in the CPT Category I code set is based on whether the procedure or service is consistent with contemporary medical practice and is performed by many practitioners in clinical practice in multiple locations. Inclusion in the CPT code set of a procedure or service, or proprietary name, does not represent endorsement by the American Medical Association (AMA) of any particular diagnostic or therapeutic procedure or service or proprietary test or manufacturer. Inclusion or exclusion of a procedure or service, or proprietary name, does not imply any health insurance coverage or reimbursement policy.

The main body of the Category I section is listed in six sections. Each section is divided into subsections with anatomic, procedural, condition, or descriptor subheadings. The procedures and services with their identifying codes are presented in numeric order with the exception of the resequenced codes and the entire **Evaluation and Management** section (99202-99499), which appears at the beginning of the listed procedures. The evaluation and management codes are used by most physicians in reporting a significant portion of their services.

Instructions for Use of the CPT Codebook

▶Select the CPT code of the procedure or service that accurately identifies the procedure or service performed. Do not select a CPT code that merely approximates the procedure or service provided. If no such specific code exists, then report the procedure or service using the appropriate unlisted procedure or service code. When using an unlisted code, any modifying or extenuating circumstances should be adequately and accurately documented in the medical record.◀

It is equally important to recognize that as techniques in medicine and surgery have evolved, new types of services, including minimally invasive surgery, as well as endovascular, percutaneous, and endoscopic interventions have challenged the traditional distinction of Surgery vs Medicine. Thus, the listing of a service or procedure in a

specific section of this book should not be interpreted as strictly classifying the service or procedure as "surgery" or "not surgery" for insurance or other purposes. The placement of a given service in a specific section of the book may reflect historical or other considerations (eg, placement of the percutaneous peripheral vascular endovascular interventions in the Surgery/Cardiovascular System section, while the percutaneous coronary interventions appear in the Medicine/Cardiovascular section).

When advanced practice nurses and physician assistants are working with physicians, they are considered as working in the exact same specialty and subspecialty as the physician. A "physician or other qualified health care professional" is an individual who is qualified by education, training, licensure/regulation (when applicable), and facility privileging (when applicable) who performs a professional service within his/her scope of practice and independently reports that professional service. These professionals are distinct from "clinical staff." A clinical staff member is a person who works under the supervision of a physician or other qualified health care professional and who is allowed by law, regulation, and facility policy to perform or assist in the performance of a specified professional service but who does not individually report that professional service. Other policies may also affect who may report specific services.

Throughout the CPT code set the use of terms such as "physician," "qualified health care professional," or "individual" is not intended to indicate that other entities may not report the service. In selected instances, specific instructions may define a service as limited to professionals or limited to other entities (eg, hospital or home health agency).

Instructions, typically included as parenthetical notes with selected codes, indicate that a code should not be reported with another code or codes. These instructions are intended to prevent errors of significant probability and are not all inclusive. For example, the code with such instructions may be a component of another code and therefore it would be incorrect to report both codes even when the component service is performed. These instructions are not intended as a listing of all possible code combinations that should not be reported, nor do they indicate all possible code combinations that are appropriately reported. When reporting codes for services provided, it is important to assure the accuracy and quality of coding through verification of the intent of the code by use of the related guidelines, parenthetical instructions, and coding resources, including CPT Assistant and other publications resulting from collaborative efforts of the American Medical Association with the medical specialty societies (ie, Clinical Examples in Radiology).

▶Because Category I or Category III codes may incorporate multiple components (bundled) that could be reported separately with other existing codes, "unbundling" of codes into their component parts for reporting purposes or combining those components with an unlisted code is inappropriate. For example, it would be inappropriate to separately report both codes 42825, *Tonsillectomy, primary or secondary; younger than age 12,* and 42830, *Adenoidectomy, primary; younger than age 12,* for removal of the tonsils and adenoids, because these two procedures are reported together using code 42820, *Tonsillectomy and adenoidectomy; younger than age 12.* Multiple Category I or Category III codes may be reported together to describe the totality of service rendered for a given patient encounter if they represent separately reportable services. Individual components of a procedure or service specified as part of a Category I or Category III code descriptor are reported neither separately with an existing CPT code nor with an unlisted code. Procedural steps necessary to reach the operative site and to close the operative site are also not reported separately, unless otherwise instructed by CPT guidelines or parenthetical notes. For example, a laparoscopic cholecystectomy should not be reported together with a code for the incision or a code for the repair of the surgical wound because these are inherent procedural steps needed to accomplish the cholecystectomy. However, if an excision of a benign lesion requires a complex repair for closure, both the lesion excision and the complex repair code are reported separately because the Repair (Closure) Guidelines indicate that "complex repair does not include excision of benign (11400-11446) or malignant (11600-11646) lesions."◀

Rationale

In accordance with the changes for reporting unlisted procedures or services, the guidelines in the Instructions for Use of the CPT Codebook section have been revised to accommodate and synchronize the changes regarding reporting unlisted codes. The revised guideline language reiterates how Category I and Category III codes are intended to be reported, instruction regarding the use of multiple codes to identify multiple services provided, and use of a single code when multiple services have been combined and presented within a single code. The guidelines also provide instructions that warn against the use of an unlisted code to identify individual components of a larger service or procedure.

▶Audio-Video (Appendix P) and Audio-Only (Appendix T) Telemedicine Services Criteria◀

▶The following criteria are used by the Current Procedural Terminology/Health Care Professional Advisory Committee (CPT/HCPAC) and the CPT Editorial Panel for evaluating inclusion of services in Appendix P (synchronous audio-video) and Appendix T (synchronous audio-only) telemedicine services. Any request for inclusion in Appendix P and Appendix T must satisfy the following criteria:

- The totality and quality of the communication of information exchanged between the physician or other qualified health care professional (QHP) and the patient during the synchronous telemedicine service must be of an amount and a nature that would be sufficient to meet the requirements for the same service if services were to be rendered during an in-person face-to-face interaction; *and*

  o The evidence supports the benefits of performing the service through telecommunications technology. These benefits may include, but are not limited to, the following:

  o Facilitate a diagnosis or treatment plan that may reduce complications

  o Decrease diagnostic or therapeutic interventions

  o Decrease hospitalizations

  o Decrease in-person visits to the emergency department

  o Decrease in-person visits to physician or other QHP offices, including urgent care centers

  o Increase rapidity of resolution

  o Decrease quantifiable symptoms

  o Reduce recovery time

  o Enhance access to care, such as for rural and vulnerable patients; *and*

- A service is ineligible for inclusion in Appendix T without also being requested for inclusion, or has current inclusion, in Appendix P.

(For a listing of CPT codes that may be used for synchronous real-time interactive audio-video telemedicine services when appended with modifier 95, see Appendix P)

(For a listing of CPT codes that may be used for synchronous real-time interactive audio-only telemedicine services when appended with modifier 93, see Appendix T)◀

Rationale

For the CPT 2024 code set, new criteria for inclusion of CPT codes in Appendixes P and T have been established, the title of Appendix P has been revised, and a new heading in the introduction section that includes specific criteria for audio-visual (Appendix P) and audio-only (Appendix T) telemedicine services has been added. In addition, guideline changes have been made for both Appendixes P and T to clarify criteria and services necessary for reporting these codes.

As more services are performed via synchronous real-time interactive audio-visual and audio-only telemedicine, the CPT Editorial Panel (the Panel) required that objective criteria be included to determine services that may be included only in Appendix P or in both Appendixes P and T. A workgroup was formed by the Panel Chair to develop objective criteria for the Panel to use for the purpose of maintaining the list of CPT codes listed in Appendixes P and T.

The changes to these sections include:

- Addition of new criteria for inclusion of services in Appendix P (synchronous audio-video) and Appendix T (synchronous audio-only) telemedicine services

- Revisions to Appendixes P and T to include adding "are typically rendered in-person but"

- Revisions to the Appendix P heading to include "Real-Time Interactive Audio-Video"

- Addition of the term "audio-visual" throughout the code set to align with the revision of the Appendix P heading.

Unlisted Procedure or Service

▶Category I and Category III codes describe the vast majority of procedures and services currently performed in the United States and should be used to report these procedures and services that are accurately described in existing CPT codes. It is recognized that there may be services or procedures performed by physicians or other qualified health care professionals (QHPs) that are not found in the CPT code set. Therefore, a number of specific code numbers have been designated for reporting unlisted procedures. When an unlisted procedure code is used, the service or procedure should be described (see specific section guidelines). Each of these unlisted codes (with the appropriate accompanying topical entry) relates to a specific section of the code set and is presented in the guidelines of that section.

The CPT code set's instructions to use an unlisted procedure code do not preclude the reporting of an appropriate code that may be found elsewhere in the CPT code set. It may be appropriate to report multiple Category I or Category III codes together to describe the totality of a service rendered for a given patient encounter, provided each code represents a separately reportable service. Similarly, it is appropriate to report an unlisted code together with a Category I or Category III code(s) for the same patient encounter on the same date of service when a separately reportable portion of a provided procedure or service is not described by an existing CPT code(s).

Example

Reporting unlisted code(s) with Category I code(s): When both radiofrequency ablation of the greater saphenous vein and stab phlebectomy using less than 10 incisions are performed in the same operative session, both codes 36475, *Endovenous ablation therapy of incompetent vein, extremity, inclusive of all imaging guidance and monitoring, percutaneous, radiofrequency; first vein treated,* and 37799, *Unlisted procedure, vascular surgery,* may be reported because there is no code for stab phlebectomy with less than 10 incisions.

While uncommon, if multiple separately reportable unlisted services are performed on the same patient on the same date of service by the same physician or other QHP, then multiple unlisted codes may be reported. If the two procedures are performed in the same anatomic region, then multiple units of the same unlisted code may be reported with modifier 59 appended to the additional unit(s). If two unlisted services are performed in two different anatomic regions, then two different unlisted codes may be reported.

Example

Reporting multiple separately reportable unlisted services: If two unlisted arthroscopic procedures are performed on two separate joints by the same surgeon on the same date of service, then two units of 29999, *Unlisted procedure, arthroscopy,* may be reported with modifier 59 appended to the second unit.

Note that unlisted codes are not used to separately report component(s) of an existing Category I or Category III service.

Example

It would not be appropriate to use 39599, *Unlisted procedure, diaphragm,* to separately report suturing of the diaphragm performed as a component of a paraesophageal hernia repair, which is reported with code 43281, *Laparoscopy, surgical, repair of paraesophageal hernia, includes fundoplasty, when performed; without implantation of mesh.*

Because unlisted codes do not include descriptor language that specifies the components of a particular service, modifiers that describe alteration of a service or procedure may not be used. For example, it would not be appropriate to append modifier 52, *Reduced Services,* to an unlisted code. However, modifiers to indicate laterality (ie, modifier 50, *Bilateral Procedure*); distinction (ie, modifier 59, *Distinct Procedural Service*); assistant-at-surgery (modifier 80, *Assistant Surgeon*); and place of service (eg, modifier 95, *Synchronous Telemedicine Service Rendered Via a Real-Time Interactive Audio and Video Telecommunications System;* modifier 93, *Synchronous telemedicine service rendered via telephone or other real-time interactive audio-only telecommunications system*), may be used, when indicated.◀

Rationale

Several changes have been made regarding the reporting of unlisted procedures, including the number of times the codes may be used, what the codes may be reported with, and how the codes may be reported. In addition, separate instructions have been included within separate subsections of the code set to accommodate direction regarding reporting.

Historically, unlisted codes have been used solely as a mechanism for reporting a procedure that was undescribed by any existing Category I or Category III codes. This included all procedural work performed during the session.

However, over time, medicine and procedures have evolved. As a result, mechanisms for reporting procedures that are not specifically identified within the CPT code set have changed as well. This includes development of updated methods of reporting unlisted services when separate work effort is performed for two or more procedures that do not have a specific CPT code. It also involves allowance of reporting undescribed work in conjunction with service(s) that may have specific CPT codes, whether it is Category I or Category III. Lastly, on many occasions, it may be appropriate to report multiple unlisted codes together and existing modifiers to further explain the circumstances for reporting. The revisions included in the code set address these issues.

Revisions to the Unlisted Procedure or Service guidelines reflect: (1) addition of language that reiterates intended use of the Category I and Category III codes (including how to report multiple Category I or Category III codes together); (2) revision to language to reiterate that unlisted codes are used only when no existing Category I or Category III code exists for the service or procedure; (3) allowance for the use of unlisted codes in conjunction with Category I or Category III services (with examples regarding reporting); and (4) an explanation regarding when modifiers may or may not be used in conjunction with unlisted codes. In addition, guidelines within certain subsections in the Pathology and Laboratory section have

been updated to direct users to the appropriate Category I, Category III, or unlisted code(s), depending on the services performed.

Time

▶The CPT code set contains many codes with a time basis for code selection. The following standards shall apply to time measurement, unless there are code or code-range–specific instructions in guidelines, parenthetical instructions, or code descriptors to the contrary. Time is the face-to-face time with the patient. Phrases such as "interpretation and report" in the code descriptor are not intended to indicate in all cases that report writing is part of the reported time. A unit of time is attained when the mid-point is passed. For example, an hour is attained when 31 minutes have elapsed (more than midway between zero and 60 minutes). A second hour is attained when a total of 91 minutes has elapsed. The evaluation and management (E/M) codes that use total time on the date of the encounter have a required time threshold for time-based reporting; therefore, the mid-point concept does not apply. See also the **Evaluation and Management (E/M) Services Guidelines**. When another service is performed concurrently with a time-based service, the time associated with the concurrent service should not be included in the time used for reporting the time-based service. Some services measured in units other than days extend across calendar dates. When this occurs, a continuous service does not reset and create a first hour. However, any disruption in the service does create a new initial service. For example, if intravenous hydration (96360, 96361) is given from 11 pm to 2 am, 96360 would be reported once and 96361 twice. For facility reporting on a single date of service or for continuous services that last beyond midnight (ie, over a range of dates), report the total units of time provided continuously.◀

Rationale

In accordance with the revision of changing the time range associated with each code to a time threshold that must be met or exceeded for codes 99202-99205 and 99212-99215, the Time guidelines in the Instructions for Use of the CPT Codebook have been revised to reflect these changes.

Refer to the codebook and the Rationale for codes 99202-99205 and 99212-99215 for a full discussion of these changes.

★ = Telemedicine   ◀ = Audio-only   ✚ = Add-on code   ⟋ = FDA approval pending   # = Resequenced code   ⊘ = Modifier 51 exempt

Evaluation and Management

Summary of Additions, Deletions, and Revisions

The summary of changes shows the actual changes that have been made to the code descriptors.

New codes appear with a bullet (●) and are indicated as "Code added." Revised codes are preceded with a triangle (▲). Within revised codes, or if a code symbol has been deleted, the deleted language and code symbol appear with a ~~strikethrough~~, while new text appears <u>underlined</u>.

The ⟋ symbol is used to identify codes for vaccines that are pending FDA approval. The # symbol is used to identify codes that have been resequenced. CPT add-on codes are annotated by the ✚ symbol. The ⊘ symbol is used to identify codes that are exempt from the use of modifier 51. The ★ symbol is used to identify codes that may be used for reporting telemedicine services. The ✕ is used to identify proprietary laboratory analyses (PLA) test that has an identical descriptor as another PLA test. A PLA code that satisfies Category I code criteria and has been accepted by the CPT Editorial Panel is annotated with the ↑↓ symbol. The ◀ symbol is used to identify codes that may be used to report audio-only telemedicine services when appended by modifier 93 (see Appendix T).

Code	Description
★▲99202	**Office or other outpatient visit** for the evaluation and management of a new patient, which requires a medically appropriate history and/or examination and straightforward medical decision making. When using <u>total</u> time <u>on the date of the encounter</u> for code selection, 15-~~29 minutes of total time is spent on the date of the encounter~~ <u>minutes must be met or exceeded</u>.
★▲99203	**Office or other outpatient visit** for the evaluation and management of a new patient, which requires a medically appropriate history and/or examination and low level of medical decision making. When using <u>total</u> time <u>on the date of the encounter</u> for code selection, 30-~~44 minutes of total time is spent on the date of the encounter~~ <u>minutes must be met or exceeded</u>.
★▲99204	**Office or other outpatient visit** for the evaluation and management of a new patient, which requires a medically appropriate history and/or examination and moderate level of medical decision making. When using <u>total</u> time <u>on the date of the encounter</u> for code selection, 45-~~59 minutes of total time is spent on the date of the encounter~~ <u>minutes must be met or exceeded</u>.
★▲99205	**Office or other outpatient visit** for the evaluation and management of a new patient, which requires a medically appropriate history and/or examination and high level of medical decision making. When using <u>total</u> time <u>on the date of the encounter</u> for code selection, 60-~~74 minutes of total time is spent on the date of the encounter~~ <u>minutes must be met or exceeded</u>.
★▲99212	**Office or other outpatient visit** for the evaluation and management of an established patient, which requires a medically appropriate history and/or examination and straightforward medical decision making. When using <u>total</u> time <u>on the date of the encounter</u> for code selection, 10-~~19 minutes of total time is spent on the date of the encounter~~ <u>minutes must be met or exceeded</u>.
★▲99213	**Office or other outpatient visit** for the evaluation and management of an established patient, which requires a medically appropriate history and/or examination and low level of medical decision making. When using <u>total</u> time <u>on the date of the encounter</u> for code selection, 20-~~29 minutes of total time is spent on the date of the encounter~~ <u>minutes must be met or exceeded</u>.

Code	Description
★▲99214	**Office or other outpatient visit** for the evaluation and management of an established patient, which requires a medically appropriate history and/or examination and moderate level of medical decision making.
	When using <u>total</u> time <u>on the date of the encounter</u> for code selection, 30~~-39 minutes of total time is spent on the date of the encounter~~ <u>minutes must be met or exceeded</u>.
★▲99215	**Office or other outpatient visit** for the evaluation and management of an established patient, which requires a medically appropriate history and/or examination and high level of medical decision making.
	When using <u>total</u> time <u>on the date of the encounter</u> for code selection, 40~~-54 minutes of total time is spent on the date of the encounter~~ <u>minutes must be met or exceeded</u>.
▲99306	Initial nursing facility care, per day, for the evaluation and management of a patient, which requires a medically appropriate history and/or examination and high level of medical decision making.
	When using total time on the date of the encounter for code selection, ~~45~~<u>50</u> minutes must be met or exceeded.
★▲99308	Subsequent nursing facility care, per day, for the evaluation and management of a patient, which requires a medically appropriate history and/or examination and low level of medical decision making.
	When using total time on the date of the encounter for code selection, ~~15~~<u>20</u> minutes must be met or exceeded.
#+●99459	Code added

★=Telemedicine   ◀=Audio-only   +=Add-on code   ✒=FDA approval pending   #=Resequenced code   ⃠=Modifier 51 exempt

Evaluation and Management (E/M) Services Guidelines

Classification of Evaluation and Management (E/M) Services

Initial and Subsequent Services

Some categories apply to both new and established patients (eg, hospital inpatient or observation care). These categories differentiate services by whether the service is the initial service or a subsequent service. For the purpose of distinguishing between initial or subsequent visits, professional services are those face-to-face services rendered by physicians and other qualified health care professionals who may report evaluation and management services. An initial service is when the patient has not received any professional services from the physician or other qualified health care professional or another physician or other qualified health care professional of the exact same specialty and subspecialty who belongs to the same group practice, during the inpatient, observation, or nursing facility admission and stay.

A subsequent service is when the patient has received professional service(s) from the physician or other qualified health care professional or another physician or other qualified health care professional of the exact same specialty and subspecialty who belongs to the same group practice, during the admission and stay.

In the instance when a physician or other qualified health care professional is on call for or covering for another physician or other qualified health care professional, the patient's encounter will be classified as it would have been by the physician or other qualified health care professional who is not available. When advanced practice nurses and physician assistants are working with physicians, they are considered as working in the exact same specialty and subspecialty as the physician.

For reporting hospital inpatient or observation care services, a stay that includes a transition from observation to inpatient is a single stay. For reporting nursing facility services, a stay that includes transition(s) between skilled nursing facility and nursing facility level of care is the same stay.

▶Split or Shared Visits◀

▶Physician(s) and other qualified health care professional(s) (QHP[s]) may act as a team in providing care for the patient, working together during a single E/M service. The split or shared visits guidelines are applied to determine which professional may report the service. If the physician or other QHP performs a substantive portion of the encounter, the physician or other QHP may report the service. If code selection is based on total time on the date of the encounter, the service is reported by the professional who spent the majority of the face-to-face or non-face-to-face time performing the service. For the purpose of reporting E/M services within the context of team-based care, performance of a substantive part of the MDM requires that the physician(s) or other QHP(s) made or approved the management plan for the *number and complexity of problems addressed at the encounter* and takes responsibility for that plan with its inherent *risk of complications and/or morbidity or mortality of patient management*. By doing so, a physician or other QHP has performed two of the three elements used in the selection of the code level based on MDM. If *the amount and/or complexity of data to be reviewed and analyzed* is used by the physician or other QHP to determine the reported code level, assessing an independent historian's narrative and the ordering or review of tests or documents do not have to be personally performed by the physician or other QHP, because the relevant items would be considered in formulating the management plan. Independent interpretation of tests and discussion of management plan or test interpretation must be personally performed by the physician or other QHP if these are used to determine the reported code level by the physician or other QHP.◀

Rationale

A new subsection, "Split or Shared Visits," has been added to the Classification of Evaluation and Management (E/M) Services subsection. Discussion of split or shared visits was initially added to the E/M guidelines in the CPT 2021 code set, which addressed reporting split or shared visits using time for code-level selection; however, it did not address code-level selection using medical decision making (MDM). In 2024, the instructions for split or shared E/M visits have been expanded to clarify appropriate reporting of split or shared visits using either time or MDM for code-level selection. In addition, the revised reporting instructions are now consistent with the Centers for Medicare & Medicaid Services (CMS) policy to reduce the administrative burden for physicians and other qualified health care professionals (QHPs).

When time is used for code selection for an E/M service at which two professionals (ie, physicians and other QHPs) act as a team, the E/M service is reported by the professional who spent the majority of the time (ie, the substantive portion of the time) performing the service. When MDM is used for code selection, the professional who made or approved the patient's management plan for the *number and complexity of problems addressed at the encounter* and takes responsibility for that plan with its inherent *risk of complications and/or morbidity or mortality of patient management* (ie, the substantive part of the MDM) should report the E/M service.

►Multiple Evaluation and Management Services on the Same Date◄

►The following guidelines apply to services that a patient may receive for hospital inpatient care, observation care, or nursing facility care. For instructions regarding transitions to these settings from the office or outpatient, home or residence, or emergency department setting, see guidelines for **Hospital Inpatient and Observation Care Services** or **Nursing Facility Services**.

A patient may receive E/M services in more than one setting on a calendar date. A patient may also have more than one visit in the same setting on a calendar date. The guidelines for multiple E/M services on the same date address circumstances in which the patient has received multiple visits or services from the same physician or other QHP or another physician or other QHP of the exact same specialty and subspecialty who belongs to the same group practice.

Per day: The hospital inpatient and observation care services and the nursing facility services are "per day" services. When multiple visits occur over the course of a single calendar date in the same setting, a single service is reported. When using MDM for code level selection, use the aggregated MDM over the course of the calendar date. When using time for code level selection, sum the time over the course of the day using the guidelines for reporting time.

Multiple encounters in different settings or facilities: A patient may be seen and treated in different facilities (eg, a hospital-to-hospital transfer). When more than one primary E/M service is reported and time is used to select the code level for either service, only the time spent providing that individual service may be allocated to the code level selected for reporting that service. No time may be counted twice when reporting more than one E/M service. Prolonged services are also based on the same allocation and their relationship to the primary service. The designation of the facility may be defined by

licensure or regulation. Transfer from a hospital bed to a nursing facility bed in a hospital with nursing facility beds is considered as two services in two facilities because there is a discharge from one type of designation to another. An intra-facility transfer for a different level of care (eg, from a routine unit to a critical care unit) does not constitute a new stay, nor does it constitute a transfer to a different facility.

Emergency department (ED) and services in other settings (same or different facilities): Time spent in an ED by a physician or other QHP who provides subsequent E/M services may be included in calculating total time on the date of the encounter when ED services are not reported and another E/M service is reported (eg, hospital inpatient and observation care services).

Discharge services and services in other facilities: Each service may be reported separately as long as any time spent on the discharge service is not counted towards the total time of a subsequent service in which code level selection for the subsequent service is based on time. This includes any hospital inpatient or observation care services (including admission and discharge services) time (99234, 99235, 99236) because these services may be selected based on MDM or time. When these services are reported with another E/M service on the same calendar date, time related to the hospital inpatient or observation care service (including admission and discharge services) may not be used for code selection of the subsequent service.

Discharge services and services in the same facility: If the patient is discharged and readmitted to the same facility on the same calendar date, report a subsequent care service instead of a discharge or initial service. For the purpose of E/M reporting, this is a single stay.

Discharge services and services in a different facility: If the patient is admitted to another facility, for the purpose of E/M reporting this is considered a different stay. Discharge and initial services may be reported as long as time spent on the discharge service is not counted towards the total time of the subsequent service reported when code level selection is based on time.

Critical care services (including neonatal intensive care services and pediatric and neonatal critical care): Reporting guidelines for intensive and critical care services that are performed on the same calendar date as another E/M service are described in the service specific section guidelines.

Transitions between office or other outpatient, home or residence, or emergency department and hospital inpatient or observation or nursing facility: See the guidelines for **Hospital Inpatient and Observation Care Services** or **Nursing Facility Services.** If the patient is seen in two settings and only one service is reported, the total time on the date of the encounter or the aggregated MDM is used for determining the level of the single reported service. If prolonged services are reported, use the prolonged services code that is appropriate for the primary service reported, regardless of where the patient was located when the prolonged services time threshold was met. The choice of the primary service is at the discretion of the reporting physician or other QHP.◀

Rationale

A new subsection, "Multiple Evaluation and Management Services on the Same Date," has been added to the Classification of Evaluation and Management (E/M) Services subsection. The new guidelines for multiple E/M services rendered on the same date provide definitions and reporting instructions when more than one E/M service is provided by the same physician or other QHP or another physician or other QHP of the exact same specialty and subspecialty who belongs to the same practice to a patient in different settings or facilities on the same date.

Hospital inpatient or observation services codes and nursing facility services codes are per-day codes; therefore, they may be reported only once per day, even if the physician or other QHP provides more than one of these services in the same setting. However, when multiple services are provided in *different* settings or facilities on the same date by the same physician or other QHP, each of the services may be reported. The new guidelines provide reporting instructions for the following circumstances in which multiple E/M services are provided to a patient *on the same date:*

- Multiple services in the same setting or facility

- Multiple services in different settings or facilities

- Emergency department (ED) services and services in other settings

- Discharge and readmission to the same facility

- Discharge from one facility and admission to another facility

- Critical care services with other E/M services

- Transition between outpatient, home, or ED and hospital inpatient and observation care services or nursing facility services

The addition of the new subsection is part of the overall effort to provide further reporting clarification in the E/M guidelines.

Levels of E/M Services

Guidelines for Selecting Level of Service Based on Medical Decision Making

Four types of MDM are recognized: straightforward, low, moderate, and high. The concept of the level of MDM does not apply to 99211, 99281.

MDM includes establishing diagnoses, assessing the status of a condition, and/or selecting a management option. MDM is defined by three elements. The elements are:

- *The number and complexity of problem(s) that are addressed during the encounter.*

- *The amount and/or complexity of data to be reviewed and analyzed.* These data include medical records, tests, and/or other information that must be obtained, ordered, reviewed, and analyzed for the encounter. This includes information obtained from multiple sources or interprofessional communications that are not reported separately and interpretation of tests that are not reported separately. Ordering a test is included in the category of test result(s) and the review of the test result is part of the encounter and not a subsequent encounter. Ordering a test may include those considered but not selected after shared decision making. For example, a patient may request diagnostic imaging that is not necessary for their condition and discussion of the lack of benefit may be required. Alternatively, a test may normally be performed, but due to the risk for a specific patient it is not ordered. These considerations must be documented. Data are divided into three categories:

- Tests, documents, orders, or independent historian(s). (Each unique test, order, or document is counted to meet a threshold number.)

- Independent interpretation of tests (not separately reported).

- Discussion of management or test interpretation with external physician or other qualified health care professional or appropriate source (not separately reported).

- *The risk of complications and/or morbidity or mortality of patient management.* This includes decisions made at the encounter associated with diagnostic procedure(s) and treatment(s). This includes the possible management options selected and those considered but not selected after shared decision making with the patient and/or family. For example, a decision about hospitalization includes consideration of alternative levels of care. Examples may include a psychiatric patient with a sufficient degree of support in the outpatient setting or the decision to not hospitalize a patient with advanced dementia with an acute condition that would generally warrant inpatient care, but for whom the goal is palliative treatment.

Shared decision making involves eliciting patient and/or family preferences, patient and/or family education, and explaining risks and benefits of management options.

MDM may be impacted by role and management responsibility.

When the physician or other qualified health care professional is reporting a separate CPT code that includes interpretation and/or report, the interpretation and/or report is not counted toward the MDM when selecting a level of E/M services. When the physician or other qualified health care professional is reporting a separate service for discussion of management with a physician or another qualified health care professional, the discussion is not counted toward the MDM when selecting a level of E/M services.

The Levels of Medical Decision Making (MDM) table (Table 1) is a guide to assist in selecting the level of MDM for reporting an E/M services code. The table includes the four levels of MDM (ie, straightforward, low, moderate, high) and the three elements of MDM (ie, number and complexity of problems addressed at the encounter, amount and/or complexity of data reviewed

and analyzed, and risk of complications and/or morbidity or mortality of patient management). To qualify for a particular level of MDM, two of the three elements for that level of MDM must be met or exceeded.

Examples in the table may be more or less applicable to specific settings of care. For example, the decision to hospitalize applies to the outpatient or nursing facility encounters, whereas the decision to escalate hospital level of care (eg, transfer to ICU) applies to the hospitalized or observation care patient. See also the introductory guidelines of each code family section.

▶The elements listed in Table 1, Levels of Medical Decision Making, are defined in the guidelines for number and complexity of problems addressed at the encounter, amount and/or complexity of data to be reviewed and analyzed, and risk of complications and/or morbidity or mortality of patient management.◀

▶Table 1: Levels of Medical Decision Making (MDM)◀

	▶Elements of Medical Decision Making		
Level of MDM (Based on 2 out of 3 Elements of MDM)	**Number and Complexity of Problems Addressed at the Encounter**	**Amount and/or Complexity of Data to Be Reviewed and Analyzed** *Each unique test, order, or document contributes to the combination of 2 or combination of 3 in Category 1 below.*	**Risk of Complications and/or Morbidity or Mortality of Patient Management**
Straightforward	**Minimal** ■ **1** self-limited or minor problem	**Minimal or none**	**Minimal risk of morbidity from additional diagnostic testing or treatment**
Low	**Low** ■ **2** or more self-limited or minor problems; or ■ **1** stable, chronic illness; or ■ **1** acute, uncomplicated illness or injury; or ■ **1** stable, acute illness; or ■ **1** acute, uncomplicated illness or injury requiring hospital inpatient or observation level of care	**Limited** *(Must meet the requirements of at least 1 out of 2 categories)* **Category 1: Tests and documents** ■ **Any combination of 2 from the following:** • Review of prior external note(s) from each unique source*; • Review of the result(s) of each unique test*; • Ordering of each unique test* **or** **Category 2: Assessment requiring an independent historian(s)** *(For the categories of independent interpretation of tests and discussion of management or test interpretation, see moderate or high)*	**Low risk of morbidity from additional diagnostic testing or treatment**

Elements of Medical Decision Making

Level of MDM (Based on 2 out of 3 Elements of MDM)	Number and Complexity of Problems Addressed at the Encounter	Amount and/or Complexity of Data to Be Reviewed and Analyzed *Each unique test, order, or document contributes to the combination of 2 or combination of 3 in Category 1 below.*	Risk of Complications and/or Morbidity or Mortality of Patient Management
Moderate	**Moderate** ■ **1** or more chronic illnesses with exacerbation, progression, or side effects of treatment; **or** ■ **2** or more stable, chronic illnesses; **or** ■ **1** undiagnosed new problem with uncertain prognosis; **or** ■ **1** acute illness with systemic symptoms; **or** ■ **1** acute, complicated injury	**Moderate** *(Must meet the requirements of at least 1 out of 3 categories)* **Category 1: Tests, documents, or independent historian(s)** ■ **Any combination of 3 from the following:** • Review of prior external note(s) from each unique source*; • Review of the result(s) of each unique test*; • Ordering of each unique test*; • Assessment requiring an independent historian(s) **or** **Category 2: Independent interpretation of tests** ■ Independent interpretation of a test performed by another physician/other qualified health care professional (not separately reported); **or** **Category 3: Discussion of management or test interpretation** ■ Discussion of management or test interpretation with external physician/other qualified health care professional/appropriate source (not separately reported)	**Moderate risk of morbidity from additional diagnostic testing or treatment** *Examples only:* ■ Prescription drug management ■ Decision regarding minor surgery with identified patient or procedure risk factors ■ Decision regarding elective major surgery without identified patient or procedure risk factors ■ Diagnosis or treatment significantly limited by social determinants of health
High	**High** ■ **1** or more chronic illnesses with severe exacerbation, progression, or side effects of treatment; **or** ■ **1** acute or chronic illness or injury that poses a threat to life or bodily function	**Extensive** *(Must meet the requirements of at least 2 out of 3 categories)* **Category 1: Tests, documents, or independent historian(s)** ■ **Any combination of 3 from the following:** • Review of prior external note(s) from each unique source*; • Review of the result(s) of each unique test*; • Ordering of each unique test*; • Assessment requiring an independent historian(s) **or** **Category 2: Independent interpretation of tests** ■ Independent interpretation of a test performed by another physician/other qualified health care professional (not separately reported); **or** **Category 3: Discussion of management or test interpretation** ■ Discussion of management or test interpretation with external physician/other qualified health care professional/appropriate source (not separately reported)	**High risk of morbidity from additional diagnostic testing or treatment** *Examples only:* ■ Drug therapy requiring intensive monitoring for toxicity ■ Decision regarding elective major surgery with identified patient or procedure risk factors ■ Decision regarding emergency major surgery ■ Decision regarding hospitalization or escalation of hospital-level care ■ Decision not to resuscitate or to de-escalate care because of poor prognosis ■ Decision regarding parenteral controlled substances ◄

Evaluation / Management 99202-99499

Rationale

Two editorial changes have been made to Table 1: Levels of Medical Decision Making (MDM). An introductory sentence has been added to inform users that definitions for the elements listed in the table are provided in the E/M Guidelines. In addition, the example, "Parenteral controlled substances," has been revised to "*Decision regarding* parenteral controlled substances," so it is consistent with the other listed examples in the "High risk of morbidity from additional diagnostic testing or treatment" column. These changes are part of the overall effort to provide further reporting clarification in the E/M guidelines.

Number and Complexity of Problems Addressed at the Encounter

One element used in selecting the level of service is the number and complexity of the problems that are addressed at the encounter. Multiple new or established conditions may be addressed at the same time and may affect MDM. Symptoms may cluster around a specific diagnosis and each symptom is not necessarily a unique condition. Comorbidities and underlying diseases, in and of themselves, are not considered in selecting a level of E/M services **unless** they are addressed, and their presence increases the amount and/or complexity of data to be reviewed and analyzed or the risk of complications and/or morbidity or mortality of patient management. The final diagnosis for a condition does not, in and of itself, determine the complexity or risk, as extensive evaluation may be required to reach the conclusion that the signs or symptoms do not represent a highly morbid condition. Therefore, presenting symptoms that are likely to represent a highly morbid condition may "drive" MDM even when the ultimate diagnosis is not highly morbid. The evaluation and/or treatment should be consistent with the likely nature of the condition. Multiple problems of a lower severity may, in the aggregate, create higher risk due to interaction.

▶The term "risk" as used in the definition of this element relates to risk from the condition. While condition risk and management risk may often correlate, the risk from the condition is distinct from the risk of the management.◀

Problem: A problem is a disease, condition, illness, injury, symptom, sign, finding, complaint, or other matter addressed at the encounter, with or without a diagnosis being established at the time of the encounter.

Rationale

The guidelines for the number and complexity of problems addressed at the encounter have been editorially revised to clarify that the term "risk" relates to risk from the patient's condition as it relates to this MDM element (ie, the number and complexity of problems addressed at the encounter). This change is part of the overall effort to provide further reporting clarification in the E/M guidelines.

Risk of Complications and/or Morbidity or Mortality of Patient Management

One element used in selecting the level of service is the risk of complications and/or morbidity or mortality of patient management at an encounter. This is distinct from the risk of the condition itself.

Risk: The probability and/or consequences of an event. The assessment of the level of risk is affected by the nature of the event under consideration. For example, a low probability of death may be high risk, whereas a high chance of a minor, self-limited adverse effect of treatment may be low risk. Definitions of risk are based upon the usual behavior and thought processes of a physician or other qualified health care professional in the same specialty. Trained clinicians apply common language usage meanings to terms such as high, medium, low, or minimal risk and do not require quantification for these definitions (though quantification may be provided when evidence-based medicine has established probabilities). For the purpose of MDM, level of risk is based upon consequences of the problem(s) addressed at the encounter when appropriately treated. Risk also includes MDM related to the need to initiate or forego further testing, treatment, and/or hospitalization. The risk of patient management criteria applies to the patient management decisions made by the reporting physician or other qualified health care professional as part of the reported encounter.

Morbidity: A state of illness or functional impairment that is expected to be of substantial duration during which function is limited, quality of life is impaired, or there is organ damage that may not be transient despite treatment.

Social determinants of health: Economic and social conditions that influence the health of people and communities. Examples may include food or housing insecurity.

Surgery (minor or major, elective, emergency, procedure or patient risk):

Surgery—Minor or Major: The classification of surgery into minor or major is based on the common meaning of such terms when used by trained clinicians, similar to the use of the term "risk." These terms are not defined by a surgical package classification.

Surgery—Elective or Emergency: Elective procedures and emergent or urgent procedures describe the timing of a procedure when the timing is related to the patient's condition. An elective procedure is typically planned in advance (eg, scheduled for weeks later), while an emergent procedure is typically performed immediately or with minimal delay to allow for patient stabilization. Both elective and emergent procedures may be minor or major procedures.

Surgery—Risk Factors, Patient or Procedure: Risk factors are those that are relevant to the patient and procedure. Evidence-based risk calculators may be used, but are not required, in assessing patient and procedure risk.

Drug therapy requiring intensive monitoring for toxicity: A drug that requires intensive monitoring is a therapeutic agent that has the potential to cause serious morbidity or death. The monitoring is performed for assessment of these adverse effects and not primarily for assessment of therapeutic efficacy. The monitoring should be that which is generally accepted practice for the agent but may be patient-specific in some cases. Intensive monitoring may be long-term or short-term. Long-term intensive monitoring is not performed less than quarterly. The monitoring may be performed with a laboratory test, a physiologic test, or imaging. Monitoring by history or examination does not qualify. The monitoring affects the level of MDM in an encounter in which it is considered in the management of the patient. An example may be monitoring for cytopenia in the use of an antineoplastic agent between dose cycles. Examples of monitoring that do not qualify include monitoring glucose levels during insulin therapy, as the primary reason is the therapeutic effect (unless severe hypoglycemia is a current, significant concern); or annual electrolytes and renal function for a patient on a diuretic, as the frequency does not meet the threshold.

▶**Parenteral controlled substances:** The level of risk is based on the usual behavior and thought processes of a physician or other qualified health care professional in the same specialty and subspecialty and not simply based on the presence of an order for parenteral controlled substances.◀

Rationale

The guidelines for risk of complications and/or morbidity or mortality of patient management have been editorially revised with the addition of a definition for parenteral controlled substances, which is listed in an example in Table 1: Levels of Medical Decision Making (MDM). This change is part of the overall effort to provide further reporting clarification in the E/M guidelines.

Guidelines for Selecting Level of Service Based on Time

Certain categories of time-based E/M codes that do not have levels of services based on MDM (eg, Critical Care Services) in the E/M section use time differently. It is important to review the instructions for each category.

Time is **not** a descriptive component for the emergency department levels of E/M services because emergency department services are typically provided on a variable intensity basis, often involving multiple encounters with several patients over an extended period of time.

When time is used for reporting E/M services codes, the time defined in the service descriptors is used for selecting the appropriate level of services. The E/M services for which these guidelines apply require a face-to-face encounter with the physician or other qualified health care professional and the patient and/or family/caregiver. For office or other outpatient services, if the physician's or other qualified health care professional's time is spent in the supervision of clinical staff who perform the face-to-face services of the encounter, use 99211.

For coding purposes, time for these services is the total time on the date of the encounter. It includes both the face-to-face time with the patient and/or family/caregiver and non-face-to-face time personally spent by the physician and/or other qualified health care professional(s) on the day of the encounter (includes time in activities that require the physician or other qualified health care professional and does not include time in activities normally performed by clinical staff). It includes time regardless of the location of the physician or other qualified health care professional (eg, whether on or off the inpatient unit or in or out of the outpatient office). It does not include any time spent in the performance of other separately reported service(s).

▶Each service that may be reported using time for code level selection has a required time threshold. The concept of attaining a mid-point between levels does not apply. A full 15 minutes is required to report any unit of prolonged services codes 99417, 99418.

Physician(s) and other qualified health care professional(s) may each provide a portion of the face-to-face and non-face-to-face work related to the service. When time is being used to select the appropriate level of services for which time-based reporting is allowed, the time personally spent by the physician(s) and other qualified health care professional(s) assessing and managing the patient and/or counseling, educating, communicating results to the patient/family/caregiver on the date of the encounter is summed to define total time. Only distinct time should be summed (ie, when two or more individuals jointly meet with or discuss the patient, only the time of one individual should be counted). ◄

When prolonged time occurs, the appropriate prolonged services code may be reported. The total time on the date of the encounter spent caring for the patient should be documented in the medical record when it is used as the basis for code selection.

Physician or other qualified health care professional time includes the following activities, when performed:

- preparing to see the patient (eg, review of tests)

- obtaining and/or reviewing separately obtained history

- performing a medically appropriate examination and/or evaluation

- counseling and educating the patient/family/caregiver

- ordering medications, tests, or procedures

- referring and communicating with other health care professionals (when not separately reported)

- documenting clinical information in the electronic or other health record

- independently interpreting results (not separately reported) and communicating results to the patient/family/caregiver

- care coordination (not separately reported)

Do not count time spent on the following:

- the performance of other services that are reported separately

- travel

- teaching that is general and not limited to discussion that is required for the management of a specific patient

►For split or shared visits, see the split or shared visits guidelines. ◄

Rationale

The time ranges in codes 99202-99205 and 99212-99215 have been changed to minimum of total time, ie, a time threshold that must be met or exceeded. In accordance with the changes, the guidelines for selecting a level of service based on time have been revised to reflect these changes.

Refer to the codebook and the Rationale for codes 99202-99205 and 99212-99215 for a full discussion of these changes.

Similarly, in accordance with the new guidelines for split or shared visits, the guidelines for selecting a level of service based on time have been revised to reflect these changes.

Refer to the codebook and the Rationale for the new split or shared visits guidelines for a full discussion of these changes.

Evaluation and Management

Office or Other Outpatient Services

New Patient

★▲ **99202**   **Office or other outpatient visit** for the evaluation and management of a new patient, which requires a medically appropriate history and/or examination and straightforward medical decision making.

When using total time on the date of the encounter for code selection, 15 minutes must be met or exceeded.

★▲ **99203**   **Office or other outpatient visit** for the evaluation and management of a new patient, which requires a medically appropriate history and/or examination and low level of medical decision making.

When using total time on the date of the encounter for code selection, 30 minutes must be met or exceeded.

★▲ **99204**   **Office or other outpatient visit** for the evaluation and management of a new patient, which requires a medically appropriate history and/or examination and moderate level of medical decision making.

When using total time on the date of the encounter for code selection, 45 minutes must be met or exceeded.

★▲ **99205**   **Office or other outpatient visit** for the evaluation and management of a new patient, which requires a medically appropriate history and/or examination and high level of medical decision making.

When using total time on the date of the encounter for code selection, 60 minutes must be met or exceeded.

(For services 75 minutes or longer, use prolonged services code 99417)

Established Patient

★ **99211**   **Office or other outpatient visit** for the evaluation and management of an established patient that may not require the presence of a physician or other qualified health care professional

★▲ **99212**   **Office or other outpatient visit** for the evaluation and management of an established patient, which requires a medically appropriate history and/or examination and straightforward medical decision making.

When using total time on the date of the encounter for code selection, 10 minutes must be met or exceeded.

★▲ **99213**   **Office or other outpatient visit** for the evaluation and management of an established patient, which requires a medically appropriate history and/or examination and low level of medical decision making.

When using total time on the date of the encounter for code selection, 20 minutes must be met or exceeded.

★▲ **99214**   **Office or other outpatient visit** for the evaluation and management of an established patient, which requires a medically appropriate history and/or examination and moderate level of medical decision making.

When using total time on the date of the encounter for code selection, 30 minutes must be met or exceeded.

★▲ **99215**   **Office or other outpatient visit** for the evaluation and management of an established patient, which requires a medically appropriate history and/or examination and high level of medical decision making.

When using total time on the date of the encounter for code selection, 40 minutes must be met or exceeded.

(For services 55 minutes or longer, use prolonged services code 99417)

Rationale

Office or other outpatient codes 99202-99205 (new patient) and 99212-99215 (established patient) have been revised by replacing total time ranges with minimum of total time that must be met or exceeded.

In the CPT 2021 code set, time was redefined for office or other outpatient services as *total time spent on the date of the encounter* in which codes 99202-99205 and 99212-99215 were revised accordingly with a time range assigned to each code. However, in Medicare's Final Rule for 2023, CMS removed time ranges from codes 99202-99205 and 99212-99215 in their reporting rules and applied the time requirement of other E/M codes (eg, hospital inpatient or observation codes 99221-99223, 99231-99233) so that total time on the date of the encounter must meet or exceed a specific number of minutes.

Therefore, the changes in codes 99202-99205 and 99212-99215 for the CPT 2024 code set will provide consistency with CMS policy to reduce the administrative burden for physicians and other QHPs.

Hospital Inpatient and Observation Care Services

The following codes are used to report initial and subsequent evaluation and management services provided to hospital inpatients and to patients designated as hospital outpatient "observation status." Hospital inpatient or observation care codes are also used to report partial hospitalization services.

For patients designated/admitted as "observation status" in a hospital, it is not necessary that the patient be located in an observation area designated by the hospital. If such an area does exist in a hospital (as a separate unit in the hospital, in the emergency department, etc), these codes may be utilized if the patient is placed in such an area.

For a patient admitted and discharged from hospital inpatient or observation status on the same date, report 99234, 99235, 99236, as appropriate.

►Total time on the date of the encounter is by calendar date. When using MDM or total time for code selection, a continuous visit that spans the transition of two calendar dates is a single service and is reported on one calendar date. If the service is continuous before and through midnight, all the time may be applied to the reported date of the service.◄

Rationale

The Hospital Inpatient and Observation Care Services guidelines have been editorially revised by replacing the term "continuous service" with "continuous visit." This change is part of an overall effort to provide further reporting clarification in the E/M guidelines.

Initial Hospital Inpatient or Observation Care

New or Established Patient

The following codes are used to report the first hospital inpatient or observation status encounter with the patient.

An initial service may be reported when the patient has not received any professional services from the physician or other qualified health care professional or another physician or other qualified health care professional of the exact same specialty and subspecialty who belongs to the same group practice during the stay. When advanced practice nurses and physician assistants are working with physicians, they are considered as working in the exact same specialty and subspecialty as the physician.

For admission services for the neonate (28 days of age or younger) requiring intensive observation, frequent interventions, and other intensive care services, see 99477.

When the patient is admitted to the hospital as an inpatient or to observation status in the course of an encounter in another site of service (eg, hospital emergency department, office, nursing facility), the services in the initial site may be separately reported. Modifier 25 may be added to the other evaluation and management service to indicate a significant, separately identifiable service by the same physician or other qualified health care professional was performed on the same date.

In the case when the services in a separate site are reported and the initial inpatient or observation care service is a consultation service, do not report 99221, 99222, 99223, 99252, 99253, 99254, 99255. The consultant reports the subsequent hospital inpatient or observation care codes 99231, 99232, 99233 for the second service on the same date.

►If a consultation is performed in anticipation of, or related to, an admission by another physician or other qualified health care professional, and then the same consultant performs an encounter once the patient is admitted by the other physician or other qualified health care professional, report the consultant's inpatient encounter with the appropriate subsequent care code (99231, 99232, 99233). It applies for consultations reported with any appropriate code (eg, office or other outpatient visit or office or other outpatient consultation).◄

For a patient admitted and discharged from hospital inpatient or observation status on the same date, report 99234, 99235, 99236, as appropriate.

For the purpose of reporting an initial hospital inpatient or observation care service, a transition from observation level to inpatient does not constitute a new stay.

99221 **Initial hospital inpatient or observation care,** per day, for the evaluation and management of a patient, which requires a medically appropriate history and/or examination and straightforward or low level medical decision making.

When using total time on the date of the encounter for code selection, 40 minutes must be met or exceeded.

★ = Telemedicine ◀ = Audio-only ✚ = Add-on code ✗ = FDA approval pending # = Resequenced code ⊘ = Modifier 51 exempt

Rationale

The Initial Hospital Inpatient or Observation Care/New or Established Patient guidelines have been revised by removing, "This instruction applies whether the consultation occurred on the date of the admission or a date previous to the admission." This change is part of an overall effort to provide further reporting clarification in the E/M guidelines.

Hospital Inpatient or Observation Care Services (Including Admission and Discharge Services)

▶The following codes are used to report hospital inpatient or observation care services provided to patients admitted and discharged on the same date of service when the stay is more than eight hours. These services are only used by the physician or other qualified health care professional team who performs both the initial and discharge services. Other physicians and other qualified health care professionals may report 99221, 99222, 99223, as appropriate.

When a patient receives hospital inpatient or observation care for fewer than eight hours, only the initial hospital inpatient or observation care codes (99221, 99222, 99223) may be reported for the date of admission. Hospital or observation discharge day management codes (99238, 99239) may not be reported. When a patient receives hospital inpatient or observation care for a minimum of eight hours and is discharged on the same calendar date, observation or inpatient care services (including admission and discharge services) codes (99234, 99235, 99236) may be reported. Codes 99238, 99239 are not reported.◀

For patients admitted to hospital inpatient or observation care and discharged on a different date, see 99221, 99222, 99223, 99231, 99232, 99233, 99238, 99239.

▶Codes 99234, 99235, 99236 require two or more visits on the same date of which one of these visits is an initial admission and another being a discharge. For a patient admitted and discharged at the same visit (ie, one visit), see 99221, 99222, 99223. Do not report 99238, 99239 in conjunction with 99221, 99222, 99223 for admission and discharge services performed on the same date.◀

▶Length of Stay	Discharged On	Report Codes
<8 hours	Same calendar date as initial hospital inpatient or observation care service	99221, 99222, 99223
8 or more hours	Same calendar date as initial hospital inpatient or observation care service	99234, 99235, 99236
<8 hours	Different calendar date as initial hospital inpatient or observation care service	99221, 99222, 99223
8 or more hours	Different calendar date as initial hospital inpatient or observation care service	99221, 99222, 99223 and 99238, 99239◀

(For discharge services provided to newborns admitted and discharged on the same date, use 99463)

99234 **Hospital inpatient or observation care,** for the evaluation and management of a patient including admission and discharge on the same date, which requires a medically appropriate history and/or examination and straightforward or low level of medical decision making.

When using total time on the date of the encounter for code selection, 45 minutes must be met or exceeded.

99235 **Hospital inpatient or observation care,** for the evaluation and management of a patient including admission and discharge on the same date, which requires a medically appropriate history and/or examination and moderate level of medical decision making.

When using total time on the date of the encounter for code selection, 70 minutes must be met or exceeded.

99236 **Hospital inpatient or observation care,** for the evaluation and management of a patient including admission and discharge on the same date, which requires a medically appropriate history and/or examination and high level of medical decision making.

When using total time on the date of the encounter for code selection, 85 minutes must be met or exceeded.

(For services of 100 minutes or longer, use prolonged services code 99418)

Rationale

The Hospital Inpatient or Observation Care Services (Including Admission and Discharge Services) guidelines have been revised.

In Medicare's Final Rule for 2023, CMS established instructions for reporting codes 99234-99236 and included a table illustrating when to report codes 99221-99223, 99234-99236, 99238, and 99239 based on the number of hours of the length of stay and whether discharge occurred on the calendar date of admission or on a different calendar date than the admission.

To reduce the administrative burden for physicians and other QHPs, the guidelines have been revised to be consistent with CMS policy. The revised guidelines clarify that codes 99234-99236 are reported only when the length of stay is more than 8 hours and when the same physician or other QHP team performs both the initial hospital inpatient or observation care and the discharge services. The revised guidelines also clarify how to report lengths of stay that are less than 8 hours. In addition, the table that was included in Medicare's Final Rule for 2023 has been replicated in the Hospital Inpatient or Observation Care Services (Including Admission and Discharge Services) guidelines.

The guidelines also have been revised by replacing "encounter" with "visits" for a more accurate context of these services and as part of the overall effort to provide further reporting clarification in the E/M guidelines.

Hospital Inpatient or Observation Discharge Services

99238   **Hospital inpatient or observation discharge day management**; 30 minutes or less on the date of the encounter

99239   more than 30 minutes on the date of the encounter

(For hospital inpatient or observation care including the admission and discharge of the patient on the same date, see 99234, 99235, 99236)

(For discharge services provided to newborns admitted and discharged on the same date, use 99463)

▶(Do not report 99238, 99239 in conjunction with 99221, 99222, 99223 for admission and discharge services performed on the same date)◀

Rationale

In accordance with the revisions to the Hospital Inpatient or Observation Care Services (Including Admission and Discharge Services) guidelines, an exclusionary parenthetical note has been added following codes 99238 and 99239, restricting their use with codes 99221-99223 for admission and discharge services performed on the same date.

Refer to the codebook and the Rationale for the Hospital Inpatient or Observation Care Services (Including Admission and Discharge Services) guidelines for a full discussion of these changes.

Nursing Facility Services

Initial Nursing Facility Care

New or Established Patient

99304   Initial nursing facility care, per day, for the evaluation and management of a patient, which requires a medically appropriate history and/or examination and straightforward or low level of medical decision making.

When using total time on the date of the encounter for code selection, 25 minutes must be met or exceeded.

99305   Initial nursing facility care, per day, for the evaluation and management of a patient, which requires a medically appropriate history and/or examination and moderate level of medical decision making.

When using total time on the date of the encounter for code selection, 35 minutes must be met or exceeded.

▲ **99306**   Initial nursing facility care, per day, for the evaluation and management of a patient, which requires a medically appropriate history and/or examination and high level of medical decision making.

When using total time on the date of the encounter for code selection, 50 minutes must be met or exceeded.

▶(For services 65 minutes or longer, use prolonged services code 99418)◀

Rationale

Initial nursing facility care code 99306 has been revised. Prior to 2024, 45 minutes of total time has to be met or exceeded to report code 99306 when using total time for code-level selection. Effective in 2024, the total-time threshold for code 99306 has been revised to 50 minutes based on feedback from the AMA/Specialty Society Relative Value Scale (RVS) Update Committee (RUC).

★ = Telemedicine   ◀ = Audio-only   ✚ = Add-on code   ✗ = FDA approval pending   # = Resequenced code   ⦸ = Modifier 51 exempt

In accordance with the revision to total time in code 99306, the time requirement for reporting prolonged nursing facility care services has been changed from 60 minutes to 65 minutes. As such, the prolonged services instructional parenthetical note following code 99306 has been revised to reflect the 65-minute time requirement.

Subsequent Nursing Facility Care

★ **99307**   Subsequent nursing facility care, per day, for the evaluation and management of a patient, which requires a medically appropriate history and/or examination and straightforward medical decision making.

When using total time on the date of the encounter for code selection, 10 minutes must be met or exceeded.

★▲ **99308**   Subsequent nursing facility care, per day, for the evaluation and management of a patient, which requires a medically appropriate history and/or examination and low level of medical decision making.

When using total time on the date of the encounter for code selection, 20 minutes must be met or exceeded.

★ **99309**   Subsequent nursing facility care, per day, for the evaluation and management of a patient, which requires a medically appropriate history and/or examination and moderate level of medical decision making.

When using total time on the date of the encounter for code selection, 30 minutes must be met or exceeded.

★ **99310**   Subsequent nursing facility care, per day, for the evaluation and management of a patient, which requires a medically appropriate history and/or examination and high level of medical decision making.

When using total time on the date of the encounter for code selection, 45 minutes must be met or exceeded.

(For services 60 minutes or longer, use prolonged services code 99418)

Rationale

Subsequent nursing facility care code 99308 has been revised. Prior to 2024, 15 minutes of total time has to be met or exceeded to report code 99308 when using total time for code-level selection. Effective in 2024, the total time threshold for code 99308 has been revised to 20 minutes based on feedback from RUC.

Prolonged Services

►Prolonged Service Without Direct Patient Contact on Date Other Than the Face-to-Face Evaluation and Management Service◄

Codes 99358 and 99359 are used when a prolonged service is provided on a date other than the date of a face-to-face evaluation and management encounter with the patient and/or family/caregiver. Codes 99358, 99359 may be reported for prolonged services in relation to any evaluation and management service on a date other than the face-to-face service, whether or not time was used to select the level of the face-to-face service.

This service is to be reported in relation to other physician or other qualified health care professional services, including evaluation and management services at any level, on a date other than the face-to-face service to which it is related. Prolonged service without direct patient contact may only be reported when it occurs on a **date other than** the date of the evaluation and management service. For example, extensive record review may relate to a previous evaluation and management service performed at an earlier date. However, it must relate to a service or patient in which (face-to-face) patient care has occurred or will occur and relate to ongoing patient management.

Codes 99358 and 99359 are used to report the total duration of non-face-to-face time spent by a physician or other qualified health care professional on a given date providing prolonged service, even if the time spent by the physician or other qualified health care professional on that date is not continuous. Code 99358 is used to report the first hour of prolonged service on a given date regardless of the place of service. It should be used only once per date.

Prolonged service of less than 30 minutes total duration on a given date is not separately reported.

Code 99359 is used to report each additional 30 minutes beyond the first hour. It may also be used to report the final 15 to 30 minutes of prolonged service on a given date.

Prolonged service of less than 15 minutes beyond the first hour or less than 15 minutes beyond the final 30 minutes is not reported separately.

Do not report 99358, 99359 for time without direct patient contact reported in other services, such as care plan oversight services (99374-99380), chronic care management by a physician or other qualified health care professional (99437, 99491), principal care management by a physician or other qualified health care professional (99424, 99425, 99426, 99427), home and outpatient INR monitoring (93792, 93793), medical team conferences (99366-99368), interprofessional telephone/Internet/electronic health record consultations (99446, 99447, 99448, 99449, 99451, 99452), or online digital evaluation and management services (99421, 99422, 99423).

99358 **Prolonged evaluation and management service**
before and/or after direct patient care; first hour

Rationale

The Prolonged Service on Date Other Than the Face-to-Face Evaluation and Management Service Without Direct Patient Contact subsection heading has been revised to "Prolonged Service Without Direct Patient Contact on Date Other Than the Face-to-Face Evaluation and Management Service." "Without Direct Patient Contact" has been transposed to the beginning of the title to make it clear that codes 99358 and 99359 are reported for prolonged services on a date other than the date of a face-to-face E/M encounter. This revision is part of the overall effort to provide further reporting clarification for E/M services and guidelines.

Prolonged Service With or Without Direct Patient Contact on the Date of an Evaluation and Management Service

▶Code 99417 is used to report prolonged total time (ie, combined time with and without direct patient contact) provided by the physician or other qualified health care professional on the date of office or other outpatient services, office consultation, or other outpatient evaluation and management services (ie, 99205, 99215, 99245, 99345, 99350, 99483). Code 99418 is used to report prolonged total time (ie, combined time with and without direct patient contact) provided by the physician or other qualified health care professional on the date of an inpatient evaluation and management service (ie, 99223, 99233, 99236, 99255, 99306, 99310). Prolonged total time is time that is 15 minutes beyond the time threshold required to report the highest-level primary service. Codes 99417, 99418 are only used when the primary service has been selected using time alone as the basis and only after the time required to report the highest-level service has been exceeded by 15 minutes. Cognitive assessment and care plan services code 99483 does not have a required time threshold, and 99417 may be reported when the typical time has been exceeded by 15 minutes. To report a unit of 99417, 99418, 15 minutes of prolonged services time must have been attained. Do not report 99417, 99418 for any time increment of less than 15 minutes.

When reporting 99417, 99418, the initial time unit of 15 minutes may be added once the time threshold required for the primary E/M code has been surpassed by 15 minutes. For example, to report the initial unit of 99417 for a new patient encounter (99205), do not report 99417 until at least 15 minutes of time have been accumulated beyond 60 minutes (ie, 75 minutes) on the date of the encounter. For an established patient encounter (99215), do not report 99417 until at least 15 minutes of time have been accumulated beyond 40 minutes (ie, 55 minutes) on the date of the encounter.◀

Time spent performing separately reported services other than the primary E/M service and prolonged E/M service is not counted toward the primary E/M and prolonged services time.

For prolonged services on a date other than the date of a face-to-face evaluation and management encounter with the patient and/or family/caregiver, see 99358, 99359. For E/M services that require prolonged clinical staff time and may include face-to-face services by the physician or other qualified health care professional, see 99415, 99416. Do not report 99417, 99418 in conjunction with 99358, 99359, 99415, 99416.

#★✛ 99417 Prolonged outpatient evaluation and management service(s) time with or without direct patient contact beyond the required time of the primary service when the primary service level has been selected using total time, each 15 minutes of total time (List separately in addition to the code of the outpatient **Evaluation and Management** service)

(Use 99417 in conjunction with 99205, 99215, 99245, 99345, 99350, 99483)

▶(Use 99417 in conjunction with 99483, when the total time on the date of the encounter exceeds the typical time of 99483 by 15 minutes or more)◀

(Do not report 99417 on the same date of service as 90833, 90836, 90838, 99358, 99359, 99415, 99416)

(Do not report 99417 for any time unit less than 15 minutes)

#★✛ 99418 Prolonged inpatient or observation evaluation and management service(s) time with or without direct patient contact beyond the required time of the primary service when the primary service level has been selected using total time, each 15 minutes of total time (List separately in addition to the code of the inpatient and observation **Evaluation and Management** service)

(Use 99418 in conjunction with 99223, 99233, 99236, 99255, 99306, 99310)

(Do not report 99418 on the same date of service as 90833, 90836, 90838, 99358, 99359)

(Do not report 99418 for any time unit less than 15 minutes)

▶**Example of initial and multiple units of prolonged service(s)**

Total Duration of New Patient Office or Other Outpatient Services (use with 99205)	Code(s)
less than 75 minutes	Not reported separately
75-89 minutes	99205 X 1 and 99417 X 1
90-104 minutes	99205 X 1 and 99417 X 2
105 minutes or more	99205 X 1 and 99417 X 3 or more for each additional 15 minutes

Reporting Prolonged Services

Primary Code	Prolonged Services Code	Total Time to Report Initial Unit of Prolonged Services	Total Time to Report Second Unit of Prolonged Services
99205	99417	75	90
99215	99417	55	70
99223	99418	90	105
99233	99418	65	80
99236	99418	100	115
99245	99417	70	85
99255	99418	95	110
99306	99418	65	80
99310	99418	60	75
99345	99417	90	105
99350	99417	75	90
99483	99417	75	90 ◀

Rationale

In accordance with the revision of time range to time threshold that must be met or exceeded in codes 99202-99205 and 99212-99215, revisions have been made to the Prolonged Service With or Without Direct Patient Contact on the Date of an Evaluation and Management Service guidelines, and a new table, "Reporting Prolonged Services," has been added following code 99418 to reflect these changes.

Refer to the codebook and the Rationale for codes 99202-99205 and 99212-99215 for a full discussion of these changes.

In addition, the guidelines have been revised to clarify that cognitive assessment and care plan services code 99483 does not have a required time threshold and code 99417 may be reported when the typical time has been exceeded by 15 minutes. An inclusionary parenthetical note has been added following code 99417 to clarify the appropriate reporting of code 99417 with code 99483.

To provide further reporting clarification, the Total Duration of New Patient Office or Other Outpatient Services table has been simplified by removing the entries for code 99215. The revised table includes only examples for code 99205.

Preventive Medicine Services

▶Vaccine/toxoid products, immunization administrations, ancillary studies involving laboratory, radiology, other procedures, or screening tests (eg, vision, hearing, developmental) identified with a specific CPT code are reported separately. For immunization administration and vaccine risk/benefit counseling, see 90460, 90461, 90471-90474, 0001A, 0002A, 0003A, 0004A, 0011A, 0012A, 0013A, 0021A, 0022A, 0031A, 0034A, 0041A, 0042A, 0044A, 0051A, 0052A, 0053A, 0054A, 0064A, 0071A, 0072A, 0073A, 0074A, 0081A, 0082A, 0083A, 0091A, 0092A, 0093A, 0094A, 0104A, 0111A, 0112A, 0113A, 0121A, 0124A, 0134A, 0141A, 0142A, 0144A, 0151A, 0154A, 0164A, 0171A, 0172A, 0173A, 0174A. For vaccine/toxoid products, see 90476-90759, 91300-91317.◀

Rationale

To accommodate the addition of multiple coronavirus disease 2019 (COVID-19) administration codes, the guidelines for the Preventive Medicine Services subsection have been updated to reflect all new administration codes and product codes for COVID-19 vaccinations for the CPT 2024 code set.

Refer to the codebook and the Rationale regarding COVID-19 codes for a full discussion of these changes.

Non-Face-to-Face Services

Digitally Stored Data Services/ Remote Physiologic Monitoring

 # 99453   Remote monitoring of physiologic parameter(s) (eg, weight, blood pressure, pulse oximetry, respiratory flow rate), initial; set-up and patient education on use of equipment

(Do not report 99453 more than once per episode of care)

(Do not report 99453 for monitoring of less than 16 days)

▶(Do not report 99453 in conjunction with 0811T)◀

Rationale

In accordance with the establishment of code 0811T, an exclusionary parenthetical note following code 99453 has been added to preclude the reporting of code 0811T with code 99453.

Refer to the codebook and the Rationale for code 0811T for a full discussion of these changes.

 # 99454   device(s) supply with daily recording(s) or programmed alert(s) transmission, each 30 days

(For physiologic monitoring treatment management services, use 99457)

(Do not report 99454 for monitoring of less than 16 days)

(Do not report 99453, 99454 in conjunction with codes for more specific physiologic parameters [eg, 93296, 94760])

▶(Do not report 99454 in conjunction with 0812T)◀

(For remote therapeutic monitoring, see 98975, 98976, 98977, 98978)

(For self-measured blood pressure monitoring, see 99473, 99474)

Rationale

In accordance with the establishment of code 0812T, an exclusionary parenthetical note following code 99454 has been added to preclude the reporting of code 0812T with code 99454.

Refer to the codebook and the Rationale for code 0812T for a full discussion of these changes.

Special Evaluation and Management Services

Work Related or Medical Disability Evaluation Services

99459   Code is out of numerical sequence. See 99497-99499

Other Evaluation and Management Services

#✚● 99459   Pelvic examination (List separately in addition to code for primary procedure)

▶(Use 99459 in conjunction with 99202, 99203, 99204, 99205, 99212, 99213, 99214, 99215, 99242, 99243, 99244, 99245, 99383, 99384, 99385, 99386, 99387, 99393, 99394, 99395, 99396, 99397)◀

99499   **Unlisted evaluation and management** service

Rationale

A new Category I add-on code 99459 has been established to report pelvic examination.

The preventive medicine services codes 99381-99397 were identified by the RUC's Relativity Assessment Workgroup as a service for potential gender-based misvaluation because these codes are valued by age, not by gender.

Code 99459 has been established to capture the additional resources during a pelvic examination that are required as part of the service for preventive medicine or the evaluation and management services for those who require pelvic examinations. Note that code 99459 is a practice-expense only code. Because code 99459 is an add-on code, an inclusionary parenthetical note has been included to direct users to the appropriate codes with which this service is reported.

Clinical Example (99459)

A 35-year-old patient presents with post-coital and irregular vaginal bleeding that has worsened over the last 6 months and is not controlled with hormonal medications. [**Note:** This is an add-on code. Only consider the additional resources related to the pelvic examination.]

Description of Procedure (99459)

N/A

★ = Telemedicine   ◀ = Audio-only   ✚ = Add-on code   ✗ = FDA approval pending   # = Resequenced code   ⃠ = Modifier 51 exempt

Surgery

Summary of Additions, Deletions, and Revisions

The summary of changes shows the actual changes that have been made to the code descriptors.

New codes appear with a bullet (●) and are indicated as "Code added." Revised codes are preceded with a triangle (▲). Within revised codes, or if a code symbol has been deleted, the deleted language and code symbol appear with a strikethrough, while new text appears underlined.

The ⚡ symbol is used to identify codes for vaccines that are pending FDA approval. The # symbol is used to identify codes that have been resequenced. CPT add-on codes are annotated by the ✚ symbol. The ⊘ symbol is used to identify codes that are exempt from the use of modifier 51. The ★ symbol is used to identify codes that may be used for reporting telemedicine services. The ✛ is used to identify proprietary laboratory analyses (PLA) test that has an identical descriptor as another PLA test. A PLA code that satisfies Category I code criteria and has been accepted by the CPT Editorial Panel is annotated with the ↕ symbol. The ◀ symbol is used to identify codes that may be used to report audio-only telemedicine services when appended by modifier 93 **(see Appendix T)**.

Code	Description
#●22836	Code added
#●22837	Code added
#●22838	Code added
●27278	Code added
▲28292	Correction, hallux valgus <u>with</u> (bunionectomy), with sesamoidectomy, when performed; with resection of proximal phalanx base, when performed, any method
▲28296	with distal metatarsal osteotomy, any method
#▲28295	with proximal metatarsal osteotomy, any method
▲28297	with first metatarsal and medial cuneiform joint arthrodesis, any method
▲28298	with proximal phalanx osteotomy, any method
▲28299	with double osteotomy, any method
#●31242	Code added
#●31243	Code added
#●33276	Code added
#✚●33277	Code added
#●33278	Code added
#●33279	Code added
#●33280	Code added
#●33281	Code added

Code	Description
#●33287	Code added
#●33288	Code added
●52284	Code added
●58580	Code added
●61889	Code added
●61891	Code added
●61892	Code added
▲63685	Insertion or replacement of spinal neurostimulator pulse generator or receiver~~, direct or inductive coupling~~, requiring pocket creation and connection between electrode array and pulse generator or receiver
▲63688	Revision or removal of implanted spinal neurostimulator pulse generator or receiver, with detachable connection to electrode array
▲64590	Insertion or replacement of peripheral, sacral, or gastric neurostimulator pulse generator or receiver, ~~direct or inductive coupling~~requiring pocket creation and connection between electrode array and pulse generator or receiver
▲64595	Revision or removal of peripheral, sacral, or gastric neurostimulator pulse generator or receiver, with detachable connection to electrode array
●64596	Code added
+●64597	Code added
●64598	Code added
●67516	Code added

★ = Telemedicine   ◀ = Audio-only   ✚ = Add-on code   ⚡ = FDA approval pending   # = Resequenced code   ⊘ = Modifier 51 exempt

Surgery 10004-68899

Surgery

Musculoskeletal System

Spine (Vertebral Column)

Arthrodesis

Spine Deformity (eg, Scoliosis, Kyphosis)

To report instrumentation procedures, see 22840-22855, 22859. (Report in addition to code[s] for the definitive procedure[s].) Do not append modifier 62 to spinal instrumentation codes 22840-22848, 22850, 22852, 22853, 22854, 22859.

To report bone graft procedures, see 20930-20938. (Report in addition to code[s] for the definitive procedure[s].) Do not append modifier 62 to bone graft codes 20900-20938.

A vertebral segment describes the basic constituent part into which the spine may be divided. It represents a single complete vertebral bone with its associated articular processes and laminae.

▶For the following codes, when two surgeons work together as primary surgeons performing distinct part(s) of an arthrodesis for spinal deformity, each surgeon should report his or her distinct operative work by appending modifier 62 to the procedure code. In this situation, modifier 62 may be appended to procedure code(s) 22800-22819 as long as both surgeons continue to work together as primary surgeons. The spinal deformity arthrodesis codes (22800, 22802, 22804, 22808, 22810, 22812) and kyphectomy codes (22818, 22819) should not be reported in conjunction with thoracic vertebral body tethering codes (22836, 22837, 22838) or lumbar or thoracolumbar vertebral body tethering codes (0656T, 0657T, 0790T).

When two surgeons work together as primary surgeons performing distinct part(s) of the thoracic vertebral body tethering, each surgeon should report his or her distinct operative work by appending modifier 62 to the procedure code. Modifier 62 may be appended to procedure code(s) 22836, 22837, 22838, as long as both surgeons continue to work together as primary surgeons.◀

Rationale

In accordance with the establishment of codes 22836-22838, revision of codes 0656T and 0657T, and addition of Category III code 0790T, the Spine Deformity (eg, Scoliosis, Kyphosis) guidelines have been revised and updated.

Refer to the codebook and the Rationale for codes 22836-22838 for a full discussion of these changes.

Exploration

22830	Exploration of spinal fusion
22836	Code is out of numerical sequence. See 22846-22849
22837	Code is out of numerical sequence. See 22846-22849
22838	Code is out of numerical sequence. See 22846-22849

Spinal Instrumentation

Segmental instrumentation is defined as fixation at each end of the construct and at least one additional interposed bony attachment.

Non-segmental instrumentation is defined as fixation at each end of the construct and may span several vertebral segments without attachment to the intervening segments.

Insertion of spinal instrumentation is reported separately and in addition to arthrodesis. Instrumentation procedure codes 22840-22848, 22853, 22854, 22859 are reported in addition to the definitive procedure(s). Do not append modifier 62 to spinal instrumentation codes 22840-22848, 22850, 22852, 22853, 22854, 22859.

To report bone graft procedures, see 20930-20938. (Report in addition to code[s] for definitive procedure[s].) Do not append modifier 62 to bone graft codes 20900-20938.

A vertebral segment describes the basic constituent part into which the spine may be divided. It represents a single complete vertebral bone with its associated articular processes and laminae. A vertebral interspace is the non-bony compartment between two adjacent vertebral bodies, which contains the intervertebral disc, and includes the nucleus pulposus, annulus fibrosus, and two cartilaginous endplates.

Codes 22849, 22850, 22852, and 22855 are subject to modifier 51 if reported with other definitive procedure(s), including arthrodesis, decompression, and exploration of fusion. Code 22849 should not be reported in conjunction with 22850, 22852, and 22855 at the same spinal levels. Only the appropriate insertion code (22840-22848) should be reported when previously placed spinal instrumentation is being removed or revised during the

---

same session where new instrumentation is inserted at levels including all or part of the previously instrumented segments. Do not report the reinsertion (22849) or removal (22850, 22852, 22855) procedures in addition to the insertion of the new instrumentation (22840-22848).

►Codes 22836, 22837, 22838 describe anterior thoracic vertebral body tethering, which corrects scoliosis without fusion using a tether (cord) to compress the vertebral growth plates on the convex side of the curve to inhibit their growth, while allowing the growth plates on the concave side of the curve to continue to grow. Codes 22836, 22837 may not be reported with anterior instrumentation codes 22845, 22846, 22847.

For the following codes, when two surgeons work together as primary surgeons performing distinct part(s) of the thoracic vertebral body tethering, each surgeon should report his or her distinct operative work by appending modifier 62 to the procedure code. Modifier 62 may be appended to procedure code(s) 22836, 22837, 22838, as long as both surgeons continue to work together as primary surgeons.

Regions of the spine include cervical, cervicothoracic, thoracic, thoracolumbar, lumbar, lumbosacral, sacral, and coccygeal.◄

+ 22845 Anterior instrumentation; 2 to 3 vertebral segments (List separately in addition to code for primary procedure)

(Use 22845 in conjunction with 22100-22102, 22110-22114, 22206, 22207, 22210-22214, 22220-22224, 22310-22327, 22532, 22533, 22548-22558, 22590-22612, 22630, 22633, 22634, 22800-22812, 63001-63030, 63040-63042, 63045-63047, 63050-63056, 63064, 63075, 63077, 63081, 63085, 63087, 63090, 63101, 63102, 63170-63290, 63300-63307)

►(For vertebral body tethering of the thoracic spine, see 22836, 22837, 22838)◄

►(For vertebral body tethering of the lumbar or thoracolumbar spine, see 0656T, 0657T, 0790T)◄

+ 22846 4 to 7 vertebral segments (List separately in addition to code for primary procedure)

(Use 22846 in conjunction with 22100-22102, 22110-22114, 22206, 22207, 22210-22214, 22220-22224, 22310-22327, 22532, 22533, 22548-22558, 22590-22612, 22630, 22633, 22634, 22800-22812, 63001-63030, 63040-63042, 63045-63047, 63050-63056, 63064, 63075, 63077, 63081, 63085, 63087, 63090, 63101, 63102, 63170-63290, 63300-63307)

►(For vertebral body tethering of the thoracic spine, see 22836, 22837, 22838)◄

►(For vertebral body tethering of the lumbar or thoracolumbar spine, see 0656T, 0657T, 0790T)◄

+ 22847 8 or more vertebral segments (List separately in addition to code for primary procedure)

(Use 22847 in conjunction with 22100-22102, 22110-22114, 22206, 22207, 22210-22214, 22220-22224, 22310-22327, 22532, 22533, 22548-22558, 22590-22612, 22630, 22633, 22634, 22800-22812, 63001-63030, 63040-63042, 63045-63047, 63050-63056, 63064, 63075, 63077, 63081, 63085, 63087, 63090, 63101, 63102, 63170-63290, 63300-63307)

►(Do not report 22845, 22846, 22847 in conjunction with 22836, 22837, 22838)◄

►(For vertebral body tethering of the thoracic spine, see 22836, 22837, 22838)◄

►(For vertebral body tethering of the lumbar or thoracolumbar spine, see 0656T, 0657T, 0790T)◄

#● 22836 Anterior thoracic vertebral body tethering, including thoracoscopy, when performed; up to 7 vertebral segments

►(For anterior lumbar or thoracolumbar vertebral body tethering, up to 7 vertebral segments, use 0656T)◄

#● 22837 8 or more vertebral segments

►(Do not report 22836, 22837 in conjunction with 22845, 22846, 22847, 32601)◄

►(For anterior lumbar or thoracolumbar vertebral body tethering, 8 or more vertebral segments, use 0657T)◄

#● 22838 Revision (eg, augmentation, division of tether), replacement, or removal of thoracic vertebral body tethering, including thoracoscopy, when performed

►(Do not report 22838 in conjunction with 22849, 22855, 32601)◄

+ 22848 Pelvic fixation (attachment of caudal end of instrumentation to pelvic bony structures) other than sacrum (List separately in addition to code for primary procedure)

(Use 22848 in conjunction with 22100-22102, 22110-22114, 22206, 22207, 22210-22214, 22220-22224, 22310-22327, 22532, 22533, 22548-22558, 22590-22612, 22630, 22633, 22634, 22800-22812, 63001-63030, 63040-63042, 63045-63047, 63050-63056, 63064, 63075, 63077, 63081, 63085, 63087, 63090, 63101, 63102, 63170-63290, 63300-63307)

Rationale

There has been increased adoption and use of vertebral body tethering (VBT) procedures in clinical practice. VBT is used to correct scoliosis without fusion with a tether (cord) that compresses the convex vertebral growth plates to inhibit their growth, while allowing the concave growth plates to grow. For this reason, the CPT 2024 code set has added three new codes (22836-22838) to report thoracic VBT. In addition, guidelines and parenthetical notes have been revised and/or added to accommodate the addition of these new codes.

Surgery / Musculoskeletal System 20100-29999

To support the establishment of the new VBT procedures, several other changes have been made in the code set. First, Category III codes 0656T and 0657T, which were added to the CPT 2022 code set, have now been revised. Code 0656T was previously intended to report anterior VBT of up to 7 vertebral segments and code 0657T to report 8 or more vertebral segments. Category III codes 0656T and 0657T have been revised to clarify their use for VBT that is limited to the lumbar or thoracolumbar spine region.

Second, a new Category III code 0790T was added to describe the work performed for revision, replacement, or removal of thoracolumbar or lumbar VBT, including thoracoscopy, when performed.

Third, the spine regions have been defined as including the "cervical, cervicothoracic, thoracic, thoracolumbar, lumbar, lumbosacral, sacral, and coccygeal" in the Spine Instrumentation guidelines.

In addition to those three revisions, several parenthetical notes have been added to provide guidance for the appropriate reporting of these new codes in the Surgery and Category III sections. Specifically, revisions have been made to the introductory guidelines in the Spine Deformity (eg, Scoliosis, Kyphosis) and Spinal Instrumentation subsections to provide instruction for the appropriate reporting of new Category I codes 22836-22838 and new Category III code 0790T, as well as reporting guidance for modifier 62 when two surgeons work together as primary surgeons to perform distinct part(s) of thoracic VBT. Guidance also has been added to restrict reporting the spinal deformity arthrodesis codes (22800, 22802, 22804, 22808, 22810, 22812) and kyphectomy codes (22818, 22819) in conjunction with thoracic VBT codes (22836-22838) or lumbar or thoracolumbar VBT codes (0656T, 0657T, 0790T).

Code 22836 is intended to describe anterior thoracic VBT of up to 7 vertebral segments, including thoracoscopy when performed. Code 22837 describes 8 or more vertebral segments and code 22838 describes the revision (eg, augmentation, division of tether), replacement, or removal of thoracic VBT, including thoracoscopy when performed. These new procedures differ from other procedures in the CPT code set because VBT does not involve arthrodesis/fusion of the spine. The other existing procedures in the code set represent arthrodesis of the anterior section/vertebral bodies of the spinal column for spinal deformity. Parenthetical notes following the new VBT codes and existing anterior instrumentation codes provide instruction regarding exclusions and directions for reporting VBT services.

Clinical Example (22836)

A 13-year-old skeletally immature female, who was diagnosed with thoracic idiopathic scoliosis, has been either unsuccessful or intolerant of bracing. The curve magnitude and remaining growth suggest likely continued progression without intervention. A vertebral body tethering construct is applied from T6 to T11 to provide initial coronal correction through tensioning.

Description of Procedure (22836)

Co-Surgeon A—Exposure: Gain surgical access through the preferred approach, which is typically thoracoscopic, which typically requires a single-lung ventilation technique and lung deflation to gain access. At each operative level, gain access to the chest by a sharp thoracostomy laterally, typically in the axillary line. Insert the scope and deflate the lung on that side to enable visualization of the lateral aspect of the vertebral body. The procedure is typically performed thoracoscopically and visualized on a video monitor. Using an ultrasonic scalpel or a thermal device, incise the parietal pleura longitudinally to identify the segmental vessels along the vertebrae to be instrumented. At the seventh vertebral segments or less, coagulate the segmental vessels and expose the lateral aspect of the vertebral bodies intended for instrumentation. Dissection to release the diaphragm is required if the construct extends distally to T12 or L1. Because all the vertebral bodies to be instrumented cannot be approached through the same thoracostomy, the procedure must be repeated as many times as it takes to access all the vertebral levels involved in the procedure.

Co-Surgeon B—Tether Placement: Confirm the trajectory and placement on the vertebral body at all levels prior to each anchor insertion, screw preparation, and screw insertion using intraoperative fluoroscopy or CT guidance. Due to smaller vertebral body size and variable venous anatomy, caution should be taken if extending instrumentation proximal to T5. At each level, secure a pronged staple to the vertebral body as needed. Then use an entry awl to create a trajectory for the screw. Insert each screw in the narrow safe zone between the spinal canal posteriorly and the great vessels anteriorly. Approach to the next level of vertebra may require another level of thoracostomy as not all levels can be approached through the same thoracostomy. Tap the hole and select and insert a screw of appropriate length and diameter. Following placement of all screws, secure a cord to the most cranial screw and segmentally tension, maintaining compression by tightening set screws at the adjacent levels to achieve correction of the spinal curvature. Applying the correct amount of tension is critical to the procedure. Following final tensioning, use intraoperative fluoroscopy or radiography to assess curve correction on anteroposterior (AP) and lateral imaging.

Co-Surgeon A—Closure: Close each thoracotomy site and place a chest tube.

Clinical Example (22837)

A 13-year-old skeletally immature female, who is diagnosed with thoracic idiopathic scoliosis, has been either unsuccessful or intolerant of bracing. The curve magnitude and remaining growth suggest likely continued progression without intervention. A vertebral body tethering construct is applied from T5 to T12 to provide initial coronal correction through tensioning.

Description of Procedure (22837)

Co-Surgeon A—Exposure: Gain surgical access through the preferred approach, which is typically thoracoscopic, which typically requires a single-lung ventilation technique and lung deflation to allow access. At each operative level, gain access to the chest by a sharp thoracostomy laterally, typically in the axillary line. Insert the scope and deflate the lung on that side to enable visualization of the lateral aspect of the vertebral body. The procedure is typically performed thoracoscopically and visualized on a video monitor. Using an ultrasonic scalpel or a thermal device, incise the parietal pleura longitudinally to identify the segmental vessels along the vertebrae to be instrumented. At the seventh vertebral segments or less, coagulate the segmental vessels and expose the lateral aspect of the vertebral bodies intended for instrumentation. Dissection to release the diaphragm is required if the construct will extend distally to T12 or L1. Because all the vertebral bodies to be instrumented cannot be approached through the same thoracostomy, the procedure must be repeated as many times as it takes to access all the vertebral levels involved in the procedure.

Co-Surgeon B—Tether Placement: Confirm the trajectory and placement on the vertebral body at all levels prior to each anchor insertion, screw preparation, and screw insertion using intraoperative fluoroscopy or CT guidance. Due to smaller vertebral body size and variable venous anatomy, caution should be taken if extending instrumentation proximal to T5. At each level, secure a pronged staple to the vertebral body as needed. Then use an entry awl to create a trajectory for the screw. Insert each screw in the narrow safe zone between the spinal canal posteriorly and the great vessels anteriorly. Approach to the next level of vertebra may require another level of thoracostomy as not all levels can be approached through the same thoracostomy. Tap the hole and select and insert a screw of appropriate length and diameter. Following placement of all screws, secure a cord to the most cranial screw and segmentally tension, maintaining compression by tightening set screws at the adjacent levels. Applying the correct amount of tension is critical to the procedure. Following final tensioning, use intraoperative fluoroscopy or radiography to assess curve correction on AP and lateral imaging.

Co-Surgeon A—Closure: Close each thoracotomy site and place a chest tube.

Clinical Example (22838)

A 15-year-old female who is 2-years post-primary-tethering procedure presents with radiographic evidence of a broken tether device and an increase in the size of the scoliosis. The patient has remaining skeletal growth. The patient is referred for removal of the broken tether and placement of a new vertebral body tethering construct to provide coronal correction.

Description of Procedure (22838)

Co-Surgeon A—Exposure: Gain surgical access through the preferred approach, which is typically thoracoscopic and typically requires a single-lung ventilation technique and lung deflation to allow access. Several levels of thoracostomy may be required to visualize and manipulate the entire construct. Using an ultrasonic scalpel or thermal device, remove pleural adhesions from the intact anterior vertebral body tethering construct.

Co-Surgeon B—Tether Removal and Replacement: Inspect the cord and assess for any areas of breakage. Remove set screws and the broken cord. Assess the vertebral body screws. Remove or replace any loose vertebral body screws. New vertebral body screws may be added at adjacent levels. Confirm the trajectory and placement on the vertebral body screws at all levels prior to anchor insertion, screw preparation, and screw insertion using fluoroscopy or CT guidance. Due to smaller vertebral body size and variable venous anatomy, caution should be taken if extending instrumentation proximal to T5. Because all the vertebral bodies to be instrumented cannot be approached through the same thoracostomy, the procedure must be repeated as many times as it takes to access all the vertebral levels involved in the procedure. When appropriate, secure a new cord to the most cranial screw and segmentally tension, maintaining compression by tightening set screws at the adjacent levels. Applying the correct amount of tension is critical to the procedure and requires careful consideration of all patient factors. Remove the broken cord segments from the thorax. Following final tensioning, use intraoperative fluoroscopy or radiography to assess curve correction on AP and lateral imaging.

Co-Surgeon A—Closure: Close each thoracotomy site and place a chest tube.

Pelvis and Hip Joint

Fracture and/or Dislocation

27235 Percutaneous skeletal fixation of femoral fracture, proximal end, neck

▶(For percutaneous injection of calcium-based biodegradable osteoconductive material, use 0814T)◀

Rationale

In support of the establishment of code 0814T, a cross-reference parenthetical note has been added following code 27235 to direct users to code 0814T for percutaneous injection of calcium-based biodegradable osteoconductive material.

Refer to the codebook and the Rationale for code 0814T for a full discussion of these changes.

Arthrodesis

▶Code 27279 describes percutaneous arthrodesis of the sacroiliac joint using a minimally invasive technique to place an internal fixation device(s) that passes through the ilium, across the sacroiliac joint and into the sacrum, thus transfixing the sacroiliac joint. Report 27278 for the percutaneous placement of an intra-articular stabilization device into the sacroiliac joint using a minimally invasive technique that does not transfix the sacroiliac joint.◀

● **27278** Arthrodesis, sacroiliac joint, percutaneous, with image guidance, including placement of intra-articular implant(s) (eg, bone allograft[s], synthetic device[s]), without placement of transfixation device

▶(For arthrodesis, sacroiliac joint, with placement of a percutaneous transfixation device, use 27279)◀

▶(For bilateral procedure, report 27278 with modifier 50)◀

27279 Arthrodesis, sacroiliac joint, percutaneous or minimally invasive (indirect visualization), with image guidance, includes obtaining bone graft when performed, and placement of transfixing device

▶(For percutaneous arthrodesis of the sacroiliac joint by intra-articular implant[s], use 27278)◀

(For bilateral procedure, report 27279 with modifier 50)

27280 Arthrodesis, sacroiliac joint, open, includes obtaining bone graft, including instrumentation, when performed

(For percutaneous/minimally invasive arthrodesis of the sacroiliac joint without fracture and/or dislocation, utilizing a transfixation device, use 27279)

(To report bilateral procedure, report 27280 with modifier 50)

Rationale

Code 0775T and associated guidelines and parenthetical notes and instructions have been deleted, and code 27278 has been added to report percutaneous arthrodesis of the sacroiliac joint (SI) using placement of an intra-articular implant without transfixation. In addition, existing guidelines and parenthetical notes have been revised to accommodate instructions for reporting the new code.

Category III code 0775T was previously used to report the percutaneous arthrodesis of the SI joint using an intra-articular implant instead of transfixation, which was released via the AMA website to be reported as part of the CPT 2023 code set. However, Category I code 27278 has been created for the CPT 2024 code set to replace code 0775T and to be used to report the percutaneous intra-articular SI joint procedure. To accommodate the conversion of Category III code 0775T to Category I code 27278, all language and instructions within the code set that previously referenced code 0775T have been updated with instructions to use code 27278 for the intra-articular procedure. This includes an update of the existing guidelines within the Surgery section to reference code 27278 instead of code 0775T. The other revision includes the deletion of the guidelines that were related to code 0775T included in the Category III section. To further differentiate reporting of intra-articular procedure from percutaneous SI joint procedures that use transfixation, a new parenthetical note has been added following code 27278 to direct users to the appropriate code for the transfixation procedure (ie, 27279). In addition, the parenthetical note following code 27279 has been revised to reflect the use of code 27278 instead of deleted code 0775T to report percutaneous arthrodesis of the SI joint by intra-articular implant. Laterality issues for reporting were also addressed within a separate parenthetical note (ie, 27278 with modifier 50 for bilateral procedures).

Several changes have been made to provide instructions for reporting percutaneous SI joint fixation. As part of the intended reporting for the CPT 2023 code set, users were originally directed to report unlisted code 27299 to identify percutaneous SI joint fixations, ie, percutaneous SI joint fixations that used both a transfixation device and intra-articular implant(s). Later in 2023, code 0809T was added and accepted for an early release to the AMA website as part of the CPT 2023 code set to report these procedures. The addition of code 0809T included revising instructions about the use of code 0809T for procedures, as well as instructions for bilateral services.

For the CPT 2024 code set, new instructions regarding the changes and instructions for reporting percutaneous SI joint fusion services have been added. These include:

- Deletion of code 0809T.

- Deletion of instructions to report code 0809T in the affected section(s), guidelines, and parenthetical notes.

- Addition of new instructions in key locations that direct users to report codes 27278 and 27279 for percutaneous arthrodesis services of the SI joint.

Clinical Example (27278)

A 51-year-old female has chronic right-sided lower back and buttock pain and presents with sacroiliac (SI) joint dysfunction. She is scheduled for a minimally invasive SI joint fusion with structural bone allograft implant.

Description of Procedure (27278)

Perform imaging in multiple obliquities to establish optimal view to access the SI joint. Use a 22-gauge 3.5- or 5-inch spinal needle to infiltrate the working site with local anesthesia from the skin to the periosteum. Mark the target location with a hemostat and surgical marker. Make a 1.5-cm incision and obtain hemostasis with electrocautery. Perform a blunt dissection down to the joint and once again establish hemostasis. Then insert a guide pin into the SI joint space and confirm on multiple oblique and lateral views. Adjust the position of the guide pin to establish optimum access to the SI joint. Next, depending on the system, advance a coaxial dilator over the guide pin to the posterior cortical line of the sacrum, which is again confirmed in the optimal view. Once alignment is confirmed, gently tap the outer working portal on the handle with a mallet until the hard stop on the outer working portal meets the posterior cortical line of the sacrum. Once the working portal is fully seated on the sacrum, remove the internal dilator and guide pin. Depending on the system used, decorticate the SI joint using either a drilling or broaching system. Carefully load the physician-prepared cortical allograft with demineralized bone matrix on the back table into a delivery insertion system. Then carefully insert the allograft and delivery system into the working portal and advance them to the decorticated area of the SI joint. Deploy the allograft using an inserter and mallet. Once the allograft position is satisfactorily established, remove the working portal. After the working portal is removed, close the wound with deep dermal suture and the skin with cyanoacrylate glue and cover with sterile dressings.

Foot and Toes

Repair, Revision, and/or Reconstruction

▲ 28292   Correction, hallux valgus with bunionectomy, with sesamoidectomy when performed; with resection of proximal phalanx base, when performed, any method

28295   Code is out of numerical sequence. See 28292-28298

▲ 28296   with distal metatarsal osteotomy, any method

#▲ 28295   with proximal metatarsal osteotomy, any method

▲ 28297   with first metatarsal and medial cuneiform joint arthrodesis, any method

▶(For first metatarsal-cuneiform joint fusion without concomitant removal of the distal medial prominence of the first metatarsal for hallux valgus correction, use 28740)◀

▲ 28298   with proximal phalanx osteotomy, any method

▲ 28299   with double osteotomy, any method

Arthrodesis

28740   Arthrodesis, midtarsal or tarsometatarsal, single joint

▶(For first metatarsal-cuneiform joint fusion without concomitant removal of the distal medial prominence of the first metatarsal for hallux valgus correction, use 28740)◀

Rationale

Codes 28292 and 28295-28299 have been revised and parenthetical notes have been added following codes 28297 and 28740 to clarify correct reporting of bunion correction performed with and without resection of bunion.

Revisions have been made to the descriptors of codes currently used to report hallux valgus correction that includes the excision or resection of the proximal phalanx base as part of the corrective measures taken to resolve bunion disorder of the foot. Previously, the descriptors for codes 28292 and 28295-28299 did not specify that bunionectomy is required for reporting these codes. As a result, many users mistakenly believed that the codes in the 28292 code family may be used if a hallux valgus correction had been performed regardless of whether a bunion was resected or not. Therefore, the addition of the term "with" to precede bunionectomy and removing the parentheses from "bunionectomy" in the main (parent) descriptor for these codes clarify that the corrective measures reported by codes 28292 and 28295-28299 should inherently include the removal of the bunion by excision or resection.

★ = Telemedicine   ◀ = Audio-only   ✚ = Add-on code   ✐ = FDA approval pending   # = Resequenced code   ⊘ = Modifier 51 exempt

To further clarify this, parenthetical notes have also been added to the code set in key locations (ie, following the codes for bunionectomy [28292, 28295-28297] and for arthrodesis [28740] of the midtarsal or tarsometatarsal joint). These parenthetical notes direct users to report code 28740 if a first metatarsal-cuneiform joint fusion is performed without concomitant removal of the distal medial prominence of the first metatarsal to correct a hallux valgus.

Respiratory System

Nose

Excision

30117 Excision or destruction (eg, laser), intranasal lesion; internal approach

30118 external approach (lateral rhinotomy)

▶(For surgical nasal/sinus endoscopy with destruction by radiofrequency ablation of posterior nasal nerve, use 31242)◀

▶(For surgical nasal/sinus endoscopy with destruction by cryoablation of posterior nasal nerve, use 31243)◀

Rationale

In accordance with the establishment of codes 31242 and 31243, two cross-reference parenthetical notes have been added following code 30118 to reflect these changes.

Refer to the codebook and the Rationale for codes 31242 and 31243 for a full discussion of these changes.

Accessory Sinuses

Endoscopy

31237 Nasal/sinus endoscopy, surgical; with biopsy, polypectomy or debridement (separate procedure)

(Do not report 31237 in conjunction with 31238, 31253, 31254, 31255, 31256, 31257, 31259, 31267, 31276, 31287, 31288, 31290, 31291, 31292, 31293, 31294, when performed on the ipsilateral side)

#● **31242** with destruction by radiofrequency ablation, posterior nasal nerve

#● **31243** with destruction by cryoablation, posterior nasal nerve

▶(Do not report 31242, 31243 in conjunction with 31231, 92511)◀

▶(31242, 31243 are used to report bilateral procedures. For unilateral procedure, use modifier 52)◀

31238 with control of nasal hemorrhage

(Do not report 31238 in conjunction with 31237, 31241, when performed on the ipsilateral side)

31239 with dacryocystorhinostomy

31240 with concha bullosa resection

31241 with ligation of sphenopalatine artery

(Do not report 31241 in conjunction with 31238, when performed on the ipsilateral side)

31242 Code is out of numerical sequence. See 31235-31239

31243 Code is out of numerical sequence. See 31235-31239

Rationale

Codes 31242 and 31243 have been established to report nasal/sinus endoscopic destruction of the posterior nasal nerve using radiofrequency ablation (31242) and cryoablation (31243).

Prior to 2024, no specific code exists for reporting energy-based destruction of the posterior nasal nerve. Existing code 30117 describes excision or destruction of an intranasal lesion using an internal approach; however, it does not include an endoscopic approach or specify radiofrequency or cryoablation of the posterior nasal nerve. Codes 31242 and 31243 describe bilateral procedures. When performed unilaterally, modifier 52 should be appended as noted in a new instructional parenthetical note following codes 31242 and 31243. An exclusionary parenthetical note has also been added to restrict the use of codes 31242 and 31243 with codes 31231 and 92511.

Clinical Example (31242)

A 68-year-old female presents with symptoms of chronic rhinitis that have been refractory to medical therapy. The patient is scheduled for endoscopic surgical energy-based neurolysis of the posterior nasal nerve, using a radiofrequency ablation probe.

Description of Procedure (31242)

Remove previously placed pledgets. Perform the following portions of the procedure under endoscopic visualization. Place additional pledgets soaked in decongestant and anesthesia more posteriorly in the middle meatus, followed by a wait time for them to take effect. Then remove the pledgets. Place pledgets soaked in decongestant and anesthesia at the lateral attachment

▲=Revised code ●=New code ▶◀=Contains new or revised text ✖=Duplicate PLA test ↕=Category I PLA American Medical Association **31**

Surgery / Respiratory System 30000-32999

site of the middle turbinate followed by a wait time for them to take effect. Inject an intranasal anesthetic or vasoconstrictive agent into the lateral attachment of middle turbinate followed by a wait time for this to take effect. Medialize the middle turbinate. Introduce the radio frequency energy delivery device into the nasal cavity. Perform multiple applications of radio frequency in the area of the posterior nasal nerve, including the lateral attachment of the middle turbinate as well as the superior aspect of the inferior turbinate. Withdraw the radio frequency delivery device. Place pledgets soaked in decongestant in the treated areas to allow for hemostasis. Then remove the pledgets. Perform the same procedure on the contralateral side.

Clinical Example (31243)

A 72-year-old female presents with symptoms of chronic rhinitis that have been refractory to medical therapy. The patient is scheduled for endoscopic surgical energy-based neurolysis of the posterior nasal nerve, using a cryoablation probe.

Description of Procedure (31243)

Remove previously placed pledgets. Perform the following parts of the procedure under endoscopic visualization. Place pledgets soaked in decongestant and anesthesia in the middle meatus followed by a wait time for them to take effect. Then remove the pledgets. Place pledgets soaked in decongestant and anesthesia at the lateral attachment site of the middle turbinate followed by a wait time for them to take effect. Inject an intranasal anesthetic or vasoconstrictive agent into the lateral attachment of middle turbinate followed by a wait time for this to take effect. Medialize the middle turbinate. Introduce the cryoablation probe into the nasal cavity. Then place the cryoablation probe at the lateral attachment of the middle turbinate and activate, initiating the freezing process. Perform cryotherapy freezing under scrupulous endoscopic observation. Once adequate cryotherapy has been applied, stop the application of cryotherapy. Ask the patient to breathe through their nose while the cryotherapy probe unfreezes from the affected mucosa. Once the cryotherapy probe unfreezes from the surrounding mucosa, withraw it. Then place pledgets soaked in decongestant in the treated areas to allow for hemostasis. Remove the pledgets. Exchange the cryoablation canister for a new one. Reorient the wand to accommodate the contralateral side. Perform the same procedure on the contralateral side.

Lungs and Pleura

Thoracoscopy (Video-assisted thoracic surgery [VATS])

32601   Thoracoscopy, diagnostic (separate procedure); lungs, pericardial sac, mediastinal or pleural space, without biopsy

▶(Do not report 32601 in conjunction with 22836, 22837, 22838)◀

32604   pericardial sac, with biopsy

(For open pericardial biopsy, use 39010)

32606   mediastinal space, with biopsy

Rationale

In accordance with the establishment of codes 22836-22838, revision of codes 0656T and 0657T, and addition of Category III code 0790T, an exclusionary parenthetical note following code 32601 has been added to restrict reporting of the new codes (22836-22838) in conjunction with diagnostic thoracoscopy services (32601).

Refer to the codebook and the Rationale for codes 22836-22838 for a full discussion of these changes.

Cardiovascular System

Heart and Pericardium

Pacemaker or Implantable Defibrillator

A pacemaker system with lead(s) includes a pulse generator containing electronics, a battery, and one or more leads. A lead consists of one or more electrodes, as well as conductor wires, insulation, and a fixation mechanism. Pulse generators are placed in a subcutaneous "pocket" created in either a subclavicular site or just above the abdominal muscles just below the ribcage. Leads may be inserted through a vein (transvenous) or they may be placed on the surface of the heart (epicardial). The epicardial location of leads requires a thoracotomy for insertion.

A single chamber pacemaker system with lead includes a pulse generator and one electrode inserted in either the atrium or ventricle. A dual chamber pacemaker system with two leads includes a pulse generator and one lead inserted in the right atrium and one lead inserted in the right ventricle. In certain circumstances, an additional lead may be required to achieve pacing of the left ventricle (bi-ventricular pacing). In this event, transvenous (cardiac vein) placement of the lead should be separately reported using code 33224 or 33225. For body surface–activation mapping to optimize electrical synchrony of a biventricular pacing or biventricular pacing-defibrillator system at the time of implant, also report 0695T with the appropriate code (ie, 33224, 33225, 33226). Epicardial placement of the lead should be separately reported using 33202, 33203.

▶A leadless cardiac pacemaker system includes a pulse generator with built-in battery and electrode for implantation in a cardiac chamber via a transvenous transcatheter approach. For implantation of a right ventricular leadless pacemaker system, use 33274. Insertion, replacement, or removal of a right ventricular leadless pacemaker system includes insertion of a catheter via transvenous access under fluoroscopic guidance into the right ventricle. For a complete dual-chamber leadless cardiac pacemaker system which is implanted in both the right ventricle and right atrium, or individual components of a dual-chamber leadless pacemaker system, see 0795T, 0796T, 0797T, 0798T, 0799T, 0800T, 0801T, 0802T, 0803T. Device evaluation at the time of leadless pacemaker insertion, replacement, or removal is included in 33274, 33275, 0795T, 0796T, 0797T, 0798T, 0799T, 0800T, 0801T, 0802T, 0803T, 0823T, 0824T, 0825T and is not separately reported. For subsequent leadless pacemaker device evaluation, see 93279, 93286, 93288, 93294, 93296, 0804T, 0826T.

For a single-chamber leadless cardiac pacemaker implanted in the right atrium that is not a component of a dual-chamber leadless pacemaker system, see 0823T, 0824T, 0825T.

Right heart catheterization (93451, 93453, 93456, 93457, 93460, 93461, 93593, 93594, 93596, 93597) may not be reported in conjunction with leadless pacemaker insertion and removal codes 33274, 33275, 0795T, 0796T, 0797T, 0798T, 0799T, 0800T, 0801T, 0802T, 0803T, 0823T, 0824T, 0825T, unless complete right heart catheterization is performed for an indication distinct from the leadless pacemaker procedure.◀

Like a pacemaker system, an implantable defibrillator system includes a pulse generator and electrodes. Three general categories of implantable defibrillators exist: transvenous implantable pacing cardioverter-defibrillator (ICD), subcutaneous implantable defibrillator (S-ICD), and substernal implantable cardioverter-defibrillator. Implantable pacing cardioverter-defibrillator devices use a combination of antitachycardia pacing, low-energy cardioversion or defibrillating shocks to treat ventricular tachycardia or ventricular fibrillation. The subcutaneous implantable defibrillator uses a single subcutaneous electrode to treat ventricular tachyarrhythmias. The substernal implantable cardioverter-defibrillator uses at least one substernal electrode to perform defibrillation, cardioversion, and antitachycardia pacing. Subcutaneous implantable defibrillators differ from transvenous

implantable pacing cardioverter-defibrillators in that subcutaneous defibrillators do not provide antitachycardia pacing or chronic pacing. Substernal implantable defibrillators differ from both subcutaneous and transvenous implantable pacing cardioverter-defibrillators in that they provide antitachycardia pacing, but not chronic pacing.

Implantable defibrillator pulse generators may be implanted in a subcutaneous infraclavicular, axillary, or abdominal pocket. Removal of an implantable defibrillator pulse generator requires opening of the existing subcutaneous pocket and disconnection of the pulse generator from its electrode(s). A thoracotomy (or laparotomy in the case of abdominally placed pulse generators) is not required to remove the pulse generator.

 # 33274   Transcatheter insertion or replacement of permanent leadless pacemaker, right ventricular, including imaging guidance (eg, fluoroscopy, venous ultrasound, ventriculography, femoral venography) and device evaluation (eg, interrogation or programming), when performed

 # 33275   Transcatheter removal of permanent leadless pacemaker, right ventricular, including imaging guidance (eg, fluoroscopy, venous ultrasound, ventriculography, femoral venography), when performed

(Do not report 33275 in conjunction with 33274)

(Do not report 33274, 33275 in conjunction with femoral venography [75820], fluoroscopy [76000, 77002], ultrasound guidance for vascular access [76937], right ventriculography [93566])

(Do not report 33274, 33275 in conjunction with 93451, 93453, 93456, 93457, 93460, 93461, 93593, 93594, 93596, 93597, 93598, unless complete right heart catheterization is performed for indications distinct from the leadless pacemaker procedure)

▶(Do not report 33274, 33275 in conjunction with dual-chamber leadless pacemaker codes 0795T, 0796T, 0797T, 0798T, 0799T, 0800T, 0801T, 0802T, 0803T)◀

▶(Do not report 33274, 33275 in conjunction with 0823T, 0824T, 0825T, for right atrial single-chamber leadless pacemaker)◀

▶(Do not report 33274, 33275 when the right ventricular single-chamber leadless pacemaker is part of a complete dual-chamber leadless pacemaker system)◀

(For insertion, replacement, repositioning, and removal of pacemaker systems with leads, see 33202, 33203, 33206, 33207, 33208, 33212, 33213, 33214, 33215, 33216, 33217, 33218, 33220, 33221, 33227, 33228, 33229, 33233, 33234, 33235, 33236, 33237)

▶(For subsequent leadless pacemaker device evaluation, see 93279, 93286, 93288, 93294, 93296, 0804T, 0826T)◀

▶(For dual-chamber leadless pacemaker, see 0795T, 0796T, 0797T, 0798T, 0799T, 0800T, 0801T, 0802T, 0803T)◀

►Procedure	System	
	Pacemaker	Implantable Defibrillator
Insert transvenous single lead only without pulse generator	33216	33216
Insert transvenous dual leads without pulse generator	33217	33217
Insert transvenous multiple leads without pulse generator	33217 + 33224	33217 + 33224
Insert subcutaneous defibrillator electrode only without pulse generator	N/A	33271
Initial pulse generator insertion only with existing single lead, includes transvenous or subcutaneous defibrillator lead	33212	33240
Initial pulse generator insertion only with existing dual leads	33213	33230
Initial pulse generator insertion only with existing multiple leads	33221	33231
Initial pulse generator insertion or replacement plus insertion of transvenous single lead	33206 (atrial) or 33207 (ventricular)	33249
Initial pulse generator insertion or replacement plus insertion of transvenous dual leads	33208	33249
Initial pulse generator insertion or replacement plus insertion of transvenous multiple leads	33208 + 33225	33249 + 33225
Initial pulse generator insertion or replacement plus insertion of subcutaneous defibrillator electrode	N/A	33270
Insertion, replacement, or removal and replacement of permanent single-chamber leadless ventricular pacemaker	33274	N/A
Insertion permanent single-chamber leadless pacemaker, right atrial	0823T	N/A
Insertion permanent dual-chamber leadless pacemaker, right atrial and right ventricular components	0795T	N/A
Insertion permanent dual-chamber leadless pacemaker, right atrial component	0796T	N/A
Insertion permanent dual-chamber leadless pacemaker, right ventricular component (when part of a dual-chamber leadless pacemaker system)	0797T	N/A
Upgrade single chamber system to dual chamber system	33214 (includes removal of existing pulse generator)	33241 + 33249
Removal pulse generator only (without replacement)	33233	33241
Removal pulse generator with replacement pulse generator only single lead system (applies to transvenous or subcutaneous defibrillator lead systems)	33227	33262
Removal pulse generator with replacement pulse generator only dual lead system (transvenous)	33228	33263
Removal pulse generator with replacement pulse generator only multiple lead system (transvenous)	33229	33264
Removal transvenous electrode only single lead system	33234	33244
Removal transvenous electrode only dual lead system	33235	33244
Removal subcutaneous defibrillator lead only	N/A	33272
Removal and replacement of pulse generator and transvenous electrodes	33233 + (33234 or 33235) + (33206, 33207 or 33208) and 33225, when appropriate	33241 + 33244 + 33249 and 33225, when appropriate

★ = Telemedicine   ◀ = Audio-only   ✚ = Add-on code   ✗ = FDA approval pending   # = Resequenced code   ⊘ = Modifier 51 exempt

Procedure	System	
	Pacemaker	Implantable Defibrillator
Removal and replacement of implantable defibrillator pulse generator and subcutaneous electrode	N/A	33272 + 33241 + 33270
Removal and replacement permanent single-chamber leadless pacemaker, right atrial	0825T	N/A
Removal and replacement permanent dual-chamber leadless pacemaker, right atrial and right ventricular components	0801T	N/A
Removal and replacement permanent dual-chamber leadless pacemaker, right atrial component	0802T	N/A
Removal and replacement permanent dual-chamber leadless pacemaker, right ventricular component (when part of a dual-chamber leadless pacemaker system)	0803T	N/A
Removal of permanent single-chamber leadless ventricular pacemaker	33275	N/A
Removal permanent single-chamber leadless right atrial pacemaker	0824T	N/A
Removal permanent dual-chamber leadless pacemaker, right atrial and right ventricular components	0798T	N/A
Removal permanent dual-chamber leadless pacemaker, right atrial component	0799T	N/A
Removal permanent dual-chamber leadless pacemaker, right ventricular component (when part of a dual-chamber leadless pacemaker system)	0800T	N/A
Conversion of existing system to bi-ventricular system (addition of LV lead and removal of current pulse generator with insertion of new pulse generator with bi-ventricular pacing capabilities)	33225 + 33228 or 33229	33225 + 33263 or 33264◄

►(For insertion or replacement of a leadless pacemaker into the right ventricle as part of a complete dual-chamber leadless pacemaker system, use 0797T)◄

►(For removal of right ventricular pacemaker component of a complete dual-chamber leadless pacemaker system, use 0800T)◄

Rationale

In accordance with the establishment of Category III codes 0795T-0804T and codes 0823T-0826T, the Pacemaker or Implantable Defibrillator guidelines have been revised to clarify the differences between leadless pacemaker codes 33274 and 33275 (right ventricular), 0795T-0804T (dual-chamber), and 0823T-0826T (right atrial). The pacemaker defibrillator procedures table has been revised to include the new Category III codes.

Two exclusionary parenthetical notes have also been added restricting the use of codes 33274 and 33275 with the new Category III codes. An instructional parenthetical note has been added to restrict reporting codes 33274 and 33275 when the right ventricular single-chamber leadless pacemaker is part of a complete dual-chamber leadless pacemaker system. The cross-reference parenthetical note

related to subsequent leadless pacemaker device evaluation has been revised to include new codes 0804T and 0826T. In addition, three other new cross-reference parenthetical notes have been added.

Refer to the codebook and the Rationale for codes 0795T-0804T, and 0823T-0826T for a full discussion of these changes.

►Phrenic Nerve Stimulation System◄

►Insertion of a phrenic nerve stimulation system includes a pulse generator (containing electronics and a battery) and one stimulation lead and is reported with 33276. Pulse generators are placed in a submuscular or subcutaneous "pocket" in the pectoral region. The stimulation lead is placed transvenously into the right brachiocephalic vein or left pericardiophrenic vein. Rarely, a separate sensing lead may be needed to augment system function and, when performed at time of system insertion, is reported with 33277. This sensing lead is placed transvenously into the azygos vein. Initial system placement includes initiation of diagnostic mode and associated system evaluation. Codes 33276, 33277,

33278, 33279, 33280, 33281, 33287, 33288 include vessel catheterization and all imaging guidance required for the procedure, when performed. For therapeutic activation of the phrenic nerve stimulation system, see 93150, 93151, 93152, 93153.◄

#● **33276** Insertion of phrenic nerve stimulator system (pulse generator and stimulating lead[s]), including vessel catheterization, all imaging guidance, and pulse generator initial analysis with diagnostic mode activation, when performed

►(Do not report 33276 in conjunction with 93150, 93151, 93152, 93153)◄

#+● **33277** Insertion of phrenic nerve stimulator transvenous sensing lead (List separately in addition to code for primary procedure)

►(Use 33277 in conjunction with 33276, 33287)◄

►(For insertion of a phrenic nerve sensing lead other than at initial insertion of the phrenic nerve stimulator system, use 33999)◄

#● **33278** Removal of phrenic nerve stimulator, including vessel catheterization, all imaging guidance, and interrogation and programming, when performed; system, including pulse generator and lead(s)

#● **33279** transvenous stimulation or sensing lead(s) only

►(Use 33279 once for removal of one or more lead[s])◄

#● **33280** pulse generator only

►(Do not report 33278, 33279, 33280 in conjunction with 33276, 33277, 33281, 33287, 33288)◄

#● **33281** Repositioning of phrenic nerve stimulator transvenous lead(s)

►(Do not report 33281 in conjunction with 33276, 33277)◄

►(Report 33281 only once per patient per day)◄

#● **33287** Removal and replacement of phrenic nerve stimulator, including vessel catheterization, all imaging guidance, and interrogation and programming, when performed; pulse generator

►(Do not report 33287 in conjunction with 33276, 33278)◄

#● **33288** transvenous stimulation or sensing lead(s)

►(Use 33288 once for removal of one or more lead[s])◄

►(Do not report 33288 in conjunction with 33277, 33279, 33281)◄

Rationale

Eight new Category I codes (33276-33281, 33287, 33288) have been established in the Surgery/Cardiovascular System/Heart and Pericardium Pacemaker or Implantable Defibrillator subsection to report insertion, removal, repositioning, and replacement of phrenic nerve stimulator system and/or its components. In addition, Category III codes 0424T-0436T have been deleted and new guidelines, headings, and parenthetical notes have been included to provide instructions regarding appropriate reporting for these services.

Codes 33276-33281, 33287, and 33288 are used to identify phrenic nerve stimulation system services. These services may be used to treat moderate to severe central sleep apnea by stimulation of the phrenic nerve to control breathing. These services include procedures for insertion (33276, 33277), removal (33278-33280), repositioning (33281), and replacement (33287, 33288) of phrenic nerve stimulation devices or their components. As stated in the guidelines, insertion of a phrenic nerve simulation system includes a pulse generator (that contains electronics and a battery) and one stimulation lead and is reported with code 33276. As noted in the code descriptor for code 33276, device placement (accomplished intravascularly), imaging guidance, and pulse generator initial analysis with diagnostic mode activation are all commonly performed when providing services for these devices. These services are inherently included as part of the procedures and not separately reported. New guidelines and exclusionary and cross-reference parenthetical notes have been established to provide instruction on the appropriate reporting. Some of the instructions include: (1) reporting when a separate sensing lead is necessary to augment system function; (2) reporting for catheterization and imaging; (3) reporting sensing lead placement when performed at a time other than initial insertion (33999); (4) restriction about reporting removal of one or more lead(s) (33279, 33288); (5) the number of times that repositioning (33281) may be reported per day; (6) restriction about reporting programming (93150-93153) that was not separately performed from the insertion procedure described by code 33276; and (7) a cross-reference to the therapeutic activation codes (93150-93153).

To accommodate these changes, Category III codes 0424T-0436T and all related references have been deleted. New parenthetical notes have been established to direct users to the appropriate codes for these services. In addition, to accommodate reporting for therapeutic activation services, four new codes (93150-93153), guidelines, and parenthetical instructions have been added within the new subsection of "Phrenic Nerve Stimulation System" located in the Medicine section.

Refer to the codebook and the Rationale for codes 93150-93153 for a full discussion of these changes.

Clinical Example (33276)

A 65-year-old male has a history of excessive daytime sleepiness and insomnia. The patient recently underwent a polysomnogram and was diagnosed with central sleep apnea with an apnea hypopnea index (AHI) of 50 events per hour.

Description of Procedure (33276)

Perform venous access into the subclavian or cephalic vein via two separate access sites. Create a subcutaneous pocket in the pectoral region using blunt dissection. Place a guiding sheath in the superior vena cava and direct to the left brachiocephalic vein. Administer a non-selective contrast injection to identify the ostia of the left pericardiophrenic vein. Once identified, place a sub-select sheath through the guiding sheath and then use a coronary guidewire to identify the left pericardiophrenic vein. Administer contrast injection at different fluoroscopic angles to identify the left pericardiophrenic vein. Once vein is identified and cannulated with a coronary angiography wire, administer a contrast injection to determine the caliber of the pericardiophrenic vein and if it is large enough to accommodate the pacing lead. Exchange the initial coronary angiography for a stiffer wire to facilitate advancing the lead to the left pericardiophrenic vein. If the stimulation lead cannot be placed in the left pericardiophrenic vein, exchange the guiding sheath for a short introducer sheath in the right subclavian vein. Place an alternate stimulation lead into the right brachiocephalic vein using standard transvenous implantation techniques. Once the stimulation lead is in position, confirm adequate stimulation and impedance characteristics using a phrenic nerve stimulation system analyzer. Rouse the patient and ask for feedback as to how closely the simulation represents a normal breath. Also ask the patient if there is any discomfort associated with stimulation. Reposition the stimulation lead if needed to ensure adequate long-term stimulation of the nerve. Stabilize the lead using suture sleeves and connect to the implantable pulse generator. At this point, determine the need for a sensing lead. Connect the leads to the pulse generator. Insert device and leads into the pocket and close the incision.

Clinical Example (33277)

A 65-year-old male with a history of excessive daytime sleepiness and insomnia recently underwent a polysomnogram and was diagnosed with central sleep apnea with an AHI of 50 events per hour. A phrenic nerve stimulator system is recommended. During system implantation, an additional sensing lead is determined to be necessary to optimize system function. [**Note:** This is an add-on code. Only consider the additional work of placing a sensing lead.]

Description of Procedure (33277)

The patient undergoes a subcutaneous implantation of a neurostimulator system and requires the additional placement of a sensing lead. Advance a guiding sheath to the superior vena cava. Utilizing contrast injections from different fluoroscopic views, a subselect sheath and a stiff guidewire, cannulate the azygos vein. In a telescoping manner, advance the subselect and then the guiding sheath over the guidewire into the azygos vein. Remove the subselect sheath and guidewire. Place a bipolar coronary sinus lead over a coronary guidewire into the guiding sheath. Advance the coronary guidewire to the intercostal vein at the level of the dome of the diaphragm and advance the lead over a guidewire. Once the sensing lead is placed, stabilize the lead using suture sleeves and connect to the implantable pulse generator.

Clinical Example (33278)

A 65-year-old male with a history of central sleep apnea was treated successfully with a phrenic nerve stimulator system. After a recent skin infection, the patient develops bacteremia that persists with signs of pocket infection; complete removal of the system is recommended.

Description of Procedure (33278)

Make an incision over the previously implanted pulse generator. Free the device and leads from the surrounding tissue and achieve hemostasis. Disconnect the lead from the pulse generator and remove the pulse generator. Free the suture collars of the leads from surrounding tissue. Insert a stylet or stiff guidewire into the lead and apply gentle traction under fluoroscopic guidance. If the lead cannot be removed with manual traction under fluoroscopic guidance, then insert a locking stylet into the lead. Next, advance a manual rotational extraction sheath or a laser sheath over the lead and use standard lead extraction techniques to remove the lead. Once the lead is removed and hemodynamic stability is verified, close the incision.

Clinical Example (33279)

A 65-year-old male with a prior history of central sleep apnea and phrenic nerve stimulator system previously had his pulse generator removed for radiation therapy. He now presents with bacteremia and infection of the abandoned stimulation lead. Complete lead removal is recommended.

Description of Procedure (33279)

Make an incision over the previously implanted pulse generator. Free the leads from the surrounding tissue and achieve hemostasis. Disconnect the lead from the pulse generator. Free the suture collars of the leads from surrounding tissue. Insert a stylet or stiff guidewire into

Surgery / Cardiovascular System 33016-39599

the lead and apply gentle traction under fluoroscopic guidance. If the lead is unable to be removed with manual traction under fluoroscopic guidance, then insert a locking stylet into the lead. Next, advance a manual rotational extraction sheath or a laser sheath over the lead and use standard lead extraction techniques to remove the lead. Once the lead is removed and hemodynamic stability is verified, close the incision.

Clinical Example (33280)

A 67-year-old male with a previously placed phrenic nerve stimulation system requires radiation therapy. The existing generator is in the planned path of the therapy beam; therefore, pulse generator removal is required.

Description of Procedure (33280)

Make an incision over the previously implanted pulse generator. Free the device and leads from the surrounding tissue and achieve hemostasis. Disconnect the lead from the pulse generator and remove the pulse generator. Once the device is removed and hemodynamic stability is verified, close the incision.

Clinical Example (33281)

A 67-year-old male, who has a phrenic nerve stimulator system for central sleep apnea, suffered a fall that caused the lead(s) to change position, which is limiting the effectiveness of the therapy. The lead(s) needs to be repositioned.

Description of Procedure (33281)

Make an incision over the previously implanted pulse generator. Free the device and leads from the surrounding tissue and achieve hemostasis. Disconnect the lead from the pulse generator. Free the suture collars of the leads from surrounding tissue. Insert a stylet or stiff guidewire into the lead and apply gentle traction under fluoroscopic guidance. Reposition the lead to a similar location in the same pericardiophrenic vein. If adequate pacing threshold or stability cannot be attained, place a new pacing lead in the right brachiocephalic vein. Once the lead is in position, confirm adequate stimulation and impedance characteristics using a neurostimulation system analyzer. Rouse the patient and ask for feedback as to how closely the simulation represents a normal breath. Also ask the patient if there is any discomfort associated with stimulation. Stabilize the lead using suture sleeves and connect to the implantable pulse generator. Place both the lead and implantable pulse generator in the subcutaneous pocket and close the incision.

Clinical Example (33287)

A 65-year-old male who has a history of central sleep apnea was treated successfully with a phrenic nerve stimulator system. The device has now reached battery depletion and requires removal of the current generator and replacement with a new generator.

Description of Procedure (33287)

Make an incision over the previously implanted pulse generator. Free the device and leads from the surrounding tissue and achieve hemostasis. Disconnect the lead from the pulse generator and remove the pulse generator. Assess the pocket for suitability to receive a new generator. Implant a new generator, reconnect the leads, and close the incision.

Clinical Example (33288)

A 65-year-old male who has a history of central sleep apnea was treated successfully with a phrenic nerve stimulator system. At a recent device check, the stimulation lead was found to have fractured and is no longer functioning. Removal of the lead and replacement with a new lead is recommended to restore normal system function.

Description of Procedure (33288)

Make an incision over the previously implanted pulse generator. Free the device and leads from the surrounding tissue and achieve hemostasis. Disconnect the lead from the pulse generator. Free the suture collars of the leads from surrounding tissue. Insert a stylet or stiff guidewire into the lead and apply gentle traction under fluoroscopic guidance. If the lead is unable to be removed with manual traction under fluoroscopic guidance, then insert a locking stylet into the lead. Next, advance a manual rotational extraction sheath or a laser sheath over the lead and use standard lead extraction techniques to remove the lead. Next, bring a new guiding sheath to the field and place into the venous system. Bring a new lead to the field and advance to the target vessel, either the left pericardiophrenic vein or the right brachiocephalic vein. Once the lead is in position, confirm adequate stimulation and impedance characteristics using a neurostimulation system analyzer. Rouse the patient and ask for feedback as to how closely the simulation represents a normal breath. Also ask the patient if there is any discomfort associated with stimulation. Stabilize the lead using suture sleeves and connect to a new implantable pulse generator. Place both the lead and implantable pulse generator in the subcutaneous pocket and close the incision.

Electrophysiologic Operative Procedures

Endoscopy

33266　　operative tissue ablation and reconstruction of atria, extensive (eg, maze procedure), without cardiopulmonary bypass

(Do not report 33265-33266 in conjunction with 32551, 33210, 33211)

33276　Code is out of numerical sequence. See 33244-33251

33277　Code is out of numerical sequence. See 33244-33251

33278　Code is out of numerical sequence. See 33244-33251

33279　Code is out of numerical sequence. See 33244-33251

33280　Code is out of numerical sequence. See 33244-33251

33281　Code is out of numerical sequence. See 33244-33251

Subcutaneous Cardiac Rhythm Monitor

33286　Removal, subcutaneous cardiac rhythm monitor

(Initial insertion includes programming. For subsequent electronic analysis and/or reprogramming, see 93285, 93291, 93298)

33287　Code is out of numerical sequence. See 33244-33251

33288　Code is out of numerical sequence. See 33244-33251

Digestive System

Stomach

Laparoscopy

43647　Laparoscopy, surgical; implantation or replacement of gastric neurostimulator electrodes, antrum

43648　　revision or removal of gastric neurostimulator electrodes, antrum

(For open approach, see 43881, 43882)

(For insertion of gastric neurostimulator pulse generator, use 64590)

(For revision or removal of gastric neurostimulator pulse generator, use 64595)

►(For electronic analysis and programming of gastric neurostimulator pulse generator, see 95980, 95981, 95982)◄

(For laparoscopic implantation, revision, or removal of gastric neurostimulator electrodes, lesser curvature [morbid obesity], use 43659)

Other Procedures

43882　Revision or removal of gastric neurostimulator electrodes, antrum, open

(For laparoscopic approach, see 43647, 43648)

(For insertion of gastric neurostimulator pulse generator, use 64590)

(For revision or removal of gastric neurostimulator pulse generator, use 64595)

►(For electronic analysis and programming of gastric neurostimulator pulse generator, see 95980, 95981, 95982)◄

►(For open implantation, revision, or removal of gastric neurostimulator electrodes, lesser curvature [morbid obesity] or vagal trunk [EGJ] neurostimulator electrodes, use 43999)◄

Rationale

The cross-reference parenthetical note following codes 43648 and 43882 regarding reporting electronic analysis and programming for gastric neurostimulator pulse generators has been editorially revised by listing all codes in the code range of 95980-95982.

Refer to the codebook and the Rationale for codes 64590-64598 for a full discussion of these changes.

The cross-reference parenthetical note following code 43882 directing users to code 43999 has been revised to also reference open implantation, revision, or removal of vagal trunk neurostimulator electrodes.

Urinary System

Bladder

Urodynamics

51736　Simple uroflowmetry (UFR) (eg, stop-watch flow rate, mechanical uroflowmeter)

►(Do not report 51736 in conjunction with 0811T, 0812T)◄

51741　Complex uroflowmetry (eg, calibrated electronic equipment)

►(Do not report 51741 in conjunction with 0811T, 0812T)◄

Rationale

In accordance with the establishment of codes 0811T and 0812T, exclusionary parenthetical notes following codes 51736 and 51741 have been added to preclude the reporting of these two new codes with codes 51736 and 51741.

Refer to the codebook and the Rationale for codes 0811T and 0812T for a full discussion of these changes.

Transurethral Surgery

Urethra and Bladder

52281   Cystourethroscopy, with calibration and/or dilation of urethral stricture or stenosis, with or without meatotomy, with or without injection procedure for cystography, male or female

►(For cystourethroscopy with mechanical urethral dilation and urethral therapeutic drug delivery by drug-coated balloon catheter for urethral stricture or stenosis, including fluoroscopy, use 52284)◄

52282   Cystourethroscopy, with insertion of permanent urethral stent

(For placement of temporary prostatic urethral stent, use 53855)

52283   Cystourethroscopy, with steroid injection into stricture

● 52284   Cystourethroscopy, with mechanical urethral dilation and urethral therapeutic drug delivery by drug-coated balloon catheter for urethral stricture or stenosis, male, including fluoroscopy, when performed

►(Do not report 52284 in conjunction with 51610, 52000, 52281, 52283, 74450, 76000)◄

Rationale

Code 0499T, *Cystourethroscopy, with mechanical dilation and urethral therapeutic drug delivery for urethral stricture or stenosis, including fluoroscopy, when performed*, has been deleted and new Category I code 52284 has been established to report cystourethroscopy with mechanical urethral dilation and therapeutic drug delivery via drug-coated balloon catheter. Several parenthetical notes have been added to provide further guidance for reporting this service.

Code 0499T has been converted to Category I code 52284 for reporting cystourethroscopy with mechanical urethral dilation and therapeutic drug delivery via drug-coated balloon catheter. New code 52284 specifically includes the drug-delivery mechanism of using a drug-coated balloon catheter. The new descriptor also specifies the procedure is specifically for a male.

Two parenthetical notes have been added in the Surgery/Urethra and Bladder subsection to provide further guidance for reporting this service. A cross-reference parenthetical note following code 52281 has been added to direct users to report new code 52284. In addition, an exclusionary parenthetical note following code 52284 has been added to restrict reporting code 52284 in conjunction with codes 51610, 52000, 52281, 52283, 74450, and 76000. In accordance with the deletion of code 0499T, a deletion parenthetical note and a cross-reference parenthetical note have been added to the Category III section.

Clinical Example (52284)

A 69-year-old male underwent a transurethral resection of the prostate (TURP) 2 years ago for benign prostatic hyperplasia (BPH). He now presents with worsening frequency, nocturia, and decreased force of stream. An office cystoscopy reveals a dense 2-cm bulbar stricture. To minimize the incidence of recurrence, patient elects to undergo urethral dilation with therapeutic drug delivery by drug-coated balloon catheter.

Description of Procedure (52284)

Position the C-arm with scout films to assure visibility. Using fluoroscopy, inject contrast solution from the urethral meatus to the bladder to identify the length and location of the stricture. After performance of retrograde urethrogram, reposition patient in dorsal lithotomy position. Place appropriate padding at knees and ankles. Prepare and drape patient in dorsal lithotomy position. Prepare and drape the penis. Place the cystoscope per urethra to the level of the stricture and pass a guidewire through the lumen into the bladder. Use fluoroscopy to confirm appropriate placement. Pass a non-drug–coated balloon over the guidewire to the level of the stricture using fluoroscopic guidance. Inflate the balloon with contrast solution under fluoroscopic guidance to predilate the stricture. Following dilation, deflate the non-drug–coated balloon and remove, leaving the guidewire in place. Place the cystoscope per urethra and position the drug-coated balloon appropriately using fluoroscopic guidance and direct visualization. Inflate the balloon and maintain inflation for a minimum of 5 minutes to allow for drug delivery. Then deflate the balloon and remove, leaving the guidewire in place. Place a 14-French council tip catheter over the guidewire into the bladder with 10 cc of sterile water placed in the balloon.

Female Genital System

Corpus Uteri

Introduction

58353   Code is out of numerical sequence. See 58578-58600

58356   Code is out of numerical sequence. See 58578-58600

Laparoscopy/Hysteroscopy

 # 58674   Laparoscopy, surgical, ablation of uterine fibroid(s) including intraoperative ultrasound guidance and monitoring, radiofrequency

▶(Do not report 58674 in conjunction with 49320, 58541-58554, 58570, 58571, 58572, 58573, 58580, 76998)◀

▶(For transcervical radiofrequency ablation of uterine fibroid[s], including intraoperative ultrasound guidance and monitoring, use 58580)◀

58579   Unlisted hysteroscopy procedure, uterus

▶Other Procedures◀

 # 58353   Endometrial ablation, thermal, without hysteroscopic guidance

(For hysteroscopic procedure, use 58563)

 # 58356   Endometrial cryoablation with ultrasonic guidance, including endometrial curettage, when performed

(Do not report 58356 in conjunction with 58100, 58120, 58340, 76700, 76856)

● 58580   Transcervical ablation of uterine fibroid(s), including intraoperative ultrasound guidance and monitoring, radiofrequency

▶(Do not report 58580 in conjunction with 58561, 58674, 76830, 76940, 76998)◀

▶(For laparoscopic radiofrequency ablation of uterine fibroid[s], including intraoperative ultrasound guidance and monitoring, use 58674)◀

Rationale

Category III code 0404T, *Transcervical uterine fibroid(s) ablation with ultrasound guidance, radiofrequency,* has been deleted, and code 58580 has been established to report transcervical radiofrequency ablation of uterine fibroid(s), including intraoperative ultrasound guidance and monitoring. Code 58580 has been placed in a new subsection, Other Procedures, of the Female Genital System section. An exclusionary parenthetical note has been added precluding the reporting of code 58580 with codes 58561, 58674, 76830, 76940, and 76998. A cross-reference parenthetical note has been added to report

code 58674 for laparoscopic radiofrequency ablation of uterine fibroid(s), including intraoperative ultrasound guidance and monitoring. Endometrial thermal ablation code 58353 and endometrial cryoablation code 58356 have been relocated from the Introduction subsection to the new Other Procedures subsection.

In code 58580, monitoring has been included in the descriptor for consistency with the other ablation codes because the physician monitors the status of the radiofrequency generator throughout the ablation procedure. Code 58580 may not be reported with code 58561 (hysteroscopic removal of leiomyomata); code 58674 (laparoscopic ablation of uterine fibroid[s]); or codes 76830, 76940, and 76998 (ultrasound guidance).

In accordance with the establishment of code 58580, the exclusionary parenthetical note following code 58674 has been revised with the addition of code 58580, and a cross-reference parenthetical note has been added directing users to code 58580 for transcervical radiofrequency ablation of uterine fibroid(s), including intraoperative ultrasound guidance and monitoring.

Clinical Example (58580)

A 38-year-old female presents with heavy menstrual bleeding for 6 months. Examination reveals an eight-week sized uterus. A human chorionic gonadotropin (hCG) test is negative and endometrial biopsy is normal. Transvaginal sonogram reveals multiple fibroids, the largest of which is a 5.2-cm x 4.5-cm x 4.6-cm transmural myoma.

Description of Procedure (58580)

Place a bi-valve speculum within the vagina and visualize the uterine cervix. Position a tenaculum on the anterior lip of the cervix and dilate the cervix to 27F. The radiofrequency handpiece, handpiece cable, and intrauterine ultrasound probe clip together to create the transcervical fibroid ablation (TFA) device (forming a single component). After adequate cervical dilatation has been achieved, insert the TFA device transcervically into the uterus. Infuse a small volume of fluid such as sterile water through the device for acoustic coupling to enhance ultrasound visualization. Leiomyomata are then visualized with the integrated intrauterine ultrasound (IUUS) probe and mapped in a systematic fashion within the uterus. Mapping with the IUUS probe is an integral and required step to view and confirm the number and location of fibroids as well as to identify other critical structures. After identifying which fibroids to treat and articulating the IUUS probe, use the graphical overlay to target and plan ablations in the fibroid. Once the size, angle, and location of the ablation have been established, advance a trocar-tipped introducer into the fibroid under guided IUUS visualization. Align the graphical overlay with the introducer tip and, as the IUUS probe rotates independently of the introducer and needle electrodes, perform an initial safety rotation by rotating the IUUS probe 360° around the introducer. Then deploy the needle electrodes, again completing a second safety rotation to confirm the position of the thermal safety border relative to the uterine serosa. After the thermal safety border has been confirmed to be within the uterine serosal margin in all adjacent ultrasound planes, activate the radiofrequency (RF) energy. During this and any subsequent ablation, monitor the status of the RF generator and hold the TFA device steady throughout the ablation time. Each treated fibroid will receive one or more ellipsoidal ablations to achieve durable symptom relief. Repeat targeting and treatment steps as required to place any additional ablations in the same fibroid (if necessary) and/or treat any additional fibroids that were previously mapped. Upon completion of the procedure, retract the needle electrodes and introducer, articulate the ultrasound to zero, and remove the TFA device. Remove the cervical tenaculum and observe the tenaculum site for bleeding. Then remove the vaginal speculum and end the procedure.

Oviduct/Ovary

Laparoscopy

58660 Laparoscopy, surgical; with lysis of adhesions (salpingolysis, ovariolysis) (separate procedure)

58661 with removal of adnexal structures (partial or total oophorectomy and/or salpingectomy)

▶(For bilateral procedure, report 58661 with modifier 50)◀

Rationale

A parenthetical note has been added to clarify that code 58661 is intended to be reported for unilateral procedures. As a result, if laparoscopic removal of adnexal structures were performed on both ovaries and/or tubes, then modifier 50 may be appended to identify that a bilateral procedure was performed during the same session. The term "structures" is intended to identify the partial or total removal of tubes and/or ovaries from one side of the anatomical location.

Nervous System

Skull, Meninges, and Brain

Neurostimulators (Intracranial)

61885 Insertion or replacement of cranial neurostimulator pulse generator or receiver, direct or inductive coupling; with connection to a single electrode array

61886 with connection to 2 or more electrode arrays

(For percutaneous placement of cranial nerve (eg, vagus, trigeminal) neurostimulator electrode(s), use 64553)

(For revision or removal of cranial nerve (eg, vagus, trigeminal) neurostimulator electrode array, use 64569)

61888 Revision or removal of cranial neurostimulator pulse generator or receiver

(Do not report 61888 in conjunction with 61885 or 61886 for the same pulse generator)

● **61889** Insertion of skull-mounted cranial neurostimulator pulse generator or receiver, including craniectomy or craniotomy, when performed, with direct or inductive coupling, with connection to depth and/or cortical strip electrode array(s)

▶(For insertion of cranial neurostimulator pulse generator or receiver other than skull mounted, see 61885, 61886)◀

● **61891** Revision or replacement of skull-mounted cranial neurostimulator pulse generator or receiver with connection to depth and/or cortical strip electrode array(s)

▶(For replacement of cranial neurostimulator pulse generator or receiver other than skull mounted, see 61885, 61886)◀

▶(For revision of cranial neurostimulator pulse generator or receiver other than skull mounted, use 61888)◀

● **61892** Removal of skull-mounted cranial neurostimulator pulse generator or receiver with cranioplasty, when performed

▶(Do not report 61892 in conjunction with 61891 for the same pulse generator)◀

▶(For removal of cranial neurostimulator pulse generator or receiver other than skull mounted, use 61888)◀

Rationale

Three new codes (61889-61892) and new parenthetical notes have been added within the Surgery/Intracranial Neurostimulators subsection to report insertion, revision, or replacement and removal of a skull-mounted neurostimulator pulse generator or receiver. Previously,

★ = Telemedicine   ◀ = Audio-only   ✛ = Add-on code   ✚ = FDA approval pending   # = Resequenced code   ⊘ = Modifier 51 exempt

there were only codes to describe implanting brain neurostimulator pulse generators subcutaneously.

Codes (61889-61892) describe skull-mounted pulse generator procedures for brain neurostimulation placed via craniectomy. Existing codes (61885, 61886, 61888) describe implanting, replacing, and removal of brain neurostimulator pulse generators typically placed in a subcutaneous pocket, most commonly in the chest or abdomen.

To provide further instruction regarding the intended use of these codes, instructional parenthetical notes have been added to differentiate between these three new codes and codes 61885, 61886, and 61888. An exclusionary parenthetical note has been added to indicate that it is not appropriate to report revision or replacement of a skull-mounted cranial neurostimulator pulse generator or receiver with connection to depth and/or cortical strip electrode array(s) (61891) and removal of skull-mounted cranial neurostimulator pulse generator or receiver with cranioplasty (61892) for the same pulse generator.

Clinical Example (61889)

A 35-year-old male has a 15-year history of poorly controlled seizures despite having tried numerous medications. Following a surgical work-up, the epileptic focus was identified in eloquent cortex, not amenable to surgical resection or laser ablation.

Description of Procedure (61889)

After making the skin incision and elevating the scalp flap, mobilize the scalp in multiple directions to allow for an appropriate tension-free closure. Use the craniectomy template to locate and mark the appropriate site for the craniectomy, taking into account the skull morphology and curvature as well as any prior bone flaps and cranial hardware (which may need to be removed/revised to accommodate the craniectomy). Create one or more burr holes using a high-speed drill, which is then used to create and appropriately size the full thickness craniectomy piece (down to the dura), which is then removed. During this process, take care to avoid violating the dura, which may be scarred to the bone from prior procedures. Obtain epidural hemostasis. Contour the craniectomy opening with the high-speed drill so that the pulse generator tray fits in securely, evenly, and completely. Individually contour the mounting arms on the tray to the determined depth for the generator tray, ensuring that they are not overly proud and that the tray is seated evenly and deeply in the craniectomy space. Secure the tray to hold the pulse generator to the skull with multiple screws. Make a separate incision as necessary to expose the previously placed cortical or deep brain stimulating electrodes. Then bring these

neurostimulator electrodes to the pulse generator and connect in the required fashion. Place the pulse generator in the previously implanted tray and secure in place with a screw, ensuring that the overall contour of the implant with respect to the skull is even and not overly proud. Arrange/coil the electrodes under the scalp flap to provide slack, minimize their risk of injury during any subsequent revision, and minimize the possibility of eroding through the scalp in delayed fashion. Drape the programming wand and bring into the field. Interrogate the generator and check the electrode connections. Spend time recording the electroencephalogram (EEG) to ensure that the previously placed electrodes are recording appropriate information. Then program the device for recording and, if necessary, stimulation. Irrigate the field and evaluate the scalp flap to ensure that the closure will be tension-free, mobilizing it further as necessary. Then close all incisions while avoiding damage to the subgaleal implants.

Clinical Example (61891)

A 40-year-old male presents with a 20-year history of seizures. Patient previously underwent implantation of a neurostimulator system with a skull-mounted cranial neurostimulator pulse generator for reduction in seizure frequency that requires revision and replacement of the pulse generator due to impending end of battery life.

Description of Procedure (61891)

Carefully open the skin incision to avoid damage to the subgaleal electrodes. Then gently mobilize the scalp flap and locate the skull-mounted generator. This is often performed without the assistance of monopolar cautery because this can cause generator malfunction. Carefully dissect the brain stimulation electrodes out of their scar and follow to the pulse generator, taking care not to damage the electrodes. Carefully mobilize the scalp flap off the pulse generator to allow for removal of the generator from its holding tray and for a tension-free closure while protecting the subgaleal electrodes from damage. Loosen the tray screw. Remove the generator from the tray. Then disconnect the cortical and/or deep brain neurostimulator electrodes from the old pulse generator and connect to the new pulse generator in the required fashion. Place the pulse generator in the tray and secure in place with the tray screw. Drape the programming wand and bring it into the field. Interrogate the generator and check the electrode connections. Spend time recording the EEG to ensure that the previously placed electrodes are recording appropriate information. Then program the device for recording and, if necessary, stimulation. Irrigate the field and evaluate the scalp flap to ensure that the closure will be tension-free, mobilizing it further as necessary. Then close all incisions while avoiding damage to the subgaleal implants.

Clinical Example (61892)

A 40-year-old male with a 20-year history of seizures previously underwent implantation of a neurostimulation system requiring a skull-mounted programmable pulse generator. He now desires removal of the generator with cranioplasty of the resulting skull defect.

Description of Procedure (61892)

Carefully open the skin incision to avoid damage to the subgaleal electrodes. Then gently mobilize the scalp flap and locate the skull-mounted generator. Carefully dissect the brain stimulation electrodes out of their scar and follow to the pulse generator. Loosen the tray screw. Remove the generator from the tray. Loosen and remove the screws mounting the tray to the skull along with the tray itself. Obtain epidural hemostasis and perform an allograft cranioplasty by appropriately shaping and sizing a piece of cranioplasty material and securing it to the skull over the craniectomy defect with screws. Irrigate the field and evaluate the scalp flap to ensure that the closure will be tension-free, mobilizing it further as necessary. Close all incisions while avoiding damage to the subgaleal implants.

Spine and Spinal Cord

Neurostimulators (Spinal)

▶For electronic analysis with programming, when performed, of spinal cord neurostimulator pulse generator or transmitters, see codes 95970, 95971, 95972. Test stimulation to confirm correct target site placement of the electrode array(s) and/or to confirm the functional status of the system is inherent to placement, and is not separately reported as electronic analysis or programming of the neurostimulator pulse generator or receiver system. Electronic analysis (95970) at the time of implantation is not separately reported.

Codes 63650, 63655, 63661, 63662, 63663, 63664 describe the operative placement, revision, replacement, or removal of the spinal neurostimulator system components to provide spinal electrical stimulation. A neurostimulator system includes an implanted pulse generator or implanted receiver with an external transmitter, a collection of contacts, electrodes (electrode array), an extension if applicable, an external controller, and an external charger, if applicable. The neurostimulator may be integrated with the electrode array (single-component implant, see 0784T, 0785T) or have a detachable connection to the electrode array (two or more component implant). Multiple contacts or electrodes (4 or more) provide the actual electrical stimulation in the epidural space.◀

For percutaneously placed neurostimulator systems (63650, 63661, 63663), the contacts are on a catheter-like lead. An array defines the collection of contacts that are on one catheter.

For systems placed via an open surgical exposure (63655, 63662, 63664), the contacts are on a plate or paddle-shaped surface.

Do not report 63661 or 63663 when removing or replacing a temporary percutaneously placed array for an external generator.

▶Codes 63650, 63661, 63663, 63685, 63688 describe insertion, replacement, revision, or removal of a percutaneous electrode array and neurostimulator requiring pocket creation and connection between electrode array and pulse generator or receiver. For insertion, replacement, revision, or removal of a percutaneous spinal cord or sacral electrode array and integrated neurostimulator, see 0784T, 0785T, 0786T, 0787T.◀

▲ **63685**   Insertion or replacement of spinal neurostimulator pulse generator or receiver, requiring pocket creation and connection between electrode array and pulse generator or receiver

   ▶(Do not report 63685 in conjunction with 63688 for the same neurostimulator pulse generator or receiver)◀

   ▶(For insertion or replacement of spinal percutaneous electrode array with integrated neurostimulator, use 0784T)◀

▲ **63688**   Revision or removal of implanted spinal neurostimulator pulse generator or receiver, with detachable connection to electrode array

   ▶(For electronic analysis with programming, when performed, of implanted spinal cord neurostimulator, see 95970, 95971, 95972)◀

   ▶(For revision or removal of spinal percutaneous electrode array and integrated neurostimulator, use 0785T)◀

   ▶(For revision or removal of sacral percutaneous electrode array and integrated neurostimulator, use 0787T)◀

Rationale

Code 63685 has been revised to reflect removal of "direct or inductive coupling" and the addition of "requiring pocket creation and connection between electrode array and pulse generator or receiver." Code 63688 has been revised to add "with detachable connection to electrode array" to better reflect the work efforts required for the services of revision/removal of implanted spinal neurostimulator pulse generators or receivers. Parenthetical notes and guidelines have also been added or revised to accommodate the revisions made to clarify the reporting of these services.

Refer to the codebook and the Rationale for codes 64590-64598 for a full discussion of these changes.

Clinical Example (63685)

A 49-year-old male with intractable back and leg pain, whose conservative treatment has been unsuccessful, has undergone a successful trial of a spinal neurostimulator electrode array. He is referred for placement of a spinal neurostimulator pulse generator and connection to the previously placed electrode array.

Description of Procedure (63685)

After induction of anesthesia, incise the skin and obtain hemostasis. Carry out dissection and develop a subcutaneous pocket for placement of the stimulator generator or, if the procedure is for replacement of a generator, dissect the old generator out of the pocket, taking care to avoid damage to the electrode arrays. Tunnel the electrode arrays to the pocket and out onto the skin or disconnect them from the pulse generator if performing a replacement. Unpack the sterile neurostimulator pulse generator, soak the generator in antibiotic solution, and then attach the generator to the lead terminals in standard fashion. Then place the generator into the fashioned subcutaneous pocket. Test each of the leads separately for impedances to verify secure connection and proper function. Track the connection and program the device to begin stimulation. Obtain hemostasis and then copiously irrigate the pocket with antibiotic solution prior to layered closure.

Clinical Example (63688)

A 50-year-old male with an implanted spinal cord stimulator requests removal of his neurostimulator pulse generator because of its waning benefit. The subcutaneous neurostimulator pulse generator is disconnected and removed from the electrode array.

Description of Procedure (63688)

Re-open the old skin incision and check the wound for hemostasis. Dissect the old generator out of its subcutaneous pocket and place on a sterile towel. Carefully disconnect the lead terminals from the expired generator. Irrigate the subcutaneous pocket with antibiotic solution and check for hemostasis. Then irrigate the wound a final time and close in three layers. Apply sterile dressing.

Extracranial Nerves, Peripheral Nerves, and Autonomic Nervous System

Neurostimulators (Peripheral Nerve)

►For electronic analysis with programming, when performed, of peripheral nerve neurostimulator pulse generator or transmitters, see codes 95970, 95971, 95972. An electrode array is a catheter or other device with more than one contact. The function of each contact may be capable of being adjusted during programming services. Test stimulation to confirm correct target site placement of the electrode array(s) and/or to confirm the functional status of the system is inherent to placement, and is not separately reported as electronic analysis or programming of the neurostimulator pulse generator or receiver system. Electronic analysis (95970) at the time of implantation is not separately reported.

A neurostimulator system includes an implanted pulse generator or implanted receiver with an external transmitter, a collection of contacts, electrodes (electrode array), an extension if applicable, an external controller, and an external charger, if applicable. The electrode array provides the actual electrical stimulation. The pulse generator or receiver may be integrated with the electrode array (single-component implant) or have a detachable connection to the electrode array (two or more component implant).◄

Codes 64553, 64555, and 64561 may be used to report both temporary and permanent placement of percutaneous electrode arrays.

►Codes 64590, 64596 describe two different approaches to placing a neurostimulator pulse generator or receiver. Code 64590 is used in conjunction with 64555, 64561 for permanent placement. Codes 64555, 64561 are used to report electrode array placement for a trial and for the permanent placement of the electrode array. Code 64590 is used to report the insertion of a neurostimulator pulse generator or receiver that requires creation of a pocket and connection between the electrode array and the neurostimulator pulse generator or receiver. Code 64596 is used to report the permanent placement of an integrated system, including the electrode array and receiver.◄

(For transcutaneous nerve stimulation [TENS], use 97014 for electrical stimulation requiring supervision only or use 97032 for electrical stimulation requiring constant attendance)

64566 Posterior tibial neurostimulation, percutaneous needle electrode, single treatment, includes programming

(Do not report 64566 in conjunction with 64555, 95970-95972)

►(For peripheral nerve transcutaneous magnetic stimulation, see 0766T, 0767T)◄

Surgery / Nervous System 61000-64999

▲● **64590** Insertion or replacement of peripheral, sacral, or gastric neurostimulator pulse generator or receiver, requiring pocket creation and connection between electrode array and pulse generator or receiver

(Do not report 64590 in conjunction with 64595)

▶(Do not report 64590 in conjunction with 64596, 64597, 64598)◀

▶(For insertion or replacement of percutaneous electrode array with integrated neurostimulator, use 64596)◀

▶(For neurostimulators without a named target nerve [eg, field stimulation], use 64999)◀

▲● **64595** Revision or removal of peripheral, sacral, or gastric neurostimulator pulse generator or receiver, with detachable connection to electrode array

▶(For revision or removal of percutaneous electrode array with integrated neurostimulator, use 64597)◀

● **64596** Insertion or replacement of percutaneous electrode array, peripheral nerve, with integrated neurostimulator, including imaging guidance, when performed; initial electrode array

+● **64597** each additional electrode array (List separately in addition to code for primary procedure)

▶(Use 64597 in conjunction with 64596)◀

▶(Do not report 64596, 64597 in conjunction with 64555, 64561, 64590, 64595)◀

▶(For percutaneous implantation of electrode array only, peripheral nerve, use 64555)◀

▶(For implantation of trial or permanent electrode arrays or pulse generators for peripheral subcutaneous field stimulation, use 64999)◀

▶(For neurostimulators without a named target nerve [eg, field stimulation], use 64999)◀

▶(For percutaneous implantation or replacement of integrated neurostimulation system for bladder dysfunction, posterior tibial nerve, use 0587T)◀

▶(For open implantation or replacement of integrated neurostimulator system, posterior tibial nerve, see 0816T, 0817T)◀

● **64598** Revision or removal of neurostimulator electrode array, peripheral nerve, with integrated neurostimulator

▶(For revision or removal of electrode array only, use 64585)◀

▶(For revision or removal of integrated neurostimulation system, posterior tibial nerve, see 0588T, 0818T, 0819T)◀

Rationale

New Category I and III codes, guidelines, and parenthetical notes have been added and/or revised to allow appropriate reporting for spinal, sacral, peripheral, and tibial nerve neurostimulator services. This includes reporting integrated neurostimulators.

The insertion or replacement, revision, and removal service codes for spinal, sacral, peripheral, and tibial neurostimulator service codes have been updated within the code set to reflect advancements in technologies that exist for insertions, replacements, revisions, removals, and programming services that are now provided for neurostimulators. This includes identification of the differences between these neurostimulators—both by explanation of what they are and by identification of the work needed to provide these services. Neurostimulator systems have common components, including a pulse generator or implanted receiver, a collection of contacts, electrodes (electrode array), an extension (if needed), and may use an external controller and an external charger. In addition, some of the neurostimulators may require the creation of a pocket for implantation, while others may be inserted percutaneously.

The codes that have been developed reflect the work necessary to perform the service. This involves not only the identification of the type of access/approach needed to place the neurostimulator system but also of the anatomic location involved in the placement. Work effort to accommodate placement of a generator or tunneling to connect electrodes are different from placement of neurostimulators that may be placed percutaneously. As a result, the guidelines, parenthetical notes, and descriptors have been written with this in mind to allow differentiation of these services.

Code 63685 is used to report insertion or replacement services, and code 63688 is used for revision or removal services for a spinal neurostimulator pulse generator or receiver that requires a pocket to be created. It also identifies the work of connecting the electrode array and pulse generator or receiver. Code 63685 has been revised by replacing "direct or inductive coupling" with language that conveys the work of pocket creation and efforts to connect the electrode array to the pulse generator or receiver once it is implanted. Code 63688 has been revised by adding "with detachable connection to electrode array" to account for the work of connecting the pulse generator or receiver to the electrode array. The parenthetical notes associated with these codes direct users to the appropriate codes to report insertion or replacement of spinal percutaneous electrode array with integrated neurostimulator (0784T) and percutaneous revision or removal of spinal (0785T) or sacral (0787T) electrode array and integrated neurostimulator.

Several editorial changes also have been made to these parenthetical notes to align with language included within the codes referenced in the parenthetical notes.

Similar changes have been made to the descriptors for codes 64590 (insertion or replacement services) and 64595 (revision or removal services) for peripheral, sacral, or gastric neurostimulator pulse generator or receivers regarding pocket creation and connections between the electrode array and pulse generator or receiver. The term "sacral" has been added to both code descriptors to confirm that the service efforts for sacral and gastric neurostimulators are comparable. For these codes, parenthetical cross-reference notes have been added that direct users to the codes for reporting insertion or replacement (64596, 64597) or revision or removal (64598) of the electrode array for an integrated neurostimulator for peripheral nerves. An exclusionary parenthetical note has also been added to restrict reporting of code 64590 in conjunction with codes 64596-64598.

An additional parenthetical note directs users to the code 64999 for reporting neurostimulators without a named target nerve (eg, field stimulation).

Codes 64596-64598 have been added to the code set for reporting the insertion or replacement (64596, 64597) and revision or removal (64598) for integrated neurostimulator electrode array services of the peripheral nerves. As is true for the aforementioned services, parenthetical notes have been added for the appropriate reporting of insertion or replacement of additional electrodes (64597); implantation of an electrode array only of the peripheral nerve (64555); implantation of a trial or permanent electrode array for peripheral subcutaneous field stimulation (64999); and percutaneous implantation or replacement of integrated neurostimulator systems for the posterior tibial nerve, ie, for bladder dysfunction (0587T). Separate instruction also redirects users to report code 64585 for revision or removal of the electrode array only and restricts reporting of codes 64596 and 64597 in conjunction with other peripheral (64555), sacral (64561), or peripheral or gastric insertion/replacement (64590) or revision/removal (64595) services.

New codes have also been added for reporting percutaneous insertion/replacement of integrated neurostimulator electrode arrays of the spine (0784T) and sacrum (0786T), as well as revisions and removals of the same (0785T, 0787T). These services include all image guidance necessary for placements, removals, and revisions. In addition, separate codes have been added within the Category III code set for all programming (simple [0788T] and complex [0789T]) for these services with exclusionary parenthetical notes that reassert these programming codes may not be used in conjunction with the placement codes because programming is inherently

included as part of the placement, replacement, and removal services. The codes for posterior tibial nerve implantation or replacement (0587T), revision or removal (0588T), and programming (0589T, 0590T) have also been revised by adding terminology to reflect their use for treatment of bladder dysfunction.

Much of the language included within the guidelines for all these services has been updated either by addition or revision to define the differences for reporting these services, differentiating the neurostimulator systems, defining the constituent components, and further directing usage of these codes via cross-references, restrictions, or editorial revision to better identify intended use and the services at issue.

In accordance with the deletion of codes 0768T and 0769T, a parenthetical note following code 64566 has been revised to reflect the deleted codes and to direct users to the appropriate codes for reporting transcutaneous magnetic stimulation.

Refer to the codebook and the Rationale for codes 0766T and 0767T for a full discussion of these changes.

Clinical Example (64590)

A 65-year-old with overactive bladder refractory to previous therapy is referred for insertion of neurostimulator pulse generator.

Description of Procedure (64590)

Identify bony landmarks and prior extension set connection to permanent lead. Confirm connection site is in an appropriate location for placement of an implantable pulse generator (IPG). Inject marked incision site with local anesthetic. Gently incise prior incision site to avoid damage to the permanent lead and carefully remove all sutures. Continue with sharp dissection for full visualization of permanent lead and connection to extension set. Remove stay suture. Enlarge incision site of the exteriorized portion of the extension set with hemostat. Unscrew extension set from permanent lead without tension on permanent lead. Gently remove liberated extension set from the connection site with gentle traction through the tunneled exit away from the connection site. Perform copious irrigation of the connection site. Ensure there is no evidence of infection. Create pocket commensurate with IPG size and confirm marked hemostasis. Introduce IPG into operative field. Secure permanent lead to IPG with screwdriver after fully seated. Manage permanent lead placement into pocket and gently place IPG in pocket. Introduce the programmer into operative field. Perform impedance evaluation of IPG in sterile fashion after positioned in pocket. Remove programmer from operative field. Close incision in two layers after securing IPG in pocket. Close prior extension set exit site in two layers. Place surgical glue on operative incision skin edges.

Clinical Example (64595)

A 65-year-old with overactive bladder refractory to previous therapy is referred for revision/removal of neurostimulator pulse generator.

Description of Procedure (64595)

Identify prior implantable pulse generator (IPG). Inject prior operative incision with local anesthetic and carefully incise prior incision site. Dissect open the prior pocket and gently exteriorize the IPG. Unscrew array set screw and remove the IPG from the array. Determine etiology of existing pocket problem. Remove debris/infectious material from pocket and copiously irrigate. Attach hemostat to array and gently retract the array to determine tunnel site to midline. Incise midline tunnel site through dermis being careful not to injure array. Use hemostat through midline incision site to elevate array through dermis. Use asepto syringe to irrigate tunnel site exit and entrance from pocket. Close the initial pocket site with multiple-layer closure and confirm hemostasis. Apply surgical glue to skin edges.

Clinical Example (64596)

A 75-year-old male with intractable knee pain after total knee replacement, who has not passed conservative treatment for management of the pain, underwent a successful trial of a percutaneously placed peripheral neurostimulator electrode array. He is now referred for exchange of the percutaneous electrode array with a subcutaneous neurostimulator that includes an electrode array placed through the same access site.

Description of Procedure (64596)

N/A

Clinical Example (64597)

A 46-year-old male presents with chronic shoulder pain. He underwent a successful trial of percutaneously placed peripheral neurostimulator electrode arrays and is now referred for placement of two separate subcutaneous neurostimulators with integrated electrode arrays. [**Note:** This is an add-on code. Only consider the additional work related to the placement of the second integrated neurostimulator that includes an electrode array.]

Description of Procedure (64597)

N/A

Clinical Example (64598)

A 46-year-old male with chronic neuropathic pain who has benefited from a peripheral nerve implanted, integrated neurostimulation system needs to have the integrated system revised due to migration.

Description of Procedure (64598)

N/A

Eye and Ocular Adnexa

Ocular Adnexa

Orbit

Other Procedures

67515 Injection of medication or other substance into Tenon's capsule

(For subconjunctival injection, use 68200)

● **67516** Suprachoroidal space injection of pharmacologic agent (separate procedure)

▶(Report medication separately)◀

Rationale

Code 0465T, *Suprachoroidal injection of a pharmacologic agent (does not include supply of medication),* has been deleted from the Category III code section, and new Category I code 67516 has been added to report suprachoroidal injection of pharmacologic agent (separate procedure). In addition, an instructional parenthetical note has been added to guide users to the appropriate reporting for this service.

Code 67516 identifies the administration of a drug into the suprachoroidal space, between the sclera and choroid, which compartmentalizes the drug within the posterior segment of the eye. This results in non-exposure of the drug to unintended targets, such as the anterior segment and vitreous. As noted in the instructional parenthetical note following the code, the supply of the medication is separately reported. In addition, as noted in the descriptor, this service is identified as a "separate procedure." Per CPT guidelines, codes designated as "separate procedure" should not be reported in addition to the code for the total procedure or service of which it is considered an integral component. Refer to the Surgery guidelines for more information on reporting codes designated as "separate procedure."

★ = Telemedicine   ◀ = Audio-only   ✛ = Add-on code   ✗ = FDA approval pending   # = Resequenced code   ⊘ = Modifier 51 exempt

Clinical Example (67516)

A 45-year-old female with macular edema associated with non-infectious uveitis in the right eye is referred for suprachoroidal space injection of a medication.

Description of Procedure (67516)

Connect the hub adapter for the needle to the vial of medication to be administered. Draw the medication up into the suprachoroidal injector. Then exchange the adapter for the 900-micron suprachoroidal needle. Remove any residual air bubbles and express any excess medication. Use a caliper to measure 4 mm posterior to the limbus and mark the injection site. Place the injector perpendicular to the sclera. Apply pressure to dimple the conjunctiva and underlying sclera. While gentle pressure is applied to the plunger, manipulate the injector to maintain perpendicularity and pressure until loss of resistance is noted. If no loss of resistance is achieved, increase pressure dimpling the sclera while continuously repositioning the injector to maintain perpendicularity and find the suprachoroidal space. If there is no success with the 900-micron needle, remove it and replace it with an 1100-micron needle and repeat the same steps. Once loss of resistance is achieved, continue a slow push until all the medication has been administered into the suprachoroidal space. Then place a cotton swab over the injection site and maintain pressure to prevent reflux of the medication. Rinse patient's eye with saline solution to remove any residual povidone-iodine solution. Remove the lid speculum.

▶(For diagnostic analysis, programming, and verification of an auditory osseointegrated sound processor, use 92622)◀

Rationale

In support of the establishment of Category I codes 92622 and 92623, a cross-reference parenthetical note has been added following code 69729 to direct users to code 92622 for diagnostic analysis, programming, and verification of an auditory osseointegrated sound processor.

Refer to the codebook and the Rationale for codes 92622 and 92623 for a full discussion of these changes.

Auditory System

Middle Ear

Osseointegrated Implants

\# **69714** Implantation, osseointegrated implant, skull; with percutaneous attachment to external speech processor

(69715 has been deleted. To report mastoidectomy performed at the same operative session as osseointegrated implant placement, revision, replacement, or removal, see 69501-69676)

\# **69716** with magnetic transcutaneous attachment to external speech processor, within the mastoid and/or resulting in removal of less than 100 sq mm surface area of bone deep to the outer cranial cortex

\# **69729** with magnetic transcutaneous attachment to external speech processor, outside of the mastoid and resulting in removal of greater than or equal to 100 sq mm surface area of bone deep to the outer cranial cortex

Notes

Radiology

Summary of Additions, Deletions, and Revisions

The summary of changes shows the actual changes that have been made to the code descriptors.

New codes appear with a bullet (●) and are indicated as "Code added." Revised codes are preceded with a triangle (▲). Within revised codes, or if a code symbol has been deleted, the deleted language and code symbol appear with a ~~strikethrough~~, while new text appears <u>underlined</u>.

The ⚡ symbol is used to identify codes for vaccines that are pending FDA approval. The # symbol is used to identify codes that have been resequenced. CPT add-on codes are annotated by the ✚ symbol. The ⊘ symbol is used to identify codes that are exempt from the use of modifier 51. The ★ symbol is used to identify codes that may be used for reporting telemedicine services. The ✣ is used to identify proprietary laboratory analyses (PLA) test that has an identical descriptor as another PLA test. A PLA code that satisfies Category I code criteria and has been accepted by the CPT Editorial Panel is annotated with the ↑↓ symbol. The ◀ symbol is used to identify codes that may be used to report audio-only telemedicine services when appended by modifier 93 (**see Appendix T**).

Code	Description
74710	~~Pelvimetry, with or without placental localization~~
●**75580**	Code added
●**76984**	Code added
●**76987**	Code added
●**76988**	Code added
●**76989**	Code added

Radiology

Diagnostic Radiology (Diagnostic Imaging)

Gynecological and Obstetrical

►(74710 has been deleted)◄

Rationale

To ensure the CPT code set reflects current clinical practice, code 74710, *Pelvimetry, with or without placental localization*, has been deleted due to low utilization. A parenthetical note has been added to indicate this deletion.

Heart

75574   Computed tomographic angiography, heart, coronary arteries and bypass grafts (when present), with contrast material, including 3D image postprocessing (including evaluation of cardiac structure and morphology, assessment of cardiac function, and evaluation of venous structures, if performed)

►(For noninvasive estimate of coronary fractional flow reserve [FFR] derived from augmentative software analysis of the data set from a coronary computed tomography angiography with interpretation and report by a physician or other qualified health care professional, use 75580)◄

(For automated quantification and characterization of coronary atherosclerotic plaque, see 0623T, 0624T, 0625T, 0626T)

● **75580**   Noninvasive estimate of coronary fractional flow reserve (FFR) derived from augmentative software analysis of the data set from a coronary computed tomography angiography, with interpretation and report by a physician or other qualified health care professional

►(Use 75580 only once per coronary computed tomography angiogram)◄

►(When noninvasive estimate of coronary FFR derived from augmentative software analysis of the data set from a coronary computed tomography angiography with interpretation and report by a physician or other qualified health care professional is performed on the same day as the coronary computed tomography angiography, use 75580 in conjunction with 75574)◄

Rationale

Category III codes 0501T-0504T, which were established in the CPT 2018 code set, have been deleted. These four codes were previously used to report noninvasive estimated coronary fractional flow reserve (FFR) derived from coronary computed tomography angiography (CCTA) data using computation fluid dynamics physiologic simulation software analysis of functional data to assess the severity of coronary artery disease. Code 75580 has been established to report noninvasive estimate of coronary FFR derived from augmentative software analysis of the data set from a CCTA.

Before 2024, those four deleted codes described the components of data preparation and transmission, analysis of fluid dynamics and simulated maximal coronary hyperemia, generation of estimated FFR model, and anatomical data review in comparison with estimated FFR model to reconcile discordant data. The monitoring and tracking since 2018 have made it evident that the procedure components should be bundled into one Category I code and described as augmentative software analysis of the data set from a CCTA. The software analysis is described as augmentative because it provides clinically meaningful output that is predicated on the standard of care for the physician to interpret. Code 75580 includes interpretation and report by a physician or other qualified health care professional.

An instructional parenthetical note has been added stating that code 75580 is reported once per CCTA. An inclusionary parenthetical note has been added to state that when the noninvasive estimate of coronary FFR derived from augmentative software analysis of the data set from a CCTA is performed on the same day as the CCTA, code 75580 may be reported with code 75574.

In accordance with the deletion of codes 0501T-0504T and the establishment of code 75580, the cross-reference parenthetical note following code 75574 has been revised to reflect these changes.

Clinical Example (75580)

A 60-year-old female, complaining of chest pains after exercising, previously underwent coronary computed tomographic angiography (CCTA) that showed coronary artery plaque and lumen narrowing of moderate severity (eg, 60% of the diameter narrowed) in the left anterior descending and right coronary arteries.

Description of Procedure (75580)

Supervise the computed tomography (CT) technologist to ensure extraction of the appropriate CCTA data and images from the picture archiving and communication system (PACS) and ensure that the appropriate conforming image subsets are identified and collected. Review the computer platform–delivered CT-derived fractional flow reserve computed tomography (FFRCT) preliminary report, which involves the transformation of the static CT images into quantitative and qualitative diagnostic information about the function of the coronary arteries, distinct from the diagnostic output of the underlying CCTA. Once the data are processed and returned to the physician, the physician accesses the web-based interactive viewer. This allows the physician to examine and query the entire model and capture noninvasive estimated coronary FFR values anywhere within the coronary tree. The physician reviews the anatomy and compares it with the estimated FFR model to reconcile discordant data, evaluate multiple and sequential lesions, and determine possible false-positive and false-negative results. This approach allows the imager and the interventional cardiologist to determine the location of the disease burden and the lesion with the most hemodynamic significance, allowing for a targeted interventional approach that yields the most benefit to patient. Prepare and notate a final report and document in patient's record. Communicate study results to patient and referring physician to facilitate appropriate patient management. Dictate the final report in PACS for patient's medical record. Enter a note into patient's chart.

Other Procedures

76000   Fluoroscopy (separate procedure), up to 1 hour physician or other qualified health care professional time

▶(Do not report 76000 in conjunction with 33274, 33275, 33957, 33958, 33959, 33962, 33963, 33964, 0515T, 0516T, 0517T, 0518T, 0519T, 0520T, 0795T, 0796T, 0797T, 0798T, 0799T, 0800T, 0801T, 0802T, 0803T, 0823T, 0824T, 0825T, 0861T, 0862T, 0863T)◀

Rationale

In accordance with the establishment of codes 0795T-0803T, 0823T-0825T, and 0861T-0863T, the exclusionary parenthetical note following code 76000 has been revised.

Refer to the codebook and the Rationale for codes 0795T-0803T, 0823T-0825T, and 0861T-0863T for a full discussion of these changes.

Diagnostic Ultrasound

Ultrasonic Guidance Procedures

+ 76937   Ultrasound guidance for vascular access requiring ultrasound evaluation of potential access sites, documentation of selected vessel patency, concurrent realtime ultrasound visualization of vascular needle entry, with permanent recording and reporting (List separately in addition to code for primary procedure)

▶(Do not report 76937 in conjunction with 33274, 33275, 36568, 36569, 36572, 36573, 36584, 36836, 36837, 37191, 37192, 37193, 37760, 37761, 76942, 0795T, 0796T, 0797T, 0798T, 0799T, 0800T, 0801T, 0802T, 0803T, 0823T, 0824T, 0825T)◀

(Do not report 76937 in conjunction with 0505T, 0620T for ultrasound guidance for vascular access)

(If extremity venous non-invasive vascular diagnostic study is performed separate from venous access guidance, see 93970, 93971)

Rationale

In accordance with the establishment of codes 0795T-0803T and 0823T-0825T, the exclusionary parenthetical note following code 76937 has been revised.

Refer to the codebook and the Rationale for codes 0795T-0803T and 0823T-0825T for a full discussion of these changes.

Other Procedures

76981   Ultrasound, elastography; parenchyma (eg, organ)

76982   first target lesion

+ 76983   each additional target lesion (List separately in addition to code for primary procedure)

(Use 76983 in conjunction with 76982)

(Report 76981 only once per session for evaluation of the same parenchymal organ)

(To report shear wave liver elastography without imaging, use 91200)

(For evaluation of a parenchymal organ and lesion[s] in the same parenchymal organ at the same session, report only 76981)

(Do not report 76981, 76982, 76983 in conjunction with 0689T)

(Do not report 76983 more than two times per organ)

● **76984**   Ultrasound, intraoperative thoracic aorta (eg, epiaortic), diagnostic

▶(For diagnostic intraoperative epicardial cardiac ultrasound [ie, echocardiography], see 76987, 76988, 76989)◀

● **76987**   Intraoperative epicardial cardiac ultrasound (ie, echocardiography) for congenital heart disease, diagnostic; including placement and manipulation of transducer, image acquisition, interpretation and report

● **76988**   placement, manipulation of transducer, and image acquisition only

● **76989**   interpretation and report only

▶(For diagnostic intraoperative thoracic aorta (eg, epiaortic) ultrasound, use 76984)◀

Rationale

Four new codes (76984-76989) have been established for reporting intraoperative ultrasound (IOUS) diagnostic procedures. To support the addition of these new codes, two parenthetical notes have been added to provide users with the appropriate reporting instructions for these services. An existing parenthetical note following code 76998 has been revised with the addition of codes 76984-76989.

Code 76998, *Ultrasonic guidance, intraoperative*, was identified by the American Medical Association (AMA)/Specialty Society Relative Value Scale (RVS) Update Committee (RUC) through a RUC screen for the Centers for Medicare & Medicaid Services/Other Source Codes as a service with Medicare utilization of over 20,000. It was determined that code 76998 is utilized by many different specialties for various procedures with significant variations in the time it takes to perform the ultrasound guidance. Therefore, specific intraoperative codes have been established to describe ultrasound of the thoracic aorta (76984) and epicardial cardiac ultrasound for congenital heart disease (76987-76989).

These codes identify diagnostic IOUS for cardiothoracic surgery according to the anatomy (thoracic aorta [eg, epiaortic] ultrasound [76984] vs cardiac epicardial echocardiography [76987-76989]). Diagnostic IOUS for these indications is used as a means of detecting aspects of the procedures that may affect the intraoperative strategy, including altering the planned procedure (eg, changing cannulation strategies, altering bypass targets, identifying additional defects).

Code 76984 is used to report diagnostic intraoperative ultrasound of the thoracic aorta (eg, epiaortic IOUS). In addition, codes 76987-76989 are used to report diagnostic intraoperative epicardial cardiac ultrasound (eg,

echocardiography) for congenital heart disease and includes placement and manipulation of the transducer and image acquisition (76988), interpretation and report (76989), or a combination of both procedures (76987).

To provide further instructions regarding the intent and use of these new codes, two instructional parenthetical notes have been added following codes 76984 and 76989. Both parenthetical notes direct users to the appropriate reporting for diagnostic intraoperative epicardial cardiac ultrasound (76987-76989) or for reporting diagnostic intraoperative thoracic aorta ultrasound (76984).

In addition, an exclusionary parenthetical note following code 76998 has been revised with the addition of the four new codes to further clarify the appropriate reporting of these codes.

Clinical Example (76984)

A 76-year-old male with prior lower extremity bypass on the left and remote stroke presents with complex coronary disease and mildly reduced left ventricular function. A preoperative X ray demonstrates calcification of the aortic knob. He is now undergoing coronary artery bypass grafting (CABG) and grade III atheroma is noted in the descending aorta by perioperative transesophageal echocardiogram (TEE). An intraoperative epiaortic ultrasound is performed and interpreted by the cardiothoracic surgeon.

Description of Procedure (76984)

The cardiothoracic surgeon holds the sterile probe drape and the anesthesiologist or technician drops the probe into the sterile drape. The surgeon secures the probe drape and places the epiaortic ultrasound probe on the thoracic aorta (which TEE cannot fully visualize during the surgery due to air in the trachea or contraindications to TEE, such as previous esophagectomy, achalasia, or stenosis). The surgeon examines the desired cannulation or grafting sites to determine if plaque or calcium is present. If plaque or calcium is found, examine alternative targets to identify a site without plaque or calcium for aortic cannulation or proximal graft placement. If the site is not suitable, alternative cannulation or grafting strategies are necessary (ie, peripheral or off-pump cardiopulmonary cannulations, elimination of aortic cross-clamp, identification of different anastomotic sites for proximal grafts) to avoid aortic dissection or cerebral/systemic embolic events. Obtain images and interpret in real time during the procedure. The cardiothoracic surgeon acquires the final digital images for subsequent transfer to archival storage. The cardiac procedures (eg, CABG, aortic dissection repair, valve repair/replacement) are reported separately.

Clinical Example (76987)

A 5-month-old male with prior repair of tracheoesophageal fistula with subsequent esophageal stricture has a complete atrioventricular (AV) septal (AV canal) defect. He is now undergoing repair of the complete AV septal defect. TEE is contraindicated. An intraoperative epicardial ultrasound is performed, the images are interpreted, and a report generated.

Description of Procedure (76987)

Prior to and at the completion of an AV septal defect repair (complete AV canal) or other cardiac procedure(s) (reported separately) and weaning patient from cardiopulmonary bypass, a sterile epicardial echocardiography probe is passed off the operative field by the cardiothoracic surgeon and connected to the echocardiography machine. The cardiothoracic surgeon performs epicardial echocardiography by carefully placing the probe directly over the epicardium on the beating heart. The cardiac surgeon manipulates the probe and the heart to obtain multiple images of different cardiac structures that might include (1) epicardial aortic valve short-axis view; (2) epicardial aortic valve long-axis view; (3) epicardial left ventricle basal short-axis view; (4) epicardial left ventricle mid-short-axis view; (5) epicardial left ventricle long-axis view; (6) epicardial two-chamber view; and (7) epicardial right ventricular outflow–tract view. The cardiothoracic surgeon reviews and interprets the images in real time in the operating room to determine if surgical plan alterations are needed or if additional repairs must be made to the heart (eg, a sizable residual ventricular septal defect [VSD] is identified along with residual regurgitation of the left AV valve). If necessary, the surgical plan is altered or, if additional repairs are required, cardiopulmonary bypass is reestablished and the repairs (eg, residual VSD and left AV valve cleft) are re-repaired. (The cardiac procedures are reported separately.) The cardiothoracic surgeon acquires the final digital images for subsequent transfer to archival storage.

Clinical Example (76988)

A 5-month-old male with prior repair of tracheoesophageal fistula with subsequent esophageal stricture has a complete AV septal (AV canal) defect. He is now undergoing repair of the complete AV septal defect. TEE is contraindicated. An intraoperative epicardial ultrasound is performed.

Description of Procedure (76988)

Prior to and at the completion of an AV septal defect repair (complete AV canal) or other cardiac procedure(s) (reported separately) and weaning patient from cardiopulmonary bypass, a sterile epicardial echocardiography transducer is passed off the operative field by the cardiothoracic surgeon and connected to the echocardiography machine. The cardiothoracic surgeon performs epicardial echocardiography by carefully placing the probe directly over the epicardium on the beating heart. The cardiac surgeon manipulates the probe and the heart as directed by the cardiologist to obtain multiple images of different cardiac structures that might include (1) epicardial aortic valve short-axis view; (2) epicardial aortic valve long-axis view; (3) epicardial left ventricle basal short-axis view; (4) epicardial left ventricle mid-short-axis view; (5) epicardial left ventricle long-axis view; (6) epicardial two-chamber view; and (7) epicardial right ventricular outflow–tract view. Upon completion of image acquisition and the cardiologist's real-time interpretation of the findings, the cardiothoracic surgeon discusses the images with the cardiologist in real time in the operating room to determine if surgical plan alterations are needed or if additional procedures or repairs need to be made to the heart (eg, a sizable residual VSD is identified along with residual regurgitation of the left AV valve). If necessary, the surgical plan is altered or, if additional repairs are required, cardiopulmonary bypass is reestablished and the repairs (eg, residual VSD and left AV valve cleft) are re-repaired. (The cardiac procedures are reported separately.)

Clinical Example (76989)

A 5-month-old male with prior repair of tracheoesophageal fistula with subsequent esophageal stricture has a complete AV septal (AV canal) defect. He is now undergoing repair of the complete AV septal defect. TEE is contraindicated. The images from an intraoperative epicardial ultrasound are interpreted and a report generated.

Description of Procedure (76989)

In the operating room, the cardiologist directs the cardiothoracic surgeon on probe manipulation to obtain multiple images of different cardiac structures relevant to the pediatric and/or congenital cardiac repair. These views might include (1) epicardial aortic valve short-axis view; (2) epicardial aortic valve long-axis view; (3) epicardial left ventricle basal short-axis view; (4) epicardial left ventricle mid-short-axis view; (5) epicardial left ventricle long-axis view; (6) epicardial two-chamber view; and (7) epicardial right ventricular outflow–tract view. Upon completion of image acquisition, the cardiologist interprets the images and discusses findings with the cardiothoracic surgeon in real time in the operating room to determine if surgical plan alterations are needed or if any additional procedures or repairs must be made to the heart based on findings (eg, a sizable residual VSD is identified along with residual regurgitation of the left AV valve). The cardiologist acquires the digital images for subsequent transfer to archival storage.

76998 Ultrasonic guidance, intraoperative

▶(Do not report 76998 in conjunction with 36475, 36479, 37760, 37761, 46948, 47370, 47371, 47380, 47381, 47382, 76984, 76987, 76988, 76989, 0515T, 0516T, 0517T, 0518T, 0519T, 0520T, 0861T, 0862T, 0863T)◀

(For ultrasound guidance for open and laparoscopic radiofrequency tissue ablation, use 76940)

Rationale

In accordance with the establishment of codes 76984-76989 and 0861T-0863T, the exclusionary parenthetical note following code 76998 has been revised to reflect these changes.

Refer to the codebook and the Rationale for codes 76984-76989 and 0861T-0863T for a full discussion of these changes.

Radiation Oncology

Hyperthermia

77600 Hyperthermia, externally generated; superficial (ie, heating to a depth of 4 cm or less)

77605 deep (ie, heating to depths greater than 4 cm)

▶(For intraoperative hyperthermic intraperitoneal chemotherapy [HIPEC], see 96547, 96548)◀

Rationale

To support appropriate reporting guidance, a cross-reference parenthetical note has been added following code 77605 to direct users to new codes 96547 and 96548 for intraoperative hyperthermic intraperitoneal chemotherapy.

Refer to the codebook and the Rationale for codes 96547 and 96548 for a full discussion of these changes.

Pathology and Laboratory

Summary of Additions, Deletions, and Revisions

The summary of changes shows the actual changes that have been made to the code descriptors.

New codes appear with a bullet (●) and are indicated as "Code added." Revised codes are preceded with a triangle (▲). Within revised codes, or if a code symbol has been deleted, the deleted language and code symbol appear with a ~~strikethrough~~, while new text appears <u>underlined</u>.

The ⊮ symbol is used to identify codes for vaccines that are pending FDA approval. The # symbol is used to identify codes that have been resequenced. CPT add-on codes are annotated by the ✚ symbol. The ⊘ symbol is used to identify codes that are exempt from the use of modifier 51. The ★ symbol is used to identify codes that may be used for reporting telemedicine services. The ✕ is used to identify proprietary laboratory analyses (PLA) test that has an identical descriptor as another PLA test. A PLA code that satisfies Category I code criteria and has been accepted by the CPT Editorial Panel is annotated with the ⇅ symbol. The ◀ symbol is used to identify codes that may be used to report audio-only telemedicine services when appended by modifier 93 (see Appendix T).

Code	Description
▲81171	*AFF2 (~~AF4/FMR2 family, member 2~~<u>ALF transcription elongation factor 2 [FMR2]</u>)* (eg, fragile X ~~mental retardation~~<u>intellectual disability</u> 2 [FRAXE]) gene analysis; evaluation to detect abnormal (eg, expanded) alleles
▲81172	characterization of alleles (eg, expanded size and methylation status)
▲81243	*FMR1 (fragile X ~~mental retardation~~ <u>messenger</u> <u>ribonucleoprotein</u> 1)* (eg, fragile X ~~mental retardation~~<u>syndrome, X-linked intellectual disability [XLID]</u>) gene analysis; evaluation to detect abnormal (eg, expanded) alleles
▲81244	characterization of alleles (eg, expanded size and promoter methylation status)
▲81403	Molecular pathology procedure, Level 4 (eg, analysis of single exon by DNA sequence analysis, analysis of >10 amplicons using multiplex PCR in 2 or more independent reactions, mutation scanning or duplication/deletion variants of 2-5 exons)
	ARX (aristaless<u>-</u>-related homeobox) (eg, X-linked lissencephaly with ambiguous genitalia, X-linked ~~mental retardation~~<u>intellectual disability</u>), duplication/deletion analysis
▲81404	Molecular pathology procedure, Level 5 (eg, analysis of 2-5 exons by DNA sequence analysis, mutation scanning or duplication/deletion variants of 6-10 exons, or characterization of a dynamic mutation disorder/triplet repeat by Southern blot analysis)
	ARX (aristaless related homeobox) (eg, X-linked lissencephaly with ambiguous genitalia, X-linked ~~mental retardation~~<u>intellectual disability</u>), full gene sequence
	ZNF41 (zinc finger protein 41) (eg, X-linked ~~mental retardation~~<u>intellectual disability</u> 89), full gene sequence
▲81405	Molecular pathology procedure, Level 6 (eg, analysis of 6-10 exons by DNA sequence analysis, mutation scanning or duplication/deletion variants of 11-25 exons, regionally targeted cytogenomic array analysis)
	FTSJ1 (FtsJ RNA ~~methyltransferase homolog 1 [E. coli]~~<u>2'-O-methyltransferase 1</u>) (eg, X-linked ~~mental retardation~~<u>intellectual disability</u> 9), duplication/deletion analysis
▲81406	Molecular pathology procedure, Level 7 (eg, analysis of 11-25 exons by DNA sequence analysis, mutation scanning or duplication/deletion variants of 26-50 exons)
	FTSJ1 (FtsJ RNA <u>2'-O-methyltransferase 1</u>~~methyltransferase homolog 1 [E. coli]~~) (eg, X-linked ~~mental retardation~~ <u>intellectual disability</u> 9), full gene sequence

Pathology and Laboratory 80047-89398, 0001U-0419U

Pathology and Laboratory 80047-89398, 0001U-0419U

Code	Description
▲81407	Molecular pathology procedure, Level 8 (eg, analysis of 26-50 exons by DNA sequence analysis, mutation scanning or duplication/deletion variants of >50 exons, sequence analysis of multiple genes on one platform) *KDM5C (lysine [K]-specific demethylase 5C)* (eg, X-linked ~~mental retardation~~intellectual disability), full gene sequence
▲81445	~~Targeted genomic sequence analysis panel, s~~Solid organ neoplasm, genomic sequence analysis panel, 5-50 genes ~~(eg, *ALK, BRAF, CDKN2A, EGFR, ERBB2, KIT, KRAS, MET, NRAS, PDGFRA, PDGFRB, PGR, PIK3CA, PTEN, RET)*,~~ interrogation for sequence variants and copy number variants or rearrangements, if performed; DNA analysis or combined DNA and RNA analysis
▲81449	RNA analysis
▲81450	~~Targeted genomic sequence analysis panel, h~~Hematolymphoid neoplasm or disorder, genomic sequence analysis panel, 5-50 genes ~~(eg, *BRAF, CEBPA, DNMT3A, EZH2, FLT3, IDH1, IDH2, JAK2, KIT, KRAS, MLL, NOTCH1, NPM1, NRAS)*,~~ interrogation for sequence variants, and copy number variants or rearrangements, or isoform expression or mRNA expression levels, if performed; DNA analysis or combined DNA and RNA analysis
▲81451	RNA analysis
▲81455	~~Targeted genomic sequence analysis panel, s~~Solid organ or hematolymphoid neoplasm or disorder, 51 or greater genes, genomic sequence analysis panel, ~~(eg, *ALK, BRAF, CDKN2A, CEBPA, DNMT3A, EGFR, ERBB2, EZH2, FLT3, IDH1, IDH2, JAK2, KIT, KRAS, MET, MLL, NOTCH1, NPM1, NRAS, PDGFRA, PDGFRB, PGR, PIK3CA, PTEN, RET)*,~~ interrogation for sequence variants and copy number variants or rearrangements, or isoform expression or mRNA expression levels, if performed; DNA analysis or combined DNA and RNA analysis
▲81456	RNA analysis
●81457	Code added
●81458	Code added
●81459	Code added
#●81462	Code added
#●81463	Code added
#●81464	Code added
●81517	Code added
●82166	Code added
#●86041	Code added
#●86042	Code added
#●86043	Code added
#●86366	Code added
●87523	Code added
●87593	Code added
▲0022U	Targeted genomic sequence analysis panel, ~~cholangiocarcinoma and~~ non-small cell lung neoplasia, DNA and RNA analysis, ~~1-~~23 genes, interrogation for sequence variants and rearrangements, reported as presence~~/~~ or absence of variants and associated therapy(ies) to consider
0053U	~~Oncology (prostate cancer), FISH analysis of 4 genes (*ASAP1, HDAC9, CHD1* and *PTEN*), needle biopsy specimen, algorithm reported as probability of higher tumor grade~~

Code	Description
0066U	~~Placental alpha-micro globulin-1 (PAMG-1), immunoassay with direct optical observation, cervico-vaginal fluid, each specimen~~
▲0095U	~~Inflammation (e~~Eosinophilic esophagitis~~),~~ ~~ELISA analysis of e~~Eotaxin-3 *([CCL26 [[C-C motif chemokine ligand 26]]])* and major basic protein *([PRG2 [[proteoglycan 2, pro eosinophil major basic protein]]])*, enzyme-linked immunosorbent assays (ELISA), specimen obtained by ~~swallowed nylon~~ esophageal string test device, algorithm reported as ~~predictive~~ probability ~~index for~~ of active or inactive eosinophilic esophagitis
0143U	~~Drug assay, definitive, 120 or more drugs or metabolites, urine, quantitative liquid chromatography with tandem mass spectrometry (LC-MS/MS) using multiple reaction monitoring (MRM), with drug or metabolite description, comments including sample validation, per date of service~~
0144U	~~Drug assay, definitive, 160 or more drugs or metabolites, urine, quantitative liquid chromatography with tandem mass spectrometry (LC-MS/MS) using multiple reaction monitoring (MRM), with drug or metabolite description, comments including sample validation, per date of service~~
0145U	~~Drug assay, definitive, 65 or more drugs or metabolites, urine, quantitative liquid chromatography with tandem mass spectrometry (LC-MS/MS) using multiple reaction monitoring (MRM), with drug or metabolite description, comments including sample validation, per date of service~~
0146U	~~Drug assay, definitive, 80 or more drugs or metabolites, urine, by quantitative liquid chromatography with tandem mass spectrometry (LC-MS/MS) using multiple reaction monitoring (MRM), with drug or metabolite description, comments including sample validation, per date of service~~
0147U	~~Drug assay, definitive, 85 or more drugs or metabolites, urine, quantitative liquid chromatography with tandem mass spectrometry (LC-MS/MS) using multiple reaction monitoring (MRM), with drug or metabolite description, comments including sample validation, per date of service~~
0148U	~~Drug assay, definitive, 100 or more drugs or metabolites, urine, quantitative liquid chromatography with tandem mass spectrometry (LC-MS/MS) using multiple reaction monitoring (MRM), with drug or metabolite description, comments including sample validation, per date of service~~
0149U	~~Drug assay, definitive, 60 or more drugs or metabolites, urine, quantitative liquid chromatography with tandem mass spectrometry (LC-MS/MS) using multiple reaction monitoring (MRM), with drug or metabolite description, comments including sample validation, per date of service~~
0150U	~~Drug assay, definitive, 120 or more drugs or metabolites, urine, quantitative liquid chromatography with tandem mass spectrometry (LC-MS/MS) using multiple reaction monitoring (MRM), with drug or metabolite description, comments including sample validation, per date of service~~
▲0269U	Hematology (autosomal dominant congenital thrombocytopenia), genomic sequence analysis of ~~14~~22 genes, blood, buccal swab, or amniotic fluid
▲0271U	Hematology (congenital neutropenia), genomic sequence analysis of ~~23~~24 genes, blood, buccal swab, or amniotic fluid
▲0272U	Hematology (genetic bleeding disorders), genomic sequence analysis of ~~51~~60 genes and duplication/deletion of *PLAU*, blood, buccal swab, or amniotic fluid, comprehensive
▲0274U	Hematology (genetic platelet disorders), genomic sequence analysis of ~~43~~62 genes and duplication/deletion of *PLAU*, blood, buccal swab, or amniotic fluid
▲0277U	Hematology (genetic platelet function disorder), genomic sequence analysis of ~~31~~40 genes and duplication/deletion of *PLAU*, blood, buccal swab, or amniotic fluid
▲0278U	Hematology (genetic thrombosis), genomic sequence analysis of ~~12~~14 genes, blood, buccal swab, or amniotic fluid
▲0308U	Cardiology (coronary artery disease [CAD]), analysis of 3 proteins (high sensitivity [hs] troponin, adiponectin, and kidney injury molecule-1 [KIM-1]) with 3 clinical parameters (age, sex, history of cardiac intervention), plasma, algorithm reported as a risk score for obstructive CAD

Code	Description
0324U	~~Oncology (ovarian), spheroid cell culture, 4-drug panel (carboplatin, doxorubicin, gemcitabine, paclitaxel), tumor chemotherapy response prediction for each drug~~
0325U	~~Oncology (ovarian), spheroid cell culture, poly (ADP-ribose) polymerase (PARP) inhibitors (niraparib, olaparib, rucaparib, velparib), tumor response prediction for each drug~~
●0355U	Code added
●0356U	Code added
0357U	~~Oncology (melanoma), artificial intelligence (AI)-enabled quantitative mass spectrometry analysis of 142 unique pairs of glycopeptide and product fragments, plasma, prognostic, and predictive algorithm reported as likely, unlikely, or uncertain benefit from immunotherapy agents~~
●0358U	Code added
●0359U	Code added
●0360U	Code added
●0361U	Code added
▲0362U	Oncology (papillary thyroid cancer), gene-expression profiling via targeted hybrid capture–enrichment RNA sequencing of 82 content genes and 10 housekeeping genes, <u>fine needle aspirate or</u> formalin-fixed paraffin-embedded (FFPE) tissue, algorithm reported as one of three molecular subtypes
●0363U	Code added
●0364U	Code added
●0365U	Code added
●0366U	Code added
●0367U	Code added
●0368U	Code added
●0369U	Code added
●0370U	Code added
●0371U	Code added
●0372U	Code added
●0373U	Code added
●0374U	Code added
●0375U	Code added
●0376U	Code added
●0377U	Code added
●0378U	Code added
●0379U	Code added
●0380U	Code added
●0381U	Code added

★ = Telemedicine   ◀ = Audio-only   ✚ = Add-on code   ⊁ = FDA approval pending   # = Resequenced code   ⊘ = Modifier 51 exempt

Code	Description
●0382U	Code added
●0383U	Code added
●0384U	Code added
●0385U	Code added
0386U	~~Gastroenterology (Barrett's esophagus), P16, RUNX3, HPP1, and FBN1 methylation analysis, prognostic and predictive algorithm reported as a risk score for progression to high-grade dysplasia or esophageal cancer~~
●0387U	Code added
●0388U	Code added
●0389U	Code added
●0390U	Code added
●0391U	Code added
●0392U	Code added
●0393U	Code added
●0394U	Code added
●0395U	Code added
●0396U	Code added
0397U	~~Oncology (non-small cell lung cancer), cell-free DNA from plasma, targeted sequence analysis of at least 109 genes, including sequence variants, substitutions, insertions, deletions, select rearrangements, and copy number variations~~
●0398U	Code added
●0399U	Code added
●0400U	Code added
●0401U	Code added
●0402U	Code added
●0403U	Code added
●0404U	Code added
●0405U	Code added
●0406U	Code added
●0407U	Code added
●0408U	Code added
●0409U	Code added
●0410U	Code added
✖●0411U	Code added
●0412U	Code added
●0413U	Code added

Code	Description
●**0414U**	Code added
●**0415U**	Code added
●**0416U**	Code added
●**0417U**	Code added
●**0418U**	Code added
●**0419U**	Code added

★ =Telemedicine   ◀ =Audio-only   ✚ =Add-on code   ✗ =FDA approval pending   # =Resequenced code   ⊘ =Modifier 51 exempt

Pathology and Laboratory 80047-89398, 0001U-0419U

Pathology and Laboratory

Urinalysis

▶Urinalysis procedures that are not specified in 81000, 81001, 81002, 81003, 81005, 81007, 81015, 81020, 81025, 81050 may be reported using either the appropriate analyte-specific code in the Chemistry (82009-84830) subsection or the unlisted urinalysis procedure code 81099, if an analyte-specific code is not available.◀

Rationale

In support of the 2024 changes for unlisted procedures and services, the Urinalysis subsection guidelines have been revised by removing "For specific analyses, see appropriate section" and adding new instructions for appropriate reporting of urinalysis procedures that are not specified in codes 81000-81003, 81005, 81007, 81015, 81020, 81025, and 81050. The new instructions indicate that either the appropriate analyte-specific code in the Chemistry subsection (82009-84830) may be reported or report code 81099, *Unlisted urinalysis procedure,* only if an analyte-specific code is not available.

Refer to the codebook and the Rationale for the Unlisted Procedure or Service subsection of the Introduction section for a full discussion of these changes.

81000	Urinalysis, by dip stick or tablet reagent for bilirubin, glucose, hemoglobin, ketones, leukocytes, nitrite, pH, protein, specific gravity, urobilinogen, any number of these constituents; non-automated, with microscopy
81001	automated, with microscopy
81002	non-automated, without microscopy

Molecular Pathology

Tier 1 Molecular Pathology Procedures

▲ 81171   *AFF2 (ALF transcription elongation factor 2 [FMR2]) (eg, fragile X intellectual disability 2 [FRAXE]) gene analysis; evaluation to detect abnormal (eg, expanded) alleles*

▲ 81172   *characterization of alleles (eg, expanded size and methylation status)*

▲ 81243   *FMR1 (fragile X messenger ribonucleoprotein 1) (eg, fragile X syndrome, X-linked intellectual disability [XLID]) gene analysis; evaluation to detect abnormal (eg, expanded) alleles*

(For evaluation to detect and characterize abnormal alleles, see 81243, 81244)

(For evaluation to detect and characterize abnormal alleles using a single assay [eg, PCR], use 81243)

▲ 81244   characterization of alleles (eg, expanded size and promoter methylation status)

Rationale

Codes 81171, 81172, 81243, and 81244 have been revised by replacing "mental retardation" with "syndrome, X-linked intellectual disability [XLID]."

In 2010, the 111th US Congress passed Rosa's Law, which is a bill to change references of "mental retardation" in federal law to "intellectual disability(ies)." Tier 1 codes list the full gene names approved by the Human Genome Organization (HUGO). The full names of the AFF2 and FMR1 genes and/or their associated proteins or diseases included "mental retardation." In accordance with Rosa's Law, HUGO has updated the full names of these genes and removed the term "mental retardation." Codes 81171, 81172, 81243, and 81244 have been revised to reflect this terminology change.

Clinical Example (81243)

A 17-year-old male with moderate intellectual disability (IQ of 50 to 60), above-average height with a long narrow face, close-set eyes, a highly arched palate, a prominent mandible, joint laxity in his fingers, and macroorchidism presents to a physician for evaluation of the etiology of his intellectual disability. Although his mother was of normal intelligence, his family history was remarkable for having an 18-year-old sister with a mild learning disability, a maternal aunt with premature ovarian failure, and a 68-year-old maternal grandfather with a progressive neurological illness characterized by development of a tremor, followed by difficulties with balance and occasional falling. A previously performed karyotype was normal. A sample of anticoagulated peripheral blood is submitted to the laboratory for FMR1 gene testing.

Description of Procedure (81243)

Upon receipt of the specimen, isolate high-quality genomic DNA. The genomic region containing the site of the CGG trinucleotide repeat region that is expanded in fragile X syndrome is amplified by using a polymerase chain reaction (PCR) technique. The amplicons are then subjected to analysis using fluorescent capillary electrophoresis. The pathologist or other qualified health care professional (QHP) examines the electropherogram and compares it to a sizing ladder to determine the number of CGG repeats within the amplicon. Based on this analysis, the pathologist or other QHP determines the patient's FMR1 allele status and whether additional characterization of alleles is necessary. The pathologist or other QHP composes a report that specifies the patient's allele status. Edit and sign the report, and communicate the results to appropriate caregivers.

Clinical Example (81244)

A 10-year-old female is reported by her mother as having unusual shyness leading to apparent social isolation, as well as occasional stereotypic behaviors, such as hand wringing, during a routine pediatric office visit. The child attends regular school classes, and her performance is somewhat below average. There is no family history of intellectual disability or other neurologic problems. Both parents are healthy and of average intelligence, and the patient has a 13-year-old brother who is otherwise healthy and performs well in school. The patient had a normal karyotype and array comparative genomic hybridization (CGH) study. FMR1 gene testing performed by gel-based PCR analysis revealed a single allele of normal CGG repeat size but did not definitely show the presence of a second allele. A sample of anticoagulated peripheral blood is sent to the laboratory for Southern blot testing for fragile X syndrome utilizing a methylation-specific enzyme.

Description of Procedure (81244)

Upon receipt of the specimen, isolate a large quantity of high-quality genomic DNA. Perform gel electrophoresis of the extracted DNA to assess DNA integrity. The DNA specimen undergoes double restriction digestion with the methylation-sensitive restriction enzyme EagI and the methylation-insensitive restriction enzyme. The genomic fragments are separated by gel electrophoresis, transferred to a nylon membrane by capillary action, and hybridized to a labeled probe. The hybridization pattern is visualized on X-ray film by autoradiography. The physician examines the image, compares the observed fragments to a sizing ladder to estimate CGG repeat numbers, and analyzes the patterns generated to assess the methylation status of the promoter region of the expanded FMR1 allele. Based on this analysis, the physician determines the patient's allele status, presence of expanded allele(s), and methylation status of the FMR1 promoter. The physician composes a report that specifies the patient's allele status, approximate allele sizes, and promoter-methylation status. Edit and sign the report and communicate the results to the appropriate caregivers.

Tier 2 Molecular Pathology Procedures

▲ 81403   Molecular pathology procedure, Level 4 (eg, analysis of single exon by DNA sequence analysis, analysis of >10 amplicons using multiplex PCR in 2 or more independent reactions, mutation scanning or duplication/deletion variants of 2-5 exons)

ANG (angiogenin, ribonuclease, RNase A family, 5) (eg, amyotrophic lateral sclerosis), full gene sequence

ARX (aristaless related homeobox) (eg, X-linked lissencephaly with ambiguous genitalia, X-linked intellectual disability), duplication/deletion analysis

CEL (carboxyl ester lipase [bile salt-stimulated lipase]) (eg, maturity-onset diabetes of the young [MODY]), targeted sequence analysis of exon 11 (eg, c.1785delC, c.1686delT)

CTNNB1 (catenin [cadherin-associated protein], beta 1, 88kDa) (eg, desmoid tumors), targeted sequence analysis (eg, exon 3)

DAZ/SRY (deleted in azoospermia and sex detƒning region Y) (eg, male infertility), common deletions (eg, AZFa, AZFb, AZFc, AZFd)

DNMT3A (DNA [cytosine-5-]-methyltransferase 3 alpha) (eg, acute myeloid leukemia), targeted sequence analysis (eg, exon 23)

EPCAM (epithelial cell adhesion molecule) (eg, Lynch syndrome), duplication/deletion analysis

F8 (coagulation factor VIII) (eg, hemophilia A), inversion analysis, intron 1 and intron 22A

F12 (coagulation factor XII [Hageman factor]) (eg, angioedema, hereditary, type III; factor XII deficiency), targeted sequence analysis of exon 9

FGFR3 (fibroblast growth factor receptor 3) (eg, isolated craniosynostosis), targeted sequence analysis (eg, exon 7)

(For targeted sequence analysis of multiple FGFR3 exons, use 81404)

GJB1 (gap junction protein, beta 1) (eg, Charcot-Marie-Tooth X-linked), full gene sequence

GNAQ (guanine nucleotide-binding protein G[q] subunit alpha) (eg, uveal melanoma), common variants (eg, R183, Q209)

Human erythrocyte antigen gene analyses (eg, SLC14A1 [Kidd blood group], BCAM [Lutheran blood group], ICAM4 [Landsteiner-Wiener blood group], SLC4A1 [Diego blood group], AQP1 [Colton blood group], ERMAP [Scianna blood group], RHCE [Rh blood group, CcEe antigens], KEL [Kell blood group], DARC [Duffy blood group], GYPA, GYPB, GYPE [MNS blood group], ART4 [Dombrock blood group]) (eg, sickle-cell disease, thalassemia, hemolytic transfusion reactions, hemolytic disease of the fetus or newborn), common variants

HRAS (v-Ha-ras Harvey rat sarcoma viral oncogene homolog) (eg, Costello syndrome), exon 2 sequence

KCNC3 (potassium voltage-gated channel, Shaw-related subfamily, member 3) (eg, spinocerebellar ataxia), targeted sequence analysis (eg, exon 2)

KCNJ2 (potassium inwardly-rectifying channel, subfamily J, member 2) (eg, Andersen-Tawil syndrome), full gene sequence

KCNJ11 (potassium inwardly-rectifying channel, subfamily J, member 11) (eg, familial hyperinsulinism), full gene sequence

Killer cell immunoglobulin-like receptor (KIR) gene family (eg, hematopoietic stem cell transplantation), genotyping of KIR family genes

Known familial variant not otherwise specified, for gene listed in Tier 1 or Tier 2, or identified during a genomic sequencing procedure, DNA sequence analysis, each variant exon

(For a known familial variant that is considered a common variant, use specific common variant Tier 1 or Tier 2 code)

MC4R (melanocortin 4 receptor) (eg, obesity), full gene sequence

MICA (MHC class I polypeptide-related sequence A) (eg, solid organ transplantation), common variants (eg, *001, *002)

MT-RNR1 (mitochondrially encoded 12S RNA) (eg, nonsyndromic hearing loss), full gene sequence

MT-TS1 (mitochondrially encoded tRNA serine 1) (eg, nonsyndromic hearing loss), full gene sequence

NDP (Norrie disease [pseudoglioma]) (eg, Norrie disease), duplication/deletion analysis

NHLRC1 (NHL repeat containing 1) (eg, progressive myoclonus epilepsy), full gene sequence

PHOX2B (paired-like homeobox 2b) (eg, congenital central hypoventilation syndrome), duplication/deletion analysis

PLN (phospholamban) (eg, dilated cardiomyopathy, hypertrophic cardiomyopathy), full gene sequence

RHD (Rh blood group, D antigen) (eg, hemolytic disease of the fetus and newborn, Rh maternal/fetal compatibility), deletion analysis (eg, exons 4, 5, and 7, pseudogene)

RHD (Rh blood group, D antigen) (eg, hemolytic disease of the fetus and newborn, Rh maternal/fetal compatibility), deletion analysis (eg, exons 4, 5, and 7, pseudogene), performed on cell-free fetal DNA in maternal blood

(For human erythrocyte gene analysis of RHD, use a separate unit of 81403)

SH2D1A (SH2 domain containing 1A) (eg, X-linked lymphoproliferative syndrome), duplication/deletion analysis

TWIST1 (twist homolog 1 [Drosophila]) (eg, Saethre-Chotzen syndrome), duplication/deletion analysis

UBA1 (ubiquitin-like modifier activating enzyme 1) (eg, spinal muscular atrophy, X-linked), targeted sequence analysis (eg, exon 15)

VHL (von Hippel-Lindau tumor suppressor) (eg, von Hippel-Lindau familial cancer syndrome), deletion/duplication analysis

VWF (von Willebrand factor) (eg, von Willebrand disease types 2A, 2B, 2M), targeted sequence analysis (eg, exon 28)

▲ 81404   Molecular pathology procedure, Level 5 (eg, analysis of 2-5 exons by DNA sequence analysis, mutation scanning or duplication/deletion variants of 6-10 exons, or characterization of a dynamic mutation disorder/triplet repeat by Southern blot analysis)

ACADS (acyl-CoA dehydrogenase, C-2 to C-3 short chain) (eg, short chain acyl-CoA dehydrogenase deficiency), targeted sequence analysis (eg, exons 5 and 6)

AQP2 (aquaporin 2 [collecting duct]) (eg, nephrogenic diabetes insipidus), full gene sequence

ARX (aristaless related homeobox) (eg, X-linked lissencephaly with ambiguous genitalia, X-linked intellectual disability), full gene sequence

AVPR2 (arginine vasopressin receptor 2) (eg, nephrogenic diabetes insipidus), full gene sequence

BBS10 (Bardet-Biedl syndrome 10) (eg, Bardet-Biedl syndrome), full gene sequence

BTD (biotinidase) (eg, biotinidase deficiency), full gene sequence

C10orf2 (chromosome 10 open reading frame 2) (eg, mitochondrial DNA depletion syndrome), full gene sequence

CAV3 (caveolin 3) (eg, CAV3-related distal myopathy, limb-girdle muscular dystrophy type 1C), full gene sequence

CD40LG (CD40 ligand) (eg, X-linked hyper IgM syndrome), full gene sequence

CDKN2A (cyclin-dependent kinase inhibitor 2A) (eg, CDKN2A-related cutaneous malignant melanoma, familial atypical mole-malignant melanoma syndrome), full gene sequence

CLRN1 (clarin 1) (eg, Usher syndrome, type 3), full gene sequence

COX6B1 (cytochrome c oxidase subunit VIb polypeptide 1) (eg, mitochondrial respiratory chain complex IV deficiency), full gene sequence

CPT2 (carnitine palmitoyltransferase 2) (eg, carnitine palmitoyltransferase II deficiency), full gene sequence

CRX (cone-rod homeobox) (eg, cone-rod dystrophy 2, Leber congenital amaurosis), full gene sequence

CYP1B1 (cytochrome P450, family 1, subfamily B, polypeptide 1) (eg, primary congenital glaucoma), full gene sequence

EGR2 (early growth response 2) (eg, Charcot-Marie-Tooth), full gene sequence

EMD (emerin) (eg, Emery-Dreifuss muscular dystrophy), duplication/deletion analysis

EPM2A (epilepsy, progressive myoclonus type 2A, Lafora disease [laforin]) (eg, progressive myoclonus epilepsy), full gene sequence

FGF23 (fibroblast growth factor 23) (eg, hypophosphatemic rickets), full gene sequence

FGFR2 (fibroblast growth factor receptor 2) (eg, craniosynostosis, Apert syndrome, Crouzon syndrome), targeted sequence analysis (eg, exons 8, 10)

FGFR3 (fibroblast growth factor receptor 3) (eg, achondroplasia, hypochondroplasia), targeted sequence analysis (eg, exons 8, 11, 12, 13)

FHL1 (four and a half LIM domains 1) (eg, Emery-Dreifuss muscular dystrophy), full gene sequence

FKRP (fukutin related protein) (eg, congenital muscular dystrophy type 1C [MDC1C], limb-girdle muscular dystrophy [LGMD] type 2I), full gene sequence

FOXG1 (forkhead box G1) (eg, Rett syndrome), full gene sequence

FSHMD1A (facioscapulohumeral muscular dystrophy 1A) (eg, facioscapulohumeral muscular dystrophy), evaluation to detect abnormal (eg, deleted) alleles

FSHMD1A (facioscapulohumeral muscular dystrophy 1A) (eg, facioscapulohumeral muscular dystrophy), characterization of haplotype(s) (ie, chromosome 4A and 4B haplotypes)

GH1 (growth hormone 1) (eg, growth hormone deficiency), full gene sequence

GP1BB (glycoprotein Ib [platelet], beta polypeptide) (eg, Bernard-Soulier syndrome type B), full gene sequence

(For common deletion variants of alpha globin 1 and alpha globin 2 genes, use 81257)

HNF1B (HNF1 homeobox B) (eg, maturity-onset diabetes of the young [MODY]), duplication/deletion analysis

HRAS (v-Ha-ras Harvey rat sarcoma viral oncogene homolog) (eg, Costello syndrome), full gene sequence

HSD3B2 (hydroxy-delta-5-steroid dehydrogenase, 3 beta- and steroid delta-isomerase 2) (eg, 3-beta-hydroxysteroid dehydrogenase type II deficiency), full gene sequence

HSD11B2 (hydroxysteroid [11-beta] dehydrogenase 2) (eg, mineralocorticoid excess syndrome), full gene sequence

HSPB1 (heat shock 27kDa protein 1) (eg, Charcot-Marie-Tooth disease), full gene sequence

INS (insulin) (eg, diabetes mellitus), full gene sequence

KCNJ1 (potassium inwardly-rectifying channel, subfamily J, member 1) (eg, Bartter syndrome), full gene sequence

KCNJ10 (potassium inwardly-rectifying channel, subfamily J, member 10) (eg, SeSAME syndrome, EAST syndrome, sensorineural hearing loss), full gene sequence

LITAF (lipopolysaccharide-induced TNF factor) (eg, Charcot-Marie-Tooth), full gene sequence

MEFV (Mediterranean fever) (eg, familial Mediterranean fever), full gene sequence

MEN1 (multiple endocrine neoplasia I) (eg, multiple endocrine neoplasia type 1, Wermer syndrome), duplication/deletion analysis

MMACHC (methylmalonic aciduria [cobalamin deficiency] cblC type, with homocystinuria) (eg, methylmalonic acidemia and homocystinuria), full gene sequence

MPV17 (MpV17 mitochondrial inner membrane protein) (eg, mitochondrial DNA depletion syndrome), duplication/deletion analysis

NDP (Norrie disease [pseudoglioma]) (eg, Norrie disease), full gene sequence

NDUFA1 (NADH dehydrogenase [ubiquinone] 1 alpha subcomplex, 1, 7.5kDa) (eg, Leigh syndrome, mitochondrial complex I deficiency), full gene sequence

NDUFAF2 (NADH dehydrogenase [ubiquinone] 1 alpha subcomplex, assembly factor 2) (eg, Leigh syndrome, mitochondrial complex I deficiency), full gene sequence

NDUFS4 (NADH dehydrogenase [ubiquinone] Fe-S protein 4, 18kDa [NADH-coenzyme Q reductase]) (eg, Leigh syndrome, mitochondrial complex I deficiency), full gene sequence

NIPA1 (non-imprinted in Prader-Willi/Angelman syndrome 1) (eg, spastic paraplegia), full gene sequence

NLGN4X (neuroligin 4, X-linked) (eg, autism spectrum disorders), duplication/deletion analysis

NPC2 (Niemann-Pick disease, type C2 [epididymal secretory protein E1]) (eg, Niemann-Pick disease type C2), full gene sequence

NR0B1 (nuclear receptor subfamily 0, group B, member 1) (eg, congenital adrenal hypoplasia), full gene sequence

PDX1 (pancreatic and duodenal homeobox 1) (eg, maturity-onset diabetes of the young [MODY]), full gene sequence

PHOX2B (paired-like homeobox 2b) (eg, congenital central hypoventilation syndrome), full gene sequence

PLP1 (proteolipid protein 1) (eg, Pelizaeus-Merzbacher disease, spastic paraplegia), duplication/deletion analysis

PQBP1 (polyglutamine binding protein 1) (eg, Renpenning syndrome), duplication/deletion analysis

PRNP (prion protein) (eg, genetic prion disease), full gene sequence

PROP1 (PROP paired-like homeobox 1) (eg, combined pituitary hormone deficiency), full gene sequence

PRPH2 (peripherin 2 [retinal degeneration, slow]) (eg, retinitis pigmentosa), full gene sequence

PRSS1 (protease, serine, 1 [trypsin 1]) (eg, hereditary pancreatitis), full gene sequence

RAF1 (v-raf-1 murine leukemia viral oncogene homolog 1) (eg, LEOPARD syndrome), targeted sequence analysis (eg, exons 7, 12, 14, 17)

RET (ret proto-oncogene) (eg, multiple endocrine neoplasia, type 2B and familial medullary thyroid carcinoma), common variants (eg, M918T, 2647_2648delinsTT, A883F)

RHO (rhodopsin) (eg, retinitis pigmentosa), full gene sequence

RP1 (retinitis pigmentosa 1) (eg, retinitis pigmentosa), full gene sequence

SCN1B (sodium channel, voltage-gated, type I, beta) (eg, Brugada syndrome), full gene sequence

SCO2 (SCO cytochrome oxidase deficient homolog 2 [SCO1L]) (eg, mitochondrial respiratory chain complex IV deficiency), full gene sequence

SDHC (succinate dehydrogenase complex, subunit C, integral membrane protein, 15kDa) (eg, hereditary paraganglioma-pheochromocytoma syndrome), duplication/deletion analysis

SDHD (succinate dehydrogenase complex, subunit D, integral membrane protein) (eg, hereditary paraganglioma), full gene sequence

SGCG (sarcoglycan, gamma [35kDa dystrophin-associated glycoprotein]) (eg, limb-girdle muscular dystrophy), duplication/deletion analysis

SH2D1A (SH2 domain containing 1A) (eg, X-linked lymphoproliferative syndrome), full gene sequence

SLC16A2 (solute carrier family 16, member 2 [thyroid hormone transporter]) (eg, specific thyroid hormone cell transporter deficiency, Allan-Herndon-Dudley syndrome), duplication/deletion analysis

SLC25A20 (solute carrier family 25 [carnitine/acylcarnitine translocase], member 20) (eg, carnitine-acylcarnitine translocase deficiency), duplication/deletion analysis

SLC25A4 (solute carrier family 25 [mitochondrial carrier; adenine nucleotide translocator], member 4) (eg, progressive external ophthalmoplegia), full gene sequence

SOD1 (superoxide dismutase 1, soluble) (eg, amyotrophic lateral sclerosis), full gene sequence

SPINK1 (serine peptidase inhibitor, Kazal type 1) (eg, hereditary pancreatitis), full gene sequence

STK11 (serine/threonine kinase 11) (eg, Peutz-Jeghers syndrome), duplication/deletion analysis

TACO1 (translational activator of mitochondrial encoded cytochrome c oxidase I) (eg, mitochondrial respiratory chain complex IV deficiency), full gene sequence

THAP1 (THAP domain containing, apoptosis associated protein 1) (eg, torsion dystonia), full gene sequence

TOR1A (torsin family 1, member A [torsin A]) (eg, torsion dystonia), full gene sequence

TTPA (tocopherol [alpha] transfer protein) (eg, ataxia), full gene sequence

TTR (transthyretin) (eg, familial transthyretin amyloidosis), full gene sequence

TWIST1 (twist homolog 1 [Drosophila]) (eg, Saethre-Chotzen syndrome), full gene sequence

TYR (tyrosinase [oculocutaneous albinism IA]) (eg, oculocutaneous albinism IA), full gene sequence

UGT1A1 (UDP glucuronosyltransferase 1 family, polypeptide A1) (eg, hereditary unconjugated hyperbilirubinemia [Crigler-Najjar syndrome]) full gene sequence

USH1G (Usher syndrome 1G [autosomal recessive]) (eg, Usher syndrome, type 1), full gene sequence

VHL (von Hippel-Lindau tumor suppressor) (eg, von Hippel-Lindau familial cancer syndrome), full gene sequence

VWF (von Willebrand factor) (eg, von Willebrand disease type 1C), targeted sequence analysis (eg, exons 26, 27, 37)

ZEB2 (zinc finger E-box binding homeobox 2) (eg, Mowat-Wilson syndrome), duplication/deletion analysis

ZNF41 (zinc finger protein 41) (eg, X-linked intellectual disability 89), full gene sequence

▲ **81405**　Molecular pathology procedure, Level 6 (eg, analysis of 6-10 exons by DNA sequence analysis, mutation scanning or duplication/deletion variants of 11-25 exons, regionally targeted cytogenomic array analysis)

ABCD1 (ATP-binding cassette, sub-family D [ALD], member 1) (eg, adrenoleukodystrophy), full gene sequence

ACADS (acyl-CoA dehydrogenase, C-2 to C-3 short chain) (eg, short chain acyl-CoA dehydrogenase deficiency), full gene sequence

ACTA2 (actin, alpha 2, smooth muscle, aorta) (eg, thoracic aortic aneurysms and aortic dissections), full gene sequence

ACTC1 (actin, alpha, cardiac muscle 1) (eg, familial hypertrophic cardiomyopathy), full gene sequence

ANKRD1 (ankyrin repeat domain 1) (eg, dilated cardiomyopathy), full gene sequence

APTX (aprataxin) (eg, ataxia with oculomotor apraxia 1), full gene sequence

ARSA (arylsulfatase A) (eg, arylsulfatase A deficiency), full gene sequence

BCKDHA (branched chain keto acid dehydrogenase E1, alpha polypeptide) (eg, maple syrup urine disease, type 1A), full gene sequence

BCS1L (BCS1-like [S. cerevisiae]) (eg, Leigh syndrome, mitochondrial complex III deficiency, GRACILE syndrome), full gene sequence

BMPR2 (bone morphogenetic protein receptor, type II [serine/threonine kinase]) (eg, heritable pulmonary arterial hypertension), duplication/deletion analysis

CASQ2 (calsequestrin 2 [cardiac muscle]) (eg, catecholaminergic polymorphic ventricular tachycardia), full gene sequence

CASR (calcium-sensing receptor) (eg, hypocalcemia), full gene sequence

CDKL5 (cyclin-dependent kinase-like 5) (eg, early infantile epileptic encephalopathy), duplication/deletion analysis

CHRNA4 (cholinergic receptor, nicotinic, alpha 4) (eg, nocturnal frontal lobe epilepsy), full gene sequence

CHRNB2 (cholinergic receptor, nicotinic, beta 2 [neuronal]) (eg, nocturnal frontal lobe epilepsy), full gene sequence

COX10 (COX10 homolog, cytochrome c oxidase assembly protein) (eg, mitochondrial respiratory chain complex IV deficiency), full gene sequence

COX15 (COX15 homolog, cytochrome c oxidase assembly protein) (eg, mitochondrial respiratory chain complex IV deficiency), full gene sequence

CPOX (coproporphyrinogen oxidase) (eg, hereditary coproporphyria), full gene sequence

CTRC (chymotrypsin C) (eg, hereditary pancreatitis), full gene sequence

CYP11B1 (cytochrome P450, family 11, subfamily B, polypeptide 1) (eg, congenital adrenal hyperplasia), full gene sequence

CYP17A1 (cytochrome P450, family 17, subfamily A, polypeptide 1) (eg, congenital adrenal hyperplasia), full gene sequence

CYP21A2 (cytochrome P450, family 21, subfamily A, polypeptide2) (eg, steroid 21-hydroxylase isoform, congenital adrenal hyperplasia), full gene sequence

Cytogenomic constitutional targeted microarray analysis of chromosome 22q13 by interrogation of genomic regions for copy number and single nucleotide polymorphism (SNP) variants for chromosomal abnormalities

(When performing cytogenomic [genome-wide] analysis for constitutional chromosomal abnormalities, see 81228, 81229, 81349)

(Do not report analyte-specific molecular pathology procedures separately when the specific analytes are included as part of the microarray analysis of chromosome 22q13)

(Do not report 88271 when performing cytogenomic microarray analysis)

DBT (dihydrolipoamide branched chain transacylase E2) (eg, maple syrup urine disease, type 2), duplication/deletion analysis

DCX (doublecortin) (eg, X-linked lissencephaly), full gene sequence

DES (desmin) (eg, myofibrillar myopathy), full gene sequence

DFNB59 (deafness, autosomal recessive 59) (eg, autosomal recessive nonsyndromic hearing impairment), full gene sequence

DGUOK (deoxyguanosine kinase) (eg, hepatocerebral mitochondrial DNA depletion syndrome), full gene sequence

DHCR7 (7-dehydrocholesterol reductase) (eg, Smith-Lemli-Opitz syndrome), full gene sequence

EIF2B2 (eukaryotic translation initiation factor 2B, subunit 2 beta, 39kDa) (eg, leukoencephalopathy with vanishing white matter), full gene sequence

EMD (emerin) (eg, Emery-Dreifuss muscular dystrophy), full gene sequence

ENG (endoglin) (eg, hereditary hemorrhagic telangiectasia, type 1), duplication/deletion analysis

★ = Telemedicine　◀ = Audio-only　✚ = Add-on code　✚ = FDA approval pending　# = Resequenced code　⊘ = Modifier 51 exempt

EYA1 (eyes absent homolog 1 [Drosophila]) (eg, branchio-oto-renal [BOR] spectrum disorders), duplication/deletion analysis

FGFR1 (fibroblast growth factor receptor 1) (eg, Kallmann syndrome 2), full gene sequence

FH (fumarate hydratase) (eg, fumarate hydratase deficiency, hereditary leiomyomatosis with renal cell cancer), full gene sequence

FKTN (fukutin) (eg, limb-girdle muscular dystrophy [LGMD] type 2M or 2L), full gene sequence

FTSJ1 (FtsJ RNA 2'-O-methyltransferase 1) (eg, X-linked intellectual disability 9), duplication/deletion analysis

GABRG2 (gamma-aminobutyric acid [GABA] A receptor, gamma 2) (eg, generalized epilepsy with febrile seizures), full gene sequence

GCH1 (GTP cyclohydrolase 1) (eg, autosomal dominant dopa-responsive dystonia), full gene sequence

GDAP1 (ganglioside-induced differentiation-associated protein 1) (eg, Charcot-Marie-Tooth disease), full gene sequence

GFAP (glial fibrillary acidic protein) (eg, Alexander disease), full gene sequence

GHR (growth hormone receptor) (eg, Laron syndrome), full gene sequence

GHRHR (growth hormone releasing hormone receptor) (eg, growth hormone deficiency), full gene sequence

GLA (galactosidase, alpha) (eg, Fabry disease), full gene sequence

HNF1A (HNF1 homeobox A) (eg, maturity-onset diabetes of the young [MODY]), full gene sequence

HNF1B (HNF1 homeobox B) (eg, maturity-onset diabetes of the young [MODY]), full gene sequence

HTRA1 (HtrA serine peptidase 1) (eg, macular degeneration), full gene sequence

IDS (iduronate 2-sulfatase) (eg, mucopolysacchridosis, type II), full gene sequence

IL2RG (interleukin 2 receptor, gamma) (eg, X-linked severe combined immunodeficiency), full gene sequence

ISPD (isoprenoid synthase domain containing) (eg, muscle-eye-brain disease, Walker-Warburg syndrome), full gene sequence

KRAS (Kirsten rat sarcoma viral oncogene homolog) (eg, Noonan syndrome), full gene sequence

LAMP2 (lysosomal-associated membrane protein 2) (eg, Danon disease), full gene sequence

LDLR (low density lipoprotein receptor) (eg, familial hypercholesterolemia), duplication/deletion analysis

MEN1 (multiple endocrine neoplasia I) (eg, multiple endocrine neoplasia type 1, Wermer syndrome), full gene sequence

MMAA (methylmalonic aciduria [cobalamine deficiency] type A) (eg, MMAA-related methylmalonic acidemia), full gene sequence

MMAB (methylmalonic aciduria [cobalamine deficiency] type B) (eg, MMAA-related methylmalonic acidemia), full gene sequence

MPI (mannose phosphate isomerase) (eg, congenital disorder of glycosylation 1b), full gene sequence

MPV17 (MpV17 mitochondrial inner membrane protein) (eg, mitochondrial DNA depletion syndrome), full gene sequence

MPZ (myelin protein zero) (eg, Charcot-Marie-Tooth), full gene sequence

MTM1 (myotubularin 1) (eg, X-linked centronuclear myopathy), duplication/deletion analysis

MYL2 (myosin, light chain 2, regulatory, cardiac, slow) (eg, familial hypertrophic cardiomyopathy), full gene sequence

MYL3 (myosin, light chain 3, alkali, ventricular, skeletal, slow) (eg, familial hypertrophic cardiomyopathy), full gene sequence

MYOT (myotilin) (eg, limb-girdle muscular dystrophy), full gene sequence

NDUFS7 (NADH dehydrogenase [ubiquinone] Fe-S protein 7, 20kDa [NADH-coenzyme Q reductase]) (eg, Leigh syndrome, mitochondrial complex I deficiency), full gene sequence

NDUFS8 (NADH dehydrogenase [ubiquinone] Fe-S protein 8, 23kDa [NADH-coenzyme Q reductase]) (eg, Leigh syndrome, mitochondrial complex I deficiency), full gene sequence

NDUFV1 (NADH dehydrogenase [ubiquinone] flavoprotein 1, 51kDa) (eg, Leigh syndrome, mitochondrial complex I deficiency), full gene sequence

NEFL (neurofilament, light polypeptide) (eg, Charcot-Marie-Tooth), full gene sequence

NF2 (neurofibromin 2 [merlin]) (eg, neurofibromatosis, type 2), duplication/deletion analysis

NLGN3 (neuroligin 3) (eg, autism spectrum disorders), full gene sequence

NLGN4X (neuroligin 4, X-linked) (eg, autism spectrum disorders), full gene sequence

NPHP1 (nephronophthisis 1 [juvenile]) (eg, Joubert syndrome), deletion analysis, and duplication analysis, if performed

NPHS2 (nephrosis 2, idiopathic, steroid-resistant [podocin]) (eg, steroid-resistant nephrotic syndrome), full gene sequence

Pathology and Laboratory 80047-89398, 0001U-0419U

NSD1 (nuclear receptor binding SET domain protein 1) (eg, Sotos syndrome), duplication/deletion analysis

OTC (ornithine carbamoyltransferase) (eg, ornithine transcarbamylase deficiency), full gene sequence

PAFAH1B1 (platelet-activating factor acetylhydrolase 1b, regulatory subunit 1 [45kDa]) (eg, lissencephaly, Miller-Dieker syndrome), duplication/deletion analysis

PARK2 (Parkinson protein 2, E3 ubiquitin protein ligase [parkin]) (eg, Parkinson disease), duplication/deletion analysis

PCCA (propionyl CoA carboxylase, alpha polypeptide) (eg, propionic acidemia, type 1), duplication/deletion analysis

PCDH19 (protocadherin 19) (eg, epileptic encephalopathy), full gene sequence

PDHA1 (pyruvate dehydrogenase [lipoamide] alpha 1) (eg, lactic acidosis), duplication/deletion analysis

PDHB (pyruvate dehydrogenase [lipoamide] beta) (eg, lactic acidosis), full gene sequence

PINK1 (PTEN induced putative kinase 1) (eg, Parkinson disease), full gene sequence

PKLR (pyruvate kinase, liver and RBC) (eg, pyruvate kinase deficiency), full gene sequence

PLP1 (proteolipid protein 1) (eg, Pelizaeus-Merzbacher disease, spastic paraplegia), full gene sequence

POU1F1 (POU class 1 homeobox 1) (eg, combined pituitary hormone deficiency), full gene sequence

PRX (periaxin) (eg, Charcot-Marie-Tooth disease), full gene sequence

PQBP1 (polyglutamine binding protein 1) (eg, Renpenning syndrome), full gene sequence

PSEN1 (presenilin 1) (eg, Alzheimer disease), full gene sequence

RAB7A (RAB7A, member RAS oncogene family) (eg, Charcot-Marie-Tooth disease), full gene sequence

RAI1 (retinoic acid induced 1) (eg, Smith-Magenis syndrome), full gene sequence

REEP1 (receptor accessory protein 1) (eg, spastic paraplegia), full gene sequence

RET (ret proto-oncogene) (eg, multiple endocrine neoplasia, type 2A and familial medullary thyroid carcinoma), targeted sequence analysis (eg, exons 10, 11, 13-16)

RPS19 (ribosomal protein S19) (eg, Diamond-Blackfan anemia), full gene sequence

RRM2B (ribonucleotide reductase M2 B [TP53 inducible]) (eg, mitochondrial DNA depletion), full gene sequence

SCO1 (SCO cytochrome oxidase deficient homolog 1) (eg, mitochondrial respiratory chain complex IV deficiency), full gene sequence

SDHB (succinate dehydrogenase complex, subunit B, iron sulfur) (eg, hereditary paraganglioma), full gene sequence

SDHC (succinate dehydrogenase complex, subunit C, integral membrane protein, 15kDa) (eg, hereditary paraganglioma-pheochromocytoma syndrome), full gene sequence

SGCA (sarcoglycan, alpha [50kDa dystrophin-associated glycoprotein]) (eg, limb-girdle muscular dystrophy), full gene sequence

SGCB (sarcoglycan, beta [43kDa dystrophin-associated glycoprotein]) (eg, limb-girdle muscular dystrophy), full gene sequence

SGCD (sarcoglycan, delta [35kDa dystrophin-associated glycoprotein]) (eg, limb-girdle muscular dystrophy), full gene sequence

SGCE (sarcoglycan, epsilon) (eg, myoclonic dystonia), duplication/deletion analysis

SGCG (sarcoglycan, gamma [35kDa dystrophin-associated glycoprotein]) (eg, limb-girdle muscular dystrophy), full gene sequence

SHOC2 (soc-2 suppressor of clear homolog) (eg, Noonan-like syndrome with loose anagen hair), full gene sequence

SHOX (short stature homeobox) (eg, Langer mesomelic dysplasia), full gene sequence

SIL1 (SIL1 homolog, endoplasmic reticulum chaperone [S. cerevisiae]) (eg, ataxia), full gene sequence

SLC2A1 (solute carrier family 2 [facilitated glucose transporter], member 1) (eg, glucose transporter type 1 [GLUT 1] deficiency syndrome), full gene sequence

SLC16A2 (solute carrier family 16, member 2 [thyroid hormone transporter]) (eg, specific thyroid hormone cell transporter deficiency, Allan-Herndon-Dudley syndrome), full gene sequence

SLC22A5 (solute carrier family 22 [organic cation/carnitine transporter], member 5) (eg, systemic primary carnitine deficiency), full gene sequence

SLC25A20 (solute carrier family 25 [carnitine/acylcarnitine translocase], member 20) (eg, carnitine-acylcarnitine translocase deficiency), full gene sequence

SMAD4 (SMAD family member 4) (eg, hemorrhagic telangiectasia syndrome, juvenile polyposis), duplication/deletion analysis

SPAST (spastin) (eg, spastic paraplegia), duplication/deletion analysis

SPG7 (spastic paraplegia 7 [pure and complicated autosomal recessive]) (eg, spastic paraplegia), duplication/deletion analysis

SPRED1 (sprouty-related, EVH1 domain containing 1) (eg, Legius syndrome), full gene sequence

★ = Telemedicine   ◀ = Audio-only   ✚ = Add-on code   ✗ = FDA approval pending   # = Resequenced code   ⊘ = Modifier 51 exempt

STAT3 (signal transducer and activator of transcription 3 [acute-phase response factor]) (eg, autosomal dominant hyper-IgE syndrome), targeted sequence analysis (eg, exons 12, 13, 14, 16, 17, 20, 21)

STK11 (serine/threonine kinase 11) (eg, Peutz-Jeghers syndrome), full gene sequence

SURF1 (surfeit 1) (eg, mitochondrial respiratory chain complex IV deficiency), full gene sequence

TARDBP (TAR DNA binding protein) (eg, amyotrophic lateral sclerosis), full gene sequence

TBX5 (T-box 5) (eg, Holt-Oram syndrome), full gene sequence

TCF4 (transcription factor 4) (eg, Pitt-Hopkins syndrome), duplication/deletion analysis

TGFBR1 (transforming growth factor, beta receptor 1) (eg, Marfan syndrome), full gene sequence

TGFBR2 (transforming growth factor, beta receptor 2) (eg, Marfan syndrome), full gene sequence

THRB (thyroid hormone receptor, beta) (eg, thyroid hormone resistance, thyroid hormone beta receptor deficiency), full gene sequence or targeted sequence analysis of >5 exons

TK2 (thymidine kinase 2, mitochondrial) (eg, mitochondrial DNA depletion syndrome), full gene sequence

TNNC1 (troponin C type 1 [slow]) (eg, hypertrophic cardiomyopathy or dilated cardiomyopathy), full gene sequence

TNNI3 (troponin I, type 3 [cardiac]) (eg, familial hypertrophic cardiomyopathy), full gene sequence

TPM1 (tropomyosin 1 [alpha]) (eg, familial hypertrophic cardiomyopathy), full gene sequence

TSC1 (tuberous sclerosis 1) (eg, tuberous sclerosis), duplication/deletion analysis

TYMP (thymidine phosphorylase) (eg, mitochondrial DNA depletion syndrome), full gene sequence

VWF (von Willebrand factor) (eg, von Willebrand disease type 2N), targeted sequence analysis (eg, exons 18-20, 23-25)

WT1 (Wilms tumor 1) (eg, Denys-Drash syndrome, familial Wilms tumor), full gene sequence

ZEB2 (zinc finger E-box binding homeobox 2) (eg, Mowat-Wilson syndrome), full gene sequence

▲ **81406**　Molecular pathology procedure, Level 7 (eg, analysis of 11-25 exons by DNA sequence analysis, mutation scanning or duplication/deletion variants of 26-50 exons)

ACADVL (acyl-CoA dehydrogenase, very long chain) (eg, very long chain acyl-coenzyme A dehydrogenase deficiency), full gene sequence

ACTN4 (actinin, alpha 4) (eg, focal segmental glomerulosclerosis), full gene sequence

AFG3L2 (AFG3 ATPase family gene 3-like 2 [S. cerevisiae]) (eg, spinocerebellar ataxia), full gene sequence

AIRE (autoimmune regulator) (eg, autoimmune polyendocrinopathy syndrome type 1), full gene sequence

ALDH7A1 (aldehyde dehydrogenase 7 family, member A1) (eg, pyridoxine-dependent epilepsy), full gene sequence

ANO5 (anoctamin 5) (eg, limb-girdle muscular dystrophy), full gene sequence

ANOS1 (anosmin-1) (eg, Kallmann syndrome 1), full gene sequence

APP (amyloid beta [A4] precursor protein) (eg, Alzheimer disease), full gene sequence

ASS1 (argininosuccinate synthase 1) (eg, citrullinemia type I), full gene sequence

ATL1 (atlastin GTPase 1) (eg, spastic paraplegia), full gene sequence

ATP1A2 (ATPase, Na+/K+ transporting, alpha 2 polypeptide) (eg, familial hemiplegic migraine), full gene sequence

ATP7B (ATPase, Cu++ transporting, beta polypeptide) (eg, Wilson disease), full gene sequence

BBS1 (Bardet-Biedl syndrome 1) (eg, Bardet-Biedl syndrome), full gene sequence

BBS2 (Bardet-Biedl syndrome 2) (eg, Bardet-Biedl syndrome), full gene sequence

BCKDHB (branched-chain keto acid dehydrogenase E1, beta polypeptide) (eg, maple syrup urine disease, type 1B), full gene sequence

BEST1 (bestrophin 1) (eg, vitelliform macular dystrophy), full gene sequence

BMPR2 (bone morphogenetic protein receptor, type II [serine/threonine kinase]) (eg, heritable pulmonary arterial hypertension), full gene sequence

BRAF (B-Raf proto-oncogene, serine/threonine kinase) (eg, Noonan syndrome), full gene sequence

BSCL2 (Berardinelli-Seip congenital lipodystrophy 2 [seipin]) (eg, Berardinelli-Seip congenital lipodystrophy), full gene sequence

BTK (Bruton agammaglobulinemia tyrosine kinase) (eg, X-linked agammaglobulinemia), full gene sequence

CACNB2 (calcium channel, voltage-dependent, beta 2 subunit) (eg, Brugada syndrome), full gene sequence

CAPN3 (calpain 3) (eg, limb-girdle muscular dystrophy [LGMD] type 2A, calpainopathy), full gene sequence

CBS (cystathionine-beta-synthase) (eg, homocystinuria, cystathionine beta-synthase deficiency), full gene sequence

Pathology and Laboratory　80047-89398, 0001U-0419U

CDH1 (cadherin 1, type 1, E-cadherin [epithelial]) (eg, hereditary diffuse gastric cancer), full gene sequence

CDKL5 (cyclin-dependent kinase-like 5) (eg, early infantile epileptic encephalopathy), full gene sequence

CLCN1 (chloride channel 1, skeletal muscle) (eg, myotonia congenita), full gene sequence

CLCNKB (chloride channel, voltage-sensitive Kb) (eg, Bartter syndrome 3 and 4b), full gene sequence

CNTNAP2 (contactin-associated protein-like 2) (eg, Pitt-Hopkins-like syndrome 1), full gene sequence

COL6A2 (collagen, type VI, alpha 2) (eg, collagen type VI-related disorders), duplication/deletion analysis

CPT1A (carnitine palmitoyltransferase 1A [liver]) (eg, carnitine palmitoyltransferase 1A [CPT1A] deficiency), full gene sequence

CRB1 (crumbs homolog 1 [Drosophila]) (eg, Leber congenital amaurosis), full gene sequence

CREBBP (CREB binding protein) (eg, Rubinstein-Taybi syndrome), duplication/deletion analysis

DBT (dihydrolipoamide branched chain transacylase E2) (eg, maple syrup urine disease, type 2), full gene sequence

DLAT (dihydrolipoamide S-acetyltransferase) (eg, pyruvate dehydrogenase E2 deficiency), full gene sequence

DLD (dihydrolipoamide dehydrogenase) (eg, maple syrup urine disease, type III), full gene sequence

DSC2 (desmocollin) (eg, arrhythmogenic right ventricular dysplasia/cardiomyopathy 11), full gene sequence

DSG2 (desmoglein 2) (eg, arrhythmogenic right ventricular dysplasia/cardiomyopathy 10), full gene sequence

DSP (desmoplakin) (eg, arrhythmogenic right ventricular dysplasia/cardiomyopathy 8), full gene sequence

EFHC1 (EF-hand domain [C-terminal] containing 1) (eg, juvenile myoclonic epilepsy), full gene sequence

EIF2B3 (eukaryotic translation initiation factor 2B, subunit 3 gamma, 58kDa) (eg, leukoencephalopathy with vanishing white matter), full gene sequence

EIF2B4 (eukaryotic translation initiation factor 2B, subunit 4 delta, 67kDa) (eg, leukoencephalopathy with vanishing white matter), full gene sequence

EIF2B5 (eukaryotic translation initiation factor 2B, subunit 5 epsilon, 82kDa) (eg, childhood ataxia with central nervous system hypomyelination/vanishing white matter), full gene sequence

ENG (endoglin) (eg, hereditary hemorrhagic telangiectasia, type 1), full gene sequence

EYA1 (eyes absent homolog 1 [Drosophila]) (eg, branchio-oto-renal [BOR] spectrum disorders), full gene sequence

F8 (coagulation factor VIII) (eg, hemophilia A), duplication/deletion analysis

FAH (fumarylacetoacetate hydrolase [fumarylacetoacetase]) (eg, tyrosinemia, type 1), full gene sequence

FASTKD2 (FAST kinase domains 2) (eg, mitochondrial respiratory chain complex IV deficiency), full gene sequence

FIG4 (FIG4 homolog, SAC1 lipid phosphatase domain containing [S. cerevisiae]) (eg, Charcot-Marie-Tooth disease), full gene sequence

FTSJ1 (FtsJ RNA 2'-O-methyltransferase 1) (eg, X-linked intellectual disability 9), full gene sequence

FUS (fused in sarcoma) (eg, amyotrophic lateral sclerosis), full gene sequence

GAA (glucosidase, alpha; acid) (eg, glycogen storage disease type II [Pompe disease]), full gene sequence

GALC (galactosylceramidase) (eg, Krabbe disease), full gene sequence

GALT (galactose-1-phosphate uridylyltransferase) (eg, galactosemia), full gene sequence

GARS (glycyl-tRNA synthetase) (eg, Charcot-Marie-Tooth disease), full gene sequence

GCDH (glutaryl-CoA dehydrogenase) (eg, glutaricacidemia type 1), full gene sequence

GCK (glucokinase [hexokinase 4]) (eg, maturity-onset diabetes of the young [MODY]), full gene sequence

GLUD1 (glutamate dehydrogenase 1) (eg, familial hyperinsulinism), full gene sequence

GNE (glucosamine [UDP-N-acetyl]-2-epimerase/N-acetylmannosamine kinase) (eg, inclusion body myopathy 2 [IBM2], Nonaka myopathy), full gene sequence

GRN (granulin) (eg, frontotemporal dementia), full gene sequence

HADHA (hydroxyacyl-CoA dehydrogenase/3-ketoacyl-CoA thiolase/enoyl-CoA hydratase [trifunctional protein] alpha subunit) (eg, long chain acyl-coenzyme A dehydrogenase deficiency), full gene sequence

HADHB (hydroxyacyl-CoA dehydrogenase/3-ketoacyl-CoA thiolase/enoyl-CoA hydratase [trifunctional protein], beta subunit) (eg, trifunctional protein deficiency), full gene sequence

HEXA (hexosaminidase A, alpha polypeptide) (eg, Tay-Sachs disease), full gene sequence

HLCS (HLCS holocarboxylase synthetase) (eg, holocarboxylase synthetase deficiency), full gene sequence

HMBS (hydroxymethylbilane synthase) (eg, acute intermittent porphyria), full gene sequence

★ = Telemedicine ◀ = Audio-only ✚ = Add-on code ✚ = FDA approval pending # = Resequenced code ⊘ = Modifier 51 exempt

HNF4A (hepatocyte nuclear factor 4, alpha) (eg, maturity-onset diabetes of the young [MODY]), full gene sequence

IDUA (iduronidase, alpha-L-) (eg, mucopolysaccharidosis type I), full gene sequence

INF2 (inverted formin, FH2 and WH2 domain containing) (eg, focal segmental glomerulosclerosis), full gene sequence

IVD (isovaleryl-CoA dehydrogenase) (eg, isovaleric acidemia), full gene sequence

JAG1 (jagged 1) (eg, Alagille syndrome), duplication/deletion analysis

JUP (junction plakoglobin) (eg, arrhythmogenic right ventricular dysplasia/cardiomyopathy 11), full gene sequence

KCNH2 (potassium voltage-gated channel, subfamily H [eag-related], member 2) (eg, short QT syndrome, long QT syndrome), full gene sequence

KCNQ1 (potassium voltage-gated channel, KQT-like subfamily, member 1) (eg, short QT syndrome, long QT syndrome), full gene sequence

KCNQ2 (potassium voltage-gated channel, KQT-like subfamily, member 2) (eg, epileptic encephalopathy), full gene sequence

LDB3 (LIM domain binding 3) (eg, familial dilated cardiomyopathy, myofibrillar myopathy), full gene sequence

LDLR (low density lipoprotein receptor) (eg, familial hypercholesterolemia), full gene sequence

LEPR (leptin receptor) (eg, obesity with hypogonadism), full gene sequence

LHCGR (luteinizing hormone/choriogonadotropin receptor) (eg, precocious male puberty), full gene sequence

LMNA (lamin A/C) (eg, Emery-Dreifuss muscular dystrophy [EDMD1, 2 and 3] limb-girdle muscular dystrophy [LGMD] type 1B, dilated cardiomyopathy [CMD1A], familial partial lipodystrophy [FPLD2]), full gene sequence

LRP5 (low density lipoprotein receptor-related protein 5) (eg, osteopetrosis), full gene sequence

MAP2K1 (mitogen-activated protein kinase 1) (eg, cardiofaciocutaneous syndrome), full gene sequence

MAP2K2 (mitogen-activated protein kinase 2) (eg, cardiofaciocutaneous syndrome), full gene sequence

MAPT (microtubule-associated protein tau) (eg, frontotemporal dementia), full gene sequence

MCCC1 (methylcrotonoyl-CoA carboxylase 1 [alpha]) (eg, 3-methylcrotonyl-CoA carboxylase deficiency), full gene sequence

MCCC2 (methylcrotonoyl-CoA carboxylase 2 [beta]) (eg, 3-methylcrotonyl carboxylase deficiency), full gene sequence

MFN2 (mitofusin 2) (eg, Charcot-Marie-Tooth disease), full gene sequence

MTM1 (myotubularin 1) (eg, X-linked centronuclear myopathy), full gene sequence

MUT (methylmalonyl CoA mutase) (eg, methylmalonic acidemia), full gene sequence

MUTYH (mutY homolog [E. coli]) (eg, MYH-associated polyposis), full gene sequence

NDUFS1 (NADH dehydrogenase [ubiquinone] Fe-S protein 1, 75kDa [NADH-coenzyme Q reductase]) (eg, Leigh syndrome, mitochondrial complex I deficiency), full gene sequence

NF2 (neurofibromin 2 [merlin]) (eg, neurofibromatosis, type 2), full gene sequence

NOTCH3 (notch 3) (eg, cerebral autosomal dominant arteriopathy with subcortical infarcts and leukoencephalopathy [CADASIL]), targeted sequence analysis (eg, exons 1-23)

NPC1 (Niemann-Pick disease, type C1) (eg, Niemann-Pick disease), full gene sequence

NPHP1 (nephronophthisis 1 [juvenile]) (eg, Joubert syndrome), full gene sequence

NSD1 (nuclear receptor binding SET domain protein 1) (eg, Sotos syndrome), full gene sequence

OPA1 (optic atrophy 1) (eg, optic atrophy), duplication/deletion analysis

OPTN (optineurin) (eg, amyotrophic lateral sclerosis), full gene sequence

PAFAH1B1 (platelet-activating factor acetylhydrolase 1b, regulatory subunit 1 [45kDa]) (eg, lissencephaly, Miller-Dieker syndrome), full gene sequence

PAH (phenylalanine hydroxylase) (eg, phenylketonuria), full gene sequence

PARK2 (Parkinson protein 2, E3 ubiquitin protein ligase [parkin]) (eg, Parkinson disease), full gene sequence

PAX2 (paired box 2) (eg, renal coloboma syndrome), full gene sequence

PC (pyruvate carboxylase) (eg, pyruvate carboxylase deficiency), full gene sequence

PCCA (propionyl CoA carboxylase, alpha polypeptide) (eg, propionic acidemia, type 1), full gene sequence

PCCB (propionyl CoA carboxylase, beta polypeptide) (eg, propionic acidemia), full gene sequence

PCDH15 (protocadherin-related 15) (eg, Usher syndrome type 1F), duplication/deletion analysis

Pathology and Laboratory 80047-89398, 0001U-0419U

PCSK9 (proprotein convertase subtilisin/kexin type 9) (eg, familial hypercholesterolemia), full gene sequence

PDHA1 (pyruvate dehydrogenase [lipoamide] alpha 1) (eg, lactic acidosis), full gene sequence

PDHX (pyruvate dehydrogenase complex, component X) (eg, lactic acidosis), full gene sequence

PHEX (phosphate-regulating endopeptidase homolog, X-linked) (eg, hypophosphatemic rickets), full gene sequence

PKD2 (polycystic kidney disease 2 [autosomal dominant]) (eg, polycystic kidney disease), full gene sequence

PKP2 (plakophilin 2) (eg, arrhythmogenic right ventricular dysplasia/cardiomyopathy 9), full gene sequence

PNKD (paroxysmal nonkinesigenic dyskinesia) (eg, paroxysmal nonkinesigenic dyskinesia), full gene sequence

POLG (polymerase [DNA directed], gamma) (eg, Alpers-Huttenlocher syndrome, autosomal dominant progressive external ophthalmoplegia), full gene sequence

POMGNT1 (protein O-linked mannose beta1,2-N acetylglucosaminyltransferase) (eg, muscle-eye-brain disease, Walker-Warburg syndrome), full gene sequence

POMT1 (protein-O-mannosyltransferase 1) (eg, limb-girdle muscular dystrophy [LGMD] type 2K, Walker-Warburg syndrome), full gene sequence

POMT2 (protein-O-mannosyltransferase 2) (eg, limb-girdle muscular dystrophy [LGMD] type 2N, Walker-Warburg syndrome), full gene sequence

PPOX (protoporphyrinogen oxidase) (eg, variegate porphyria), full gene sequence

PRKAG2 (protein kinase, AMP-activated, gamma 2 non-catalytic subunit) (eg, familial hypertrophic cardiomyopathy with Wolff-Parkinson-White syndrome, lethal congenital glycogen storage disease of heart), full gene sequence

PRKCG (protein kinase C, gamma) (eg, spinocerebellar ataxia), full gene sequence

PSEN2 (presenilin 2 [Alzheimer disease 4]) (eg, Alzheimer disease), full gene sequence

PTPN11 (protein tyrosine phosphatase, non-receptor type 11) (eg, Noonan syndrome, LEOPARD syndrome), full gene sequence

PYGM (phosphorylase, glycogen, muscle) (eg, glycogen storage disease type V, McArdle disease), full gene sequence

RAF1 (v-raf-1 murine leukemia viral oncogene homolog 1) (eg, LEOPARD syndrome), full gene sequence

RET (ret proto-oncogene) (eg, Hirschsprung disease), full gene sequence

RPE65 (retinal pigment epithelium-specific protein 65kDa) (eg, retinitis pigmentosa, Leber congenital amaurosis), full gene sequence

RYR1 (ryanodine receptor 1, skeletal) (eg, malignant hyperthermia), targeted sequence analysis of exons with functionally-confirmed mutations

SCN4A (sodium channel, voltage-gated, type IV, alpha subunit) (eg, hyperkalemic periodic paralysis), full gene sequence

SCNN1A (sodium channel, nonvoltage-gated 1 alpha) (eg, pseudohypoaldosteronism), full gene sequence

SCNN1B (sodium channel, nonvoltage-gated 1, beta) (eg, Liddle syndrome, pseudohypoaldosteronism), full gene sequence

SCNN1G (sodium channel, nonvoltage-gated 1, gamma) (eg, Liddle syndrome, pseudohypoaldosteronism), full gene sequence

SDHA (succinate dehydrogenase complex, subunit A, flavoprotein [Fp]) (eg, Leigh syndrome, mitochondrial complex II deficiency), full gene sequence

SETX (senataxin) (eg, ataxia), full gene sequence

SGCE (sarcoglycan, epsilon) (eg, myoclonic dystonia), full gene sequence

SH3TC2 (SH3 domain and tetratricopeptide repeats 2) (eg, Charcot-Marie-Tooth disease), full gene sequence

SLC9A6 (solute carrier family 9 [sodium/hydrogen exchanger], member 6) (eg, Christianson syndrome), full gene sequence

SLC26A4 (solute carrier family 26, member 4) (eg, Pendred syndrome), full gene sequence

SLC37A4 (solute carrier family 37 [glucose-6-phosphate transporter], member 4) (eg, glycogen storage disease type Ib), full gene sequence

SMAD4 (SMAD family member 4) (eg, hemorrhagic telangiectasia syndrome, juvenile polyposis), full gene sequence

SOS1 (son of sevenless homolog 1) (eg, Noonan syndrome, gingival fibromatosis), full gene sequence

SPAST (spastin) (eg, spastic paraplegia), full gene sequence

SPG7 (spastic paraplegia 7 [pure and complicated autosomal recessive]) (eg, spastic paraplegia), full gene sequence

STXBP1 (syntaxin-binding protein 1) (eg, epileptic encephalopathy), full gene sequence

TAZ (tafazzin) (eg, methylglutaconic aciduria type 2, Barth syndrome), full gene sequence

TCF4 (transcription factor 4) (eg, Pitt-Hopkins syndrome), full gene sequence

★ = Telemedicine ◀ = Audio-only ✛ = Add-on code ⚡ = FDA approval pending # = Resequenced code ⃠ = Modifier 51 exempt

TH (tyrosine hydroxylase) (eg, Segawa syndrome), full gene sequence

TMEM43 (transmembrane protein 43) (eg, arrhythmogenic right ventricular cardiomyopathy), full gene sequence

TNNT2 (troponin T, type 2 [cardiac]) (eg, familial hypertrophic cardiomyopathy), full gene sequence

TRPC6 (transient receptor potential cation channel, subfamily C, member 6) (eg, focal segmental glomerulosclerosis), full gene sequence

TSC1 (tuberous sclerosis 1) (eg, tuberous sclerosis), full gene sequence

TSC2 (tuberous sclerosis 2) (eg, tuberous sclerosis), duplication/deletion analysis

UBE3A (ubiquitin protein ligase E3A) (eg, Angelman syndrome), full gene sequence

UMOD (uromodulin) (eg, glomerulocystic kidney disease with hyperuricemia and isosthenuria), full gene sequence

VWF (von Willebrand factor) (von Willebrand disease type 2A), extended targeted sequence analysis (eg, exons 11-16, 24-26, 51, 52)

WAS (Wiskott-Aldrich syndrome [eczema-thrombocytopenia]) (eg, Wiskott-Aldrich syndrome), full gene sequence

▲ **81407**   Molecular pathology procedure, Level 8 (eg, analysis of 26-50 exons by DNA sequence analysis, mutation scanning or duplication/deletion variants of >50 exons, sequence analysis of multiple genes on one platform)

ABCC8 (ATP-binding cassette, sub-family C [CFTR/MRP], member 8) (eg, familial hyperinsulinism), full gene sequence

AGL (amylo-alpha-1, 6-glucosidase, 4-alpha-glucanotransferase) (eg, glycogen storage disease type III), full gene sequence

AHI1 (Abelson helper integration site 1) (eg, Joubert syndrome), full gene sequence

APOB (apolipoprotein B) (eg, familial hypercholesterolemia type B) full gene sequence

ASPM (asp [abnormal spindle] homolog, microcephaly associated [Drosophila]) (eg, primary microcephaly), full gene sequence

CHD7 (chromodomain helicase DNA binding protein 7) (eg, CHARGE syndrome), full gene sequence

COL4A4 (collagen, type IV, alpha 4) (eg, Alport syndrome), full gene sequence

COL4A5 (collagen, type IV, alpha 5) (eg, Alport syndrome), duplication/deletion analysis

COL6A1 (collagen, type VI, alpha 1) (eg, collagen type VI-related disorders), full gene sequence

COL6A2 (collagen, type VI, alpha 2) (eg, collagen type VI-related disorders), full gene sequence

COL6A3 (collagen, type VI, alpha 3) (eg, collagen type VI-related disorders), full gene sequence

CREBBP (CREB binding protein) (eg, Rubinstein-Taybi syndrome), full gene sequence

F8 (coagulation factor VIII) (eg, hemophilia A), full gene sequence

JAG1 (jagged 1) (eg, Alagille syndrome), full gene sequence

KDM5C (lysine demethylase 5C) (eg, X-linked intellectual disability), full gene sequence

KIAA0196 (KIAA0196) (eg, spastic paraplegia), full gene sequence

L1CAM (L1 cell adhesion molecule) (eg, MASA syndrome, X-linked hydrocephaly), full gene sequence

LAMB2 (laminin, beta 2 [laminin S]) (eg, Pierson syndrome), full gene sequence

MYBPC3 (myosin binding protein C, cardiac) (eg, familial hypertrophic cardiomyopathy), full gene sequence

MYH6 (myosin, heavy chain 6, cardiac muscle, alpha) (eg, familial dilated cardiomyopathy), full gene sequence

MYH7 (myosin, heavy chain 7, cardiac muscle, beta) (eg, familial hypertrophic cardiomyopathy, Liang distal myopathy), full gene sequence

MYO7A (myosin VIIA) (eg, Usher syndrome, type 1), full gene sequence

NOTCH1 (notch 1) (eg, aortic valve disease), full gene sequence

NPHS1 (nephrosis 1, congenital, Finnish type [nephrin]) (eg, congenital Finnish nephrosis), full gene sequence

OPA1 (optic atrophy 1) (eg, optic atrophy), full gene sequence

PCDH15 (protocadherin-related 15) (eg, Usher syndrome, type 1), full gene sequence

PKD1 (polycystic kidney disease 1 [autosomal dominant]) (eg, polycystic kidney disease), full gene sequence

PLCE1 (phospholipase C, epsilon 1) (eg, nephrotic syndrome type 3), full gene sequence

SCN1A (sodium channel, voltage-gated, type 1, alpha subunit) (eg, generalized epilepsy with febrile seizures), full gene sequence

SCN5A (sodium channel, voltage-gated, type V, alpha subunit) (eg, familial dilated cardiomyopathy), full gene sequence

SLC12A1 (solute carrier family 12 [sodium/potassium/chloride transporters], member 1) (eg, Bartter syndrome), full gene sequence

Pathology and Laboratory 80047-89398, 0001U-0419U

SLC12A3 (solute carrier family 12 [sodium/chloride transporters], member 3) (eg, Gitelman syndrome), full gene sequence

SPG11 (spastic paraplegia 11 [autosomal recessive]) (eg, spastic paraplegia), full gene sequence

SPTBN2 (spectrin, beta, non-erythrocytic 2) (eg, spinocerebellar ataxia), full gene sequence

TMEM67 (transmembrane protein 67) (eg, Joubert syndrome), full gene sequence

TSC2 (tuberous sclerosis 2) (eg, tuberous sclerosis), full gene sequence

USH1C (Usher syndrome 1C [autosomal recessive, severe]) (eg, Usher syndrome, type 1), full gene sequence

VPS13B (vacuolar protein sorting 13 homolog B [yeast]) (eg, Cohen syndrome), duplication/deletion analysis

WDR62 (WD repeat domain 62) (eg, primary autosomal recessive microcephaly), full gene sequence

Rationale

Codes 81403-81407 have been revised by replacing "mental retardation" with updated terminology.

In 2010, the 111th US Congress passed Rosa's Law, which is a bill to change references of "mental retardation" in federal law to "intellectual disability(ies)." Tier 2 codes list the full gene names approved by HUGO. The full names of the ARX, FTSJ1, KDM5C, and ZNF41 genes and/or their associated proteins or diseases included "mental retardation." In accordance with Rosa's Law, HUGO has updated the full names of these genes and removed the term "mental retardation." Codes 81403-81407 have been revised to reflect this terminology change.

Genomic Sequencing Procedures and Other Molecular Multianalyte Assays

►Genomic sequencing procedures (GSPs) and other molecular multianalyte assays are DNA and/or RNA sequence analysis methods that simultaneously assay multiple genes or genetic regions relevant to a clinical situation. They may target specific combinations of genes or genetic material, or they may assay the exome or genome. The technology typically used for genomic sequencing is massively parallel sequencing (MPS) (eg, next-generation sequencing [NGS]) although other technologies may be employed. GSPs are performed on nucleic acids from germline or neoplastic samples. Examples of applications include aneuploidy analysis of cell-free circulating fetal DNA, gene panels for somatic alterations in neoplasms, and sequence analysis of the exome or genome to determine the cause of developmental delay. Exome and genome procedures are designed to evaluate the genetic material in totality or near totality. Although commonly used to identify sequence (base) changes, they can also be used to identify copy number, structural changes, and abnormal zygosity patterns, and these analyses may be performed in combination or as separate and distinct studies. Another unique feature of GSPs is the ability to "re-query" or re-evaluate the sequence data (eg, complex phenotype such as developmental delay is reassessed when new genetic knowledge is attained, or for a separate unrelated clinical indication). The analyses below are often performed using NGS/MPS technology; however, they may also be performed using molecular techniques (eg, polymerase chain reaction [PCR] methods and microarrays). These codes should be used when the components of the descriptor(s) are fulfilled regardless of the technique used for analysis, unless specifically noted in the code descriptor. When a GSP assay includes gene(s) that is listed in more than one code descriptor, the code for the most specific test for the primary disorder sought should be reported, rather than reporting multiple codes for the same gene(s). When all of the components of the descriptor are not performed, use individual Tier 1 codes, Tier 2 codes, or 81479 (Unlisted molecular pathology procedure).

Testing for somatic alterations in neoplasms may be reported differently depending on whether combined or separate methods and analyses are used for both DNA and RNA analytes. Procedures for somatic alterations in neoplasms which include DNA analysis or DNA and RNA analysis using a single combined method are reported with 81445, 81450, 81455, 81457, 81458, 81459, 81462, 81463, 81464. RNA analysis performed using a separate method is reported with 81449, 81451, 81456. When evaluation for tumor mutation burden (TMB) and/or microsatellite instability (MSI) is performed as part of the same test for somatic alterations in neoplasms, report 81458, 81459. When a genomic sequencing procedure (GSP) is performed on cell-free nucleic acid (eg, plasma), sometimes referred to as a liquid biopsy, report 81462, 81463, 81464.◄

►Definitions◄

►**Cell-free nucleic acid:** DNA or RNA released into the blood and other body fluids. Cell-free nucleic acid released from fetal cells can be sampled for non-invasive prenatal testing (NIPT) while that released from tumor cells can be sampled for cancer, sometimes referred to as tumor liquid biopsy.

Copy number variants (CNVs): structural changes in the genome which are composed of large deletions or

★ = Telemedicine   ◀ = Audio-only   ✛ = Add-on code   ✗ = FDA approval pending   # = Resequenced code   ⊘ = Modifier 51 exempt

duplications. CNVs can be found in the germline but can also occur in somatic cells. See also Duplication/Deletion (Dup/Del). Duplications may also be referred to as amplifications.

Duplication/Deletion (Dup/Del): terms that are usually used together with the "/" to refer to molecular testing, which assesses the dosage of a particular genomic region. The region tested is typically of modest to substantial size, from several dozen to several million or more nucleotides. Normal gene dosage is two copies per cell, except for the sex chromosomes (X and Y). Thus, zero or one copy represents a deletion and three (or more) copies represent a duplication.◄

Low-pass sequencing: a method of genome sequencing intended for cytogenomic analysis of chromosomal abnormalities, such as that performed for trait mapping or copy number variation, typically performed to an average depth of sequencing ranging from 0.1 to 5X.

►*Massively parallel sequencing (MPS):* high-throughput method used to determine a portion of the nucleotide sequences in an individual patient's genome, utilizing advanced (non-Sanger) sequencing technologies that are capable of processing multiple DNA and/or RNA sequences in parallel. While other technologies exist, next-generation sequencing (NGS) is a common technique used to achieve MPS.

Microsatellite instability (MSI): a type of DNA hypermutation or predisposition to mutation in which replication errors are not corrected due to defective DNA mismatch repair (dMMR) mechanism. MSI manifests as insertions or deletions in short tandem repeat (STR) (defined in the molecular pathology guidelines) alleles and can be identified by changes in the DNA repeat sequence length.

Rearrangements: structural chromosomal variations such as deletions, insertions, inversions (defined in the molecular pathology guidelines), or translocations (defined in the molecular pathology guidelines) that bring together genetic material that is not normally adjacent in the unmodified genome. It can manifest as abnormal gene expression or as an abnormal fusion product at the RNA and/or protein level. Rearrangement can also refer to the process by which immunoglobulin and T cell receptor genes are normally modified.

Tumor mutational burden (TMB): the number of somatic mutations detected per million bases (Mb) of genomic sequence investigated from a cancer specimen. It is usually obtained from analysis using a next generation sequencing method. It is considered a biomarker to guide immunotherapy decisions for patients with cancer.

►Code	Specimen Source			Nucleic Acid	Sequence Variants	Copy Number Variants	Microsatellite Instability	Tumor Mutation Burden	Rearrangements
	Solid Organ	Hematolymphoid	Cell-Free						
81445	X		No	DNA or DNA/RNA	X	X			X
81449	X		No	RNA	X				X
81450		X	No	DNA or DNA/RNA	X	X			X
81451		X	No	RNA	X				X
81455	X	X	No	DNA or DNA/RNA	X	X			X
81456	X	X	No	RNA	X				X
81457	X		No	DNA	X		X		
81458	X		No	DNA	X	X	X		
81459	X		No	DNA or DNA/RNA	X	X	X	X	X
81462	X		Yes	DNA or DNA/RNA	X	X			X
81463	X		Yes	DNA	X	X	X		
81464	X		Yes	DNA or DNA/RNA	X	X	X	X	X◄

The assays in this section represent discrete genetic values, properties, or characteristics in which the measurement or analysis of each analyte is potentially of independent medical significance or useful in medical management. In contrast to multianalyte assays with algorithmic analyses (MAAAs), the assays in this section do not represent algorithmically combined results to obtain a risk score or other value, which in itself represents a new and distinct medical property that is of independent medical significance relative to the individual, component test results.

(For cytogenomic [genome-wide] analysis for constitutional chromosomal abnormalities, see 81228, 81229, 81349, 81405, 81406)

▲ 81445   Solid organ neoplasm, genomic sequence analysis panel, 5-50 genes, interrogation for sequence variants and copy number variants or rearrangements, if performed; DNA analysis or combined DNA and RNA analysis

▲ 81449   RNA analysis

►(For copy number assessment by microarray, use 81277)◄

▲ 81450   Hematolymphoid neoplasm or disorder, genomic sequence analysis panel, 5-50 genes, interrogation for sequence variants, and copy number variants or rearrangements, or isoform expression or mRNA expression levels, if performed; DNA analysis or combined DNA and RNA analysis

▲ 81451   RNA analysis

(For copy number assessment by microarray, use 81406)

▲ 81455   Solid organ or hematolymphoid neoplasm or disorder, 51 or greater genes, genomic sequence analysis panel, interrogation for sequence variants and copy number variants or rearrangements, or isoform expression or mRNA expression levels, if performed; DNA analysis or combined DNA and RNA analysis

▲ 81456   RNA analysis

(For copy number assessment by microarray, use 81406)

►(For genomic sequence DNA analysis and RNA analysis performed separately rather than via a combined method, report 81445, 81450, 81455, 81457, 81458, 81459 for the DNA analysis and report 81449, 81451, 81456 for the RNA analysis)◄

►(For genomic sequence RNA analysis using a separate method, see 81449, 81451, 81456)◄

● 81457   Solid organ neoplasm, genomic sequence analysis panel, interrogation for sequence variants; DNA analysis, microsatellite instability

● 81458   DNA analysis, copy number variants and microsatellite instability

● 81459   DNA analysis or combined DNA and RNA analysis, copy number variants, microsatellite instability, tumor mutation burden, and rearrangements

►(For solid organ genomic sequence DNA analysis or combined DNA and RNA analysis from cell-free nucleic acid, see 81462, 81463, 81464)◄

#● 81462   Solid organ neoplasm, genomic sequence analysis panel, cell-free nucleic acid (eg, plasma), interrogation for sequence variants; DNA analysis or combined DNA and RNA analysis, copy number variants and rearrangements

#● 81463   DNA analysis, copy number variants, and microsatellite instability

#● 81464   DNA analysis or combined DNA and RNA analysis, copy number variants, microsatellite instability, tumor mutation burden, and rearrangements

81462   Code is out of numerical sequence. See 81458-81465

81463   Code is out of numerical sequence. See 81458-81465

81464   Code is out of numerical sequence. See 81458-81465

Rationale

Changes have been made to solid tumor genomic sequence analysis procedure codes in the Genomic Sequencing Procedures and Other Molecular Multianalyte Assays subsection. Codes 81445, 81449, 81450, 81451, 81455, and 81456 have been editorially revised. Six new codes (81457-81459, 81462-81464) have been established. The Genomic Sequencing Procedures and Other Molecular Multianalyte Assays guidelines have been revised. Parenthetical notes have been added and/or revised.

Since codes 81445, 81450, and 81455 were established in 2015, advances in genomic sequencing technology and analysis have become part of the current clinical practice. Examples of these advances are testing for microsatellite instability (MSI) and tumor mutational burden (TMB) in the treatment of cancer. Codes 81457-81459 and 81462-81464 have been established to reflect these advancements in genomic sequence analysis of solid organ neoplasms. Codes 81457-81459 are reported for analysis of tissue and codes 81462-81464 for analysis of cell-free nucleic acid such as plasma. Analysis that is performed on cell-free nucleic acid is also known as a liquid biopsy. In these two code families, all the codes include interrogation for sequence variants. The codes are structured based on the additional technologies used for analysis, which are listed in the following table:

★ = Telemedicine   ◄ = Audio-only   ✚ = Add-on code   ⊮ = FDA approval pending   # = Resequenced code   ⊘ = Modifier 51 exempt

Pathology and Laboratory 80047-89398, 0001U-0419U

Specimen: Tumor Tissue		Specimen: Cell-free Nucleic Acid	
81457	■ Interrogation for sequence variants ■ DNA analysis ■ MSI	81462	■ Interrogation for sequence variants ■ DNA analysis or combined DNA and RNA analysis ■ Copy number variants ■ Rearrangements
81458	■ Interrogation for sequence variants ■ DNA analysis ■ Copy number variants ■ MSI	81463	■ Interrogation for sequence variants ■ DNA analysis ■ Copy number variants ■ MSI
81459	■ Interrogation for sequence variants ■ DNA analysis or combined DNA and RNA analysis ■ Copy number variants ■ MSI ■ TMB ■ Rearrangements	81464	■ Interrogation for sequence variants ■ DNA analysis or combined DNA and RNA analysis ■ Copy number variants ■ MSI ■ TMB ■ Rearrangements

Codes 81445, 81449, 81450, 81451, 81455, and 81456 have been editorially revised to be consistent with the format of codes 81457-81459 and 81462-81464. The Genomic Sequencing Procedures and Other Molecular Multianalyte Assays guidelines have been revised to include appropriate reporting of codes 81457-81459 and 81462-81464. Definitions have been added to the guidelines for cell-free nucleic acid, copy number variants, duplication/deletion, massively parallel sequencing, MSI, rearrangements, and TMB. A table listing the appropriate code based on the specimen analyzed and the types of analyses performed has been added to the guidelines. Parenthetical notes have been added and/or revised throughout the section to provide instruction on the appropriate reporting of codes 81445, 81449, 81450, 81451, 81455, 81456, 81457-81459, and 81462-81464.

Clinical Example (81445)

A 50-year-old female presents with a thyroid nodule. Fine-needle aspiration is performed and sent for evaluation. Initial pathology review showed a follicular lesion of indeterminate diagnosis. Residual tissue is submitted for targeted genomic DNA sequence analysis of a panel of 12 genes known to be important in thyroid cancer.

Description of Procedure (81445)

Isolate high-quality DNA from the patient's tumor tissue and perform massively parallel sequencing on the tumor DNA, looking for mutations in 12 genes. Send the analytical results to a pathologist or other QHP for identification of mutations, interpretation, and preparation of a written report that specifies the patient's mutation status, which may contain information about diagnosis, prognosis, and patient management, to include information about targeted drug therapy.

Clinical Example (81449)

A 52-year-old female presents with a lung nodule. Needle biopsy is performed and sent for evaluation. Initial pathology shows a non-small cell malignancy. Residual tissue is submitted for a targeted genomic RNA sequence panel of 19 genes with common gene rearrangements and sequence variants known to be important in lung cancer.

Description of Procedure (81449)

Isolate high-quality RNA from the patient's tumor tissue and perform massively parallel sequencing on the tumor RNA, looking for mutations in 19 genes. Send the analytical results to a pathologist or other QHP for identification of mutations, interpretation, and preparation of a written report that specifies the patient's mutation status, which may contain information about diagnosis, prognosis, and patient management, to include information about targeted drug therapy.

Clinical Example (81450)

A 55-year-old male presents with an elevated white blood cell (WBC) count with 80% blasts, anemia, and thrombocytopenia. The pathologic diagnosis was acute myeloid leukemia (AML). Cytogenetic studies were normal, stratifying the patient as intermediate risk for survival. Blood is submitted for targeted genomic sequence analysis of a panel of 25 genes known to be informative in patients with AML.

Description of Procedure (81450)

Isolate high-quality DNA from the patient's blood and perform massively parallel sequencing on the DNA, looking for mutations in 25 genes. Send the analytical results to a pathologist or other QHP for identification of mutations, interpretation, and preparation of a written report that specifies the patient's mutation status, which may contain information about diagnosis, prognosis, and patient management, to include information about targeted drug therapy.

Pathology and Laboratory   80047-89398, 0001U-0419U

Clinical Example (81451)

A 45-year-old female presents with an elevated WBC count with 85% blasts, anemia, and thrombocytopenia. The pathologic diagnosis was AML. Cytogenetic studies were normal. Blood is submitted for a targeted genomic RNA sequence panel of 32 genes with recurrent gene rearrangements known to be important in patients with AML.

Description of Procedure (81451)

Isolate high-quality RNA from the patient's tumor tissue and perform massively parallel sequencing on the tumor RNA, looking for mutations in 32 genes. Send the analytical results to a pathologist or other QHP for identification of mutations, interpretation, and preparation of a written report that specifies the patient's mutation status, which may contain information about diagnosis, prognosis, and patient management, to include information about targeted drug therapy.

Clinical Example (81455)

A 65-year-old male presents with lung and liver lesions. Pathologic evaluation of biopsies of these lesions reveals a poorly differentiated neoplasm of uncertain primary origin. Tumor tissue is submitted for a targeted genomic sequence analysis of a panel of 250 genes known to be informative in a broad array of cancers.

Description of Procedure (81455)

Isolate high-quality DNA from the patient's tumor tissue and perform massively parallel sequencing on the tumor DNA, looking for mutations in 250 genes, which may be genomic targets for therapeutic management. Send the analytical results to a pathologist or other QHP for identification of mutations, interpretation, and preparation of a written report that specifies the patient's mutation status, which may contain information about diagnosis, prognosis, and patient management, to include information about targeted drug therapy.

Clinical Example (81456)

A 57-year-old male presents with colon and liver lesions. Pathologic evaluation of biopsies of these lesions reveals a poorly differentiated neoplasm of uncertain primary origin. Tumor tissue is submitted for a targeted genomic RNA sequence analysis of a panel of 70 genes with recurrent sequence variants and gene rearrangements known to be informative in a broad array of cancers.

Description of Procedure (81456)

Isolate high-quality RNA from the patient's tumor tissue and perform massively parallel sequencing on the tumor RNA, looking for mutations in 70 genes. Send the

analytical results to a pathologist or other QHP for identification of mutations, interpretation, and preparation of a written report that specifies the patient's mutation status, which may contain information about diagnosis, prognosis, and patient management, to include information about targeted drug therapy.

Clinical Example (81457)

A 40-year-old female with lung adenocarcinoma undergoes a tumor biopsy. The tissue is submitted for genetic profiling to predict response to targeted therapies and for prognosis. A tissue block is submitted for cancer-mutation testing.

Description of Procedure (81457)

Isolate high-quality genomic DNA and RNA from the tissue specimen and subject to next-generation sequencing (NGS). The pathologist or other QHP evaluates the sequencing results and composes a report. The report is edited and signed, and the results are communicated to the appropriate caregiver.

Clinical Example (81458)

A 65-year-old male with melanoma has a tumor removed and submitted for genetic profiling to predict response to targeted therapies and for prognosis. A tissue block is submitted for cancer-mutation testing.

Description of Procedure (81458)

Isolate high-quality genomic DNA and RNA from the tissue specimen and subject to NGS. The pathologist or other QHP evaluates the sequencing results and composes a report. The report is edited and signed, and the results are communicated to the appropriate caregiver.

Clinical Example (81459)

A 52-year-old female with non-small cell lung carcinoma has a tumor removed and submitted for genetic profiling to predict response to immunotherapies and targeted therapies and for prognosis. A tissue block is submitted for cancer-mutation testing.

Description of Procedure (81459)

Submit a tissue block for cancer mutation testing using NGS. Sequence variants, copy number variants, microsatellite instability, tumor-mutation burden (TMB), and rearrangements are assessed and reported by a QHP.

★ = Telemedicine   ◀ = Audio-only   ✚ = Add-on code   ✒ = FDA approval pending   # = Resequenced code   ⊘ = Modifier 51 exempt

Clinical Example (81462)

A 52-year-old male with non-small cell lung carcinoma has a blood specimen submitted for genetic profiling to predict response to immunotherapies and targeted therapies and for prognosis. A blood specimen is submitted for cancer cell-free nucleic acid–mutation testing.

Description of Procedure (81462)

Submit a blood specimen for cancer-mutation testing. Sequence variants, copy number variants, or rearrangements are assessed and reported by a QHP.

Clinical Example (81463)

A 54-year-old female with a diagnosis of breast cancer, treated, presents with metastatic disease. A fine-needle aspiration sample is taken from one of her bone lesions. The sample was small and contained just enough cells to make the diagnosis. A plasma sample was taken for a liquid biopsy (plasma sample for circulating tumor DNA).

Description of Procedure (81463)

Submit a blood specimen for cancer-mutation testing. Sequence variants, copy number variants, microsatellite instability, and rearrangements are assessed and reported by a QHP.

Clinical Example (81464)

A 65-year-old female with stage IV lung adenocarcinoma had a blood sample submitted to examine the patient's tumor genomic composition, including tumor-mutation burden and microsatellite instability.

Description of Procedure (81464)

Submit a blood specimen for cancer-mutation testing. Sequence variants, copy number variants, microsatellite instability, TMB and rearrangements are assessed and reported by a QHP.

Multianalyte Assays with Algorithmic Analyses

 # 81596   Infectious disease, chronic hepatitis C virus (HCV) infection, six biochemical assays (ALT, A2-macroglobulin, apolipoprotein A-1, total bilirubin, GGT, and haptoglobin) utilizing serum, prognostic algorithm reported as scores for fibrosis and necroinflammatory activity in liver

● 81517   Liver disease, analysis of 3 biomarkers (hyaluronic acid [HA], procollagen III amino terminal peptide [PIIINP], tissue inhibitor of metalloproteinase 1 [TIMP-1]), using immunoassays, utilizing serum, prognostic algorithm reported as a risk score and risk of liver fibrosis and liver-related clinical events within 5 years

▶(Do not report 81517 in conjunction with 83520 for identification of biomarkers included for liver disease analysis)◀

Rationale

Category III code 0014M has been deleted and code 81517 has been established to report liver disease analysis of three biomarkers for the risk assessment of liver disease progression and other liver-related events in patients with advanced fibrosis due to nonalcoholic steatohepatitis. Parenthetical notes have been added and/or revised within the Multianalyte Assays with Algorithmic Analysis (MAAAs), Chemistry, and the Administrative MAAAs subsections to accommodate the code conversion.

Code 81517 is used to report an assay that uses individual biomarkers that reflect integral extracellular matrix (ECM) components of dynamic fibrogenesis and fibrolysis processes in real time. Assessment of the active, dynamic fibrosis may be used as a prognostic marker to determine if patients with advanced fibrosis are at risk of experiencing disease progression to other liver disease states (eg, cirrhosis). The code descriptor includes the specific biomarkers assessed for the assay and notes the specimen source.

An exclusionary parenthetical note following code 81517 restricts reporting of the new code in conjunction with the more generic quantitative immunoassay for detection of analytes that are neither infectious agent antigens nor antibodies (ie, 83520) because this code identifies the specific analytes being assayed. Additional instruction added after code 83520 and following the deletion of parenthetical note for code 0014M similarly redirects users to the appropriate code to report MAAA for liver disease using analysis of three biomarkers (81517).

Clinical Example (81517)

A 45-year-old overweight male with 6 months of elevated liver function tests that are negative for hepatitis C virus infection is being evaluated for non-alcoholic fatty liver disease. Hyperechoic findings are present on recent ultrasound. Biochemical testing at 3.53 indicates advanced fibrosis.

Description of Procedure (81517)

Perform quantitative measurements of hyaluronic acid, amino-terminal propeptide of type III procollagen, and tissue inhibitor of metalloproteinase 1 on the serum sample. Analyze the quantitative results using a proprietary algorithm to arrive at a prognostic numerical risk score for cirrhosis and liver-related events.

81518   Oncology (breast), mRNA, gene expression profiling by real-time RT-PCR of 11 genes (7 content and 4 housekeeping), utilizing formalin-fixed paraffin-embedded tissue, algorithms reported as percentage risk for metastatic recurrence and likelihood of benefit from extended endocrine therapy

Chemistry

The material for examination may be from any source unless otherwise specified in the code descriptor. When an analyte is measured in multiple specimens from different sources, or in specimens that are obtained at different times, the analyte is reported separately for each source and for each specimen. The examination is quantitative unless specified. To report an organ or disease oriented panel, see codes 80048-80076.

Clinical information or mathematically calculated values, which are not specifically requested by the ordering physician and are derived from the results of other ordered or performed laboratory tests, are considered part of the ordered test procedure(s) and therefore are not separately reportable service(s).

When the requested analyte result is derived using a calculation that requires values from nonrequested laboratory analyses, only the requested analyte code should be reported.

When the calculated analyte determination requires values derived from other requested and nonrequested laboratory analyses, the requested analyte codes (including those calculated) should be reported.

An exception to the above is when an analyte (eg, urinary creatinine) is performed to compensate for variations in urine concentration (eg, microalbumin, thromboxane metabolites) in random urine samples; the appropriate CPT code is reported for both the ordered analyte and the additional required analyte. When the calculated result(s) represent an algorithmically derived numeric score or probability, see the appropriate multianalyte assay with algorithmic analyses (MAAA) code or the MAAA unlisted code (81599).

▶Analytes that are not specified by either an analyte-specific or method-specific code in the Chemistry (82009-84830) subsection may be reported using the unlisted chemistry procedure code 84999.◀

Pathology and Laboratory 80047-89398, 0001U-0419U

Rationale

In support of the changes regarding unlisted procedures and services, a new introductory guideline has been added in the Chemistry subsection to provide instruction on how to report analytes that are not specified by the use of either an analyte-specific or method-specific code within the Chemistry section (82009-84830). The new guideline instructs that code 84999 may be reported when appropriate.

Refer to the codebook and the Rationale for the Unlisted Procedure or Service subsection of the Introduction section for a full discussion of these changes.

82009   Ketone body(s) (eg, acetone, acetoacetic acid, beta-hydroxybutyrate); qualitative

82010   quantitative

82164   Angiotensin I - converting enzyme (ACE)

     (Antidiuretic hormone (ADH), use 84588)

     (Antimony, use 83015)

     (Antitrypsin, alpha-1-, see 82103, 82104)

● **82166**   Anti-mullerian hormone (AMH)

Rationale

A new Category I code (82166) has been established in the Chemistry subsection to report anti-müllerian hormone (AMH) assay. Prior to 2024, no analyte-specific code exists to describe AMH testing.

The AMH assay provides the quantitative measurement of AMH in serum. Potential clinical applications for the measurement of AMH may include the investigation of the ovarian reserve in fertility clinic patients; the perimenopausal transition in women; the detection and management of granulosa cell tumors; the diagnosis of precocious puberty and, conversely, its delayed onset in the young; the differential diagnosis of intersex disorders; the diagnosis of cryptorchidism and anorchidism; and the evaluation of male gonadal function at all ages.

This new code now provides laboratories performing this test with an analyte-specific code to report, as well as providing specificity and transparency for this test.

Clinical Example (82166)

A 37-year-old female with family history of early menopause presents for fertility workup. Anti-müllerian hormone (AMH) is ordered to assess her reproductive potential.

Description of Procedure (82166)

Test patient serum for AMH by immunoassay. Report results.

82172 Apolipoprotein, each

83516 Immunoassay for analyte other than infectious agent antibody or infectious agent antigen; qualitative or semiquantitative, multiple step method

83518   qualitative or semiquantitative, single step method (eg, reagent strip)

83519   quantitative, by radioimmunoassay (eg, RIA)

83520   quantitative, not otherwise specified

►(For multianalyte assay with algorithmic analysis [MAAA] for liver disease using analysis of 3 biomarkers, use 81517)◄

(Immunoglobulins, see 82784, 82785)

(For immunoassay of tumor antigen not elsewhere specified, use 86316)

(For immunoassays for antibodies to infectious agent antigens, see analyte and method specific codes in the **Immunology** section)

Rationale

A parenthetical note following code 83520 has been added to redirect users to the appropriate code to report MAAA for liver disease using analysis of three biomarkers (81517).

Refer to the codebook and the Rationale for code 81517 for a full discussion of this change.

Hematology and Coagulation

►Hematology and coagulation analytes/procedures that are not specified in 85002-85810 and are not in the Chemistry (82009-84830), Immunology (86015-86835), or Transfusion Medicine (86850-86985) subsections may be reported using the unlisted hematology and coagulation procedure code 85999.◄

Rationale

In support of the changes for unlisted procedures and services, a new introductory guideline has been added in the Hematology and Coagulation subsection to provide instruction on how to report analytes/procedures that are not specified in codes 85002-85810 and codes

82009-84830 (Chemistry), 86015-86835 (Immunology), or 86850-86985 (Transfusion Medicine). The new guideline instructs that code 85999 may be reported when appropriate.

Refer to the codebook and the Rationale for Unlisted Procedure or Service subsection of the Introduction section for a full discussion of these changes.

(For blood banking procedures, see **Transfusion Medicine**)

(Agglutinins, see **Immunology**)

(Antiplasmin, use 85410)

(Antithrombin III, see 85300, 85301)

85002 Bleeding time

85060 Blood smear, peripheral, interpretation by physician with written report

►(Use 0854T in conjunction with 85060, when the digitization of glass microscope slides is performed)◄

Rationale

In support of the establishment of code 0854T, a parenthetical note has been added following code 85060 to refer users to code 0854T when the digitization of glass microscope slides is performed.

Refer to the codebook and the Rationale for code 0854T for a full discussion of these changes.

85097 Bone marrow, smear interpretation

►(Use 0855T in conjunction with 85097, when the digitization of glass microscope slides is performed)◄

(For special stains, see 88312, 88313)

(For bone biopsy, see 20220, 20225, 20240, 20245, 20250, 20251)

Rationale

In support of the establishment of code 0855T, a parenthetical note has been added following code 85097 to refer users to code 0855T when the digitization of glass microscope slides is performed.

Refer to the codebook and the Rationale for code 0855T for a full discussion of these changes.

Immunology

▶Immunology analytes/procedures that are not specified in 86015-86835 and are not in the Chemistry subsection (82009-84830) may be reported using the unlisted immunology procedure code 86849.◄

Rationale

In support of the changes for unlisted procedures and services, a new introductory guideline has been added in the Immunology subsection to provide instruction on how to report analytes/procedures that are not specified in codes 86015-86835 and 82009-84830 in the Chemistry subsection. The new guideline instructs that code 86849 may be reported when appropriate.

Refer to the codebook and the Rationale for the Unlisted Procedure or Service subsection of the Introduction section for a full discussion of these changes.

#●	**86041**	Acetylcholine receptor (AChR); binding antibody
#●	**86042**	blocking antibody
#●	**86043**	modulating antibody
#	**86015**	Actin (smooth muscle) antibody (ASMA), each
		(Actinomyces, antibodies to, use 86602)
		(Adrenal cortex antibodies, see 86255, 86256)
	86003	Allergen specific IgE; quantitative or semiquantitative, crude allergen extract, each
		(For total quantitative IgE, use 82785)
	86005	qualitative, multiallergen screen (eg, disk, sponge, card)
	86008	quantitative or semiquantitative, recombinant or purified component, each
		(For total qualitative IgE, use 83518)
		(Alpha-1 antitrypsin, see 82103, 82104)
		(Alpha-1 feto-protein, see 82105, 82106)
		▶(Anti-AChR [acetylcholine receptor] antibody, see 86041, 86042, 86043)◄
		(Anticardiolipin antibody, use 86147)
		(Anti-DNA, use 86225)
		(Anti-deoxyribonuclease titer, use 86215)

Rationale

Four new Category I codes (86041-86043, 86366) have been added in the Immunology subsection for reporting testing for acetylcholine receptor antibodies (86041-86043) and muscle-specific kinase antibody (86366). In addition, a parenthetical note preceding code 86041 has been deleted, and a parenthetical note following code 86008 has been revised to accommodate the addition of the new codes.

Acetylcholine receptor (AChR) and muscle-specific kinase (MuSK) antibody testing have been reported using non-specific immunoassay (83519) and fluorescent agent antibody screening and titer procedures (86255, 86256). However, advancement in technology has allowed the use of certain specific analytes to test for specific diseases/conditions, such as myasthenia gravis and Lambert-Eaton myasthenic syndrome. As a result, codes 86041-86043 and 86366 have been added to allow specific reporting for these analytes.

Codes 86041-86043 identify AChR testing procedures for binding (86041), blocking (86042), and modulating (86043) antibodies, and code 86366 is used to identify MuSK antibodies. To provide direction for reporting, a parenthetical note following code 86008 has been revised by adding the new codes 86041-86043 for identification of AChR testing and by deleting references to "titer." A parenthetical note preceding code 86041 has also been deleted to accommodate the addition of the codes.

Clinical Example (86041)

A 45-year-old female presents with a drooping eyelid, double vision, difficulty chewing/swallowing, weak neck muscles, and difficulty walking. Acetylcholine receptor–binding antibody test is ordered.

Description of Procedure (86041)

Obtain a serum sample. Perform a quantitative measurement of acetylcholine receptor–binding antibody by a radioimmunoassay method and report the result.

Clinical Example (86042)

A 45-year-old female presents with a drooping eyelid, double vision, difficulty chewing/swallowing, weak neck muscles, and difficulty walking. Acetylcholine receptor–blocking antibody test is ordered.

Description of Procedure (86042)

Obtain a serum sample. Perform a quantitative measurement of acetylcholine receptor–blocking antibody by a radioimmunoassay method and report the result.

Clinical Example (86043)

A 45-year-old female presents with a drooping eyelid, double vision, difficulty chewing/swallowing, weak neck muscles, and difficulty walking. Acetylcholine receptor–modulating antibody test is ordered.

Description of Procedure (86043)

Obtain a serum sample. Perform a quantitative measurement of acetylcholine receptor–modulating antibody by a radioimmunoassay method and report the result.

86041	Code is out of numerical sequence. See 85810-86001
86042	Code is out of numerical sequence. See 85810-86001
86043	Code is out of numerical sequence. See 85810-86001
86300	Immunoassay for tumor antigen, quantitative; CA 15-3 (27.29)
86304	CA 125

(For measurement of serum HER-2/neu oncoprotein, see 83950)

(For hepatitis delta agent, antibody, use 86692)

►(For hepatitis delta agent, antigen, use 87380)◄

►(For hepatitis D [delta], quantification, use 87523)◄

Rationale

Parenthetical cross-reference notes following code 86304 have been added to direct users to the appropriate codes to report hepatitis D (hep D) antigen testing only (87380) and antigen testing with quantification of the viral DNA (87523).

Refer to the codebook and the Rationale for code 87523 for a full discussion of these changes.

86356	Mononuclear cell antigen, quantitative (eg, flow cytometry), not otherwise specified, each antigen

(Do not report 88187-88189 for interpretation of 86355, 86356, 86357, 86359, 86360, 86361, 86367)

#● **86366**	Muscle-specific kinase (MuSK) antibody

Rationale

Code 86366 has been established to identify testing for MuSK antibodies. Refer to the codebook and the Rationale for codes 86041-86043 for a full discussion of these changes.

Clinical Example (86366)

A 45-year-old female presents with a drooping eyelid, double vision, difficulty chewing/swallowing, weak neck muscles, and difficulty walking. A muscle-specific kinase (MuSK) antibody test is ordered.

Description of Procedure (86366)

Obtain a serum sample. Perform a quantitative measurement of MuSK by an immunoassay method and report the result.

# **86362**	Myelin oligodendrocyte glycoprotein (MOG-IgG1) antibody; cell-based immunofluorescence assay (CBA), each
# **86363**	flow cytometry (ie, fluorescence-activated cell sorting [FACS]), each
86362	Code is out of numerical sequence. See 86355-86360
86363	Code is out of numerical sequence. See 86355-86360
86364	Code is out of numerical sequence. See 86355-86360
86366	Code is out of numerical sequence. See 86355-86360
86692	hepatitis, delta agent

(For hepatitis delta agent, antigen, use 87380)

►(For hepatitis D [delta], quantification, use 87523)◄

Rationale

A parenthetical cross-reference note following code 86692 has been added to direct users to the appropriate code to report hep D quantification of viral DNA (87523).

Refer to the codebook and the Rationale for code 87523 for a full discussion of these changes.

Transfusion Medicine

▶Transfusion medicine analytes/procedures that are not specified in 86850-86985 and are not in the Chemistry (82009-84830) or Immunology (86015-86835) subsections may be reported using the unlisted transfusion medicine procedure code 86999.◀

Rationale

In support of the changes for unlisted procedures and services, a new introductory guideline has been added in the Transfusion Medicine subsection to provide instruction on how to report analytes/procedures that are not specified in codes 86850-86985 and codes 82009-84830 (Chemistry) or 86015-86835 (Immunology). The new guideline instructs that code 86999 may be reported when appropriate.

Refer to the codebook and the Rationale for the Unlisted Procedure or Service subsection of the Introduction section for a full discussion of these changes.

(For apheresis, use 36511, 36512)

(For therapeutic phlebotomy, use 99195)

86850   Antibody screen, RBC, each serum technique

Microbiology

Includes bacteriology, mycology, parasitology, and virology.

Presumptive identification of microorganisms is defined as identification by colony morphology, growth on selective media, Gram stains, or up to three tests (eg, catalase, oxidase, indole, urease). Definitive identification of microorganisms is defined as an identification to the genus or species level that requires additional tests (eg, biochemical panels, slide cultures). If additional studies involve molecular probes, nucleic acid sequencing, chromatography, or immunologic techniques, these should be separately coded using 87140-87158, in addition to definitive identification codes. The molecular diagnostic codes (eg, 81161, 81200-81408) are not to be used in combination with or instead of the procedures represented by 87140-87158. For multiple specimens/sites use modifier 59. For repeat laboratory tests performed on the same day, use modifier 91.

▶Microbiology analytes/procedures that are not specified in 87003-87912 and are not in the Chemistry (82009-84830) or Immunology (86015-86835) subsections may be reported using the unlisted microbiology procedure code 87999.◀

Rationale

In support of the changes for unlisted procedures and services, a new introductory guideline has been added in the Microbiology subsection to provide instruction on how to report analytes/procedures that are not specified in codes 87003-87912 and codes 82009-84830 (Chemistry) or 86015-86835 (Immunology). The new guideline instructs that code 87999 may be reported when appropriate.

Refer to the codebook and the Rationale for the Unlisted Procedure or Service subsection of the Introduction section for a full discussion of these changes.

87003   Animal inoculation, small animal, with observation and dissection

87301   Infectious agent antigen detection by immunoassay technique (eg, enzyme immunoassay [EIA], enzyme-linked immunosorbent assay [ELISA], fluorescence immunoassay [FIA], immunochemiluminometric assay [IMCA]), qualitative or semiquantitative; adenovirus enteric types 40/41

87380   hepatitis, delta agent

▶(For hepatitis delta agent, antibody, use 86692)◀

▶(For hepatitis D [delta], quantification, use 87523)◀

87468   Infectious agent detection by nucleic acid (DNA or RNA); Anaplasma phagocytophilum, amplified probe technique

87522   hepatitis C, quantification, includes reverse transcription when performed

● 87523   hepatitis D (delta), quantification, including reverse transcription, when performed

Rationale

Code 87523 has been established to report quantitative infectious agent antigen detection of hep D, which is a quantification of the antigen. Parenthetical notes have also been revised to accommodate the addition.

Code 87523 identifies infectious agent antigen detection for the hep D antigen. The procedure represents quantification of the viral antigen's RNA in serum or plasma and is used to confirm and quantify the presence of hep D virus. The testing for this pathogen may be used to monitor disease progression and for therapeutic purposes, such as evaluating how the patient is responding to treatment. The quantification of the antigen is what differentiates this procedure from the infectious agent detection of hep D. To exemplify this and to provide instruction regarding other hep D testing (ie, antibody), parenthetical cross-reference notes have been placed

★ = Telemedicine   ◀ = Audio-only   ✛ = Add-on code   ✗ = FDA approval pending   # = Resequenced code   ⊘ = Modifier 51 exempt

throughout the code set to direct users to the appropriate codes to report hep D antibody testing (86692), antigen testing (87380), and antigen testing with quantification of the viral DNA (87523).

Clinical Example (87523)

A 35-year-old female with known chronic hepatitis B presents with jaundice, fever, lack of appetite, and dark urine. Hepatitis D virus (HDV) antibody testing is positive. HDV RNA by quantitative PCR (qPCR) is ordered to confirm and quantify the presence of HDV.

Description of Procedure (87523)

Test patient serum for HDV RNA quantification by real-time PCR (RT-PCR). Report the results.

87525	hepatitis G, direct probe technique
87592	Neisseria gonorrhoeae, quantification
● **87593**	Orthopoxvirus (eg, monkeypox virus, cowpox virus, vaccinia virus), amplified probe technique, each

Rationale

Code 87593 was established in 2022 to report testing of orthopoxvirus, such as monkeypox virus, cowpox virus, and vaccinia virus, using amplified probe technique.

Due to a monkeypox outbreak in the US in 2022, testing for the monkeypox virus became necessary, which warranted a specific CPT code. Code 87593 was approved and released early for use in July 2022 and has been included in the *CPT 2024* codebook. Monkeypox is a transmissible disease caused by the monkeypox virus, a species of the orthopoxvirus genus. The orthopoxvirus genus includes other viruses, such as cowpox virus and vaccinia virus. As such, code 87593 describes testing for the orthopoxvirus genus and not just the monkeypox virus species. Code 87593 is reported for each species tested.

Clinical Example (87593)

A 45-year-old male presents with skin lesions, fever, and lymphadenopathy after potential exposure to monkeypox. Swabs of skin lesions are obtained for PCR testing.

Description of Procedure (87593)

Isolate DNA and perform PCR to detect orthopoxvirus genus or member species. Report results.

Anatomic Pathology

Postmortem Examination

Procedures 88000 through 88099 represent physician services only. Use modifier 90 for outside laboratory services.

▶Postmortem examination procedures that are not specified in 88000-88045 may be reported using the unlisted necropsy (autopsy) procedure code 88099.◀

Rationale

In support of the changes for unlisted procedures and services, a new introductory guideline has been added in the Anatomic Pathology subsection to provide instruction on how to report procedures that are not specified in codes 88000-88045. The new guideline instructs that code 88099 may be reported when appropriate.

Refer to the codebook and the Rationale for the Unlisted Procedure or Service subsection of the Introduction section for a full discussion of these changes.

88000	Necropsy (autopsy), gross examination only; without CNS
88005	with brain
88007	with brain and spinal cord
88012	infant with brain
88014	stillborn or newborn with brain
88016	macerated stillborn

Cytopathology

▶Cytopathology procedures that are not specified in 88104-88189 may be reported using the unlisted cytopathology procedure code 88199.◀

Rationale

In support of the changes for unlisted procedures and services, a new introductory guideline has been added in the Cytopathology subsection to provide instruction on how to report procedures that are not specified in codes 88104-88189. The new guideline instructs that code 88199 may be reported when appropriate.

Refer to the codebook and the Rationale for the Unlisted Procedure or Service subsection of the Introduction section for a full discussion of these changes.

Pathology and Laboratory 80047-89398, 0001U-0419U

88104   Cytopathology, fluids, washings or brushings, except cervical or vaginal; smears with interpretation

▶(Use 0827T in conjunction with 88104, when the digitization of glass microscope slides is performed)◀

Rationale

In support of the establishment of code 0827T, a parenthetical note has been added following code 88104 to refer users to code 0827T when the digitization of glass microscope slides is performed.

Refer to the codebook and the Rationale for code 0827T for a full discussion of these changes.

88106   simple filter method with interpretation

▶(Use 0828T in conjunction with 88106, when the digitization of glass microscope slides is performed)◀

(Do not report 88106 in conjunction with 88104)

(For nongynecological selective cellular enhancement including filter transfer techniques, use 88112)

Rationale

In support of the establishment of code 0828T, a parenthetical note has been added following code 88106 to refer users to code 0828T when the digitization of glass microscope slides is performed.

Refer to the codebook and the Rationale for code 0828T for a full discussion of these changes.

88108   Cytopathology, concentration technique, smears and interpretation (eg, Saccomanno technique)

▶(Use 0829T in conjunction with 88108, when the digitization of glass microscope slides is performed)◀

(For cervical or vaginal smears, see 88150-88155)

(For gastric intubation with lavage, see 43754, 43755)

(For x-ray localization, use 74340)

Rationale

In support of the establishment of code 0829T, a parenthetical note has been added following code 88108 to refer users to code 0829T when the digitization of glass microscope slides is performed.

Refer to the codebook and the Rationale for code 0829T for a full discussion of these changes.

88112   Cytopathology, selective cellular enhancement technique with interpretation (eg, liquid based slide preparation method), except cervical or vaginal

▶(Use 0830T in conjunction with 88112, when the digitization of glass microscope slides is performed)◀

(Do not report 88112 with 88108)

Rationale

In support of the establishment of code 0830T, a parenthetical note has been added following code 88112 to refer users to code 0830T when the digitization of glass microscope slides is performed.

Refer to the codebook and the Rationale for code 0830T for a full discussion of these changes.

88141   Cytopathology, cervical or vaginal (any reporting system), requiring interpretation by physician

(Use 88141 in conjunction with 88142, 88143, 88147, 88148, 88150, 88152, 88153, 88164-88167, 88174-88175)

▶(Use 0831T in conjunction with 88141, when the digitization of glass microscope slides is performed)◀

Rationale

In support of the establishment of code 0831T, a parenthetical note has been added following code 88141 to refer users to code 0831T when the digitization of glass microscope slides is performed.

Refer to the codebook and the Rationale for code 0831T for a full discussion of these changes.

88160   Cytopathology, smears, any other source; screening and interpretation

▶(Use 0832T in conjunction with 88160, when the digitization of glass microscope slides is performed)◀

Rationale

In support of the establishment of code 0832T, a parenthetical note has been added following code 88160 to refer users to code 0832T when the digitization of glass microscope slides is performed.

Refer to the codebook and the Rationale for code 0832T for a full discussion of these changes.

★ = Telemedicine   ◀ = Audio-only   ✚ = Add-on code   ⊁ = FDA approval pending   # = Resequenced code   ⊘ = Modifier 51 exempt

88161   preparation, screening and interpretation

▶(Use 0833T in conjunction with 88161, when the digitization of glass microscope slides is performed)◀

Rationale

In support of the establishment of code 0833T, a parenthetical note has been added following code 88161 to refer users to code 0833T when the digitization of glass microscope slides is performed.

Refer to the codebook and the Rationale for code 0833T for a full discussion of these changes.

88162   extended study involving over 5 slides and/or multiple stains

▶(Use 0834T in conjunction with 88162, when the digitization of glass microscope slides is performed)◀

(For aerosol collection of sputum, use 89220)

(For special stains, see 88312-88314)

Rationale

In support of the establishment of code 0834T, a parenthetical note has been added following code 88162 to refer users to code 0834T when the digitization of glass microscope slides is performed.

Refer to the codebook and the Rationale for code 0834T for a full discussion of these changes.

88172   Cytopathology, evaluation of fine needle aspirate; immediate cytohistologic study to determine adequacy for diagnosis, first evaluation episode, each site

▶(Use 0835T in conjunction with 88172, when the digitization of glass microscope slides is performed)◀

(The evaluation episode represents a complete set of cytologic material submitted for evaluation and is independent of the number of needle passes or slides prepared. A separate evaluation episode occurs if the proceduralist provider obtains additional material from the same site, based on the prior immediate adequacy assessment, or a separate lesion is aspirated)

Rationale

In support of the establishment of code 0835T, a parenthetical note has been added following code 88172 to refer users to code 0835T when the digitization of glass microscope slides is performed.

Refer to the codebook and the Rationale for code 0835T for a full discussion of these changes.

88173   interpretation and report

▶(Use 0837T in conjunction with 88173, when the digitization of glass microscope slides is performed)◀

(Report one unit of 88173 for the interpretation and report from each anatomic site, regardless of the number of passes or evaluation episodes performed during the aspiration procedure)

(For fine needle aspirate biopsy, see 10004, 10005, 10006, 10007, 10008, 10009, 10010, 10011, 10012, 10021)

(Do not report 88172, 88173 in conjunction with 88333 and 88334 for the same specimen)

Rationale

In support of the establishment of code 0837T, a parenthetical note has been added following code 88173 to refer users to code 0837T when the digitization of glass microscope slides is performed.

Refer to the codebook and the Rationale for code 0837T for a full discussion of these changes.

#✚ **88177**   immediate cytohistologic study to determine adequacy for diagnosis, each separate additional evaluation episode, same site (List separately in addition to code for primary procedure)

(Use 88177 in conjunction with 88172)

▶(Use 0836T in conjunction with 88177, when the digitization of glass microscope slides is performed)◀

(When repeat immediate evaluation episode(s) is required on subsequent cytologic material from the same site, eg, following determination the prior sampling that was not adequate for diagnosis, use 1 unit of 88177 for each additional evaluation episode)

Rationale

In support of the establishment of code 0836T, a parenthetical note has been added following code 88177 to refer users to code 0836T when the digitization of glass microscope slides is performed.

Refer to the codebook and the Rationale for code 0836T for a full discussion of these changes.

Cytogenetic Studies

▶Cytogenetic study procedures that are not specified in 88230-88291 and are not in the Surgical Pathology (88300-88388) subsection may be reported using the unlisted cytogenetic study code 88299.◀

Rationale

In support of the changes for unlisted procedures and services, a new introductory guideline has been added in the Cytogenetic Studies subsection to provide instruction on how to report cytogenetic study procedures that are not specified in codes 88230-88291 and 88300-88388 (Surgical Pathology). The new guideline instructs that code 88299 may be reported when appropriate.

Refer to the codebook and the Rationale for the Unlisted Procedure or Service subsection of the Introduction section for a full discussion of these changes.

Molecular pathology procedures should be reported using the appropriate code from Tier 1 (81161, 81200-81383), Tier 2 (81400-81408), Genomic Sequencing Procedures and Other Molecular Multianalyte Assays (81410-81471), or Multianalyte Assays with Algorithmic Analyses (81500-81512) sections. If no specific code exists, one of the unlisted codes (81479 or 81599) should be used.

(For acetylcholinesterase, use 82013)

(For alpha-fetoprotein, serum or amniotic fluid, see 82105, 82106)

(For laser microdissection of cells from tissue sample, see 88380)

Surgical Pathology

▶Services 88300 through 88309 include accession, examination, and reporting. They do not include the services designated in codes 88311 through 88388 and 88399, which are coded in addition when provided.◀

Rationale

The Surgical Pathology introductory guidelines have been revised by expanding the code range from "88311-88365" to "88311-88388" for services that should be reported in addition to surgical pathology services when provided.

When the fluorescence in situ hybridization (Agre) (88365, 88367, 88368) codes were revised in 2015, the Surgical Pathology introductory guidelines were not revised, which made the existing list incomplete. Therefore, this new

revision now provides a complete list of the services that are not included and that can be additionally reported (ie, 88311-88388 and 88399), when provided.

The unit of service for codes 88300 through 88309 is the specimen.

A specimen is defined as tissue or tissues that is (are) submitted for individual and separate attention, requiring individual examination and pathologic diagnosis. Two or more such specimens from the same patient (eg, separately identified endoscopic biopsies, skin lesions) are each appropriately assigned an individual code reflective of its proper level of service.

Service code 88300 is used for any specimen that in the opinion of the examining pathologist can be accurately diagnosed without microscopic examination. Service code 88302 is used when gross and microscopic examination is performed on a specimen to confirm identification and the absence of disease. Service codes 88304 through 88309 describe all other specimens requiring gross and microscopic examination, and represent additional ascending levels of physician work. Levels 88302 through 88309 are specifically defined by the assigned specimens.

Any unlisted specimen should be assigned to the code which most closely reflects the physician work involved when compared to other specimens assigned to that code.

▶Surgical pathology procedures that are not specified in 88300-88388 may be reported using the unlisted surgical pathology procedure code 88399.◀

Rationale

In support of the changes for unlisted procedures and services, a new introductory guideline has been added in the Surgical Pathology subsection to provide instruction on how to report surgical pathology procedures that are not specified in codes 88300-88388. The new guideline instructs that code 88399 may be reported when appropriate.

Refer to the codebook and the Rationale for the Unlisted Procedure or Service subsection of the Introduction section for a full discussion of these changes.

(Do not report 88302-88309 on the same specimen as part of Mohs surgery)

88321   Consultation and report on referred slides prepared elsewhere

▶(Use 0838T in conjunction with 88321, when the digitization of glass microscope slides is performed)◀

Rationale

In support of the establishment of code 0838T, a parenthetical note has been added following code 88321 to refer users to code 0838T when the digitization of glass microscope slides is performed.

Refer to the codebook and the Rationale for code 0838T for a full discussion of these changes.

88323 Consultation and report on referred material requiring preparation of slides

►(Use 0839T in conjunction with 88323, when the digitization of glass microscope slides is performed)◄

Rationale

In support of the establishment of code 0839T, a parenthetical note has been added following code 88323 to refer users to code 0839T when the digitization of glass microscope slides is performed.

Refer to the codebook and the Rationale for code 0839T for a full discussion of these changes.

88325 Consultation, comprehensive, with review of records and specimens, with report on referred material

►(Use 0840T in conjunction with 88325, when the digitization of glass microscope slides is performed)◄

Rationale

In support of the establishment of code 0840T, a parenthetical note has been added following code 88325 to refer users to code 0840T when the digitization of glass microscope slides is performed.

Refer to the codebook and the Rationale for code 0840T for a full discussion of these changes.

88329 Pathology consultation during surgery;

88331 first tissue block, with frozen section(s), single specimen

►(Use 0841T in conjunction with 88331, when the digitization of glass microscope slides is performed)◄

Rationale

In support of the establishment of code 0841T, a parenthetical note has been added following code 88331

to refer users to code 0841T when the digitization of glass microscope slides is performed.

Refer to the codebook and the Rationale for code 0841T for a full discussion of these changes.

+ 88332 each additional tissue block with frozen section(s) (List separately in addition to code for primary procedure)

(Use 88332 in conjunction with 88331)

►(Use 0842T in conjunction with 88332, when the digitization of glass microscope slides is performed)◄

Rationale

In support of the establishment of code 0842T, a parenthetical note has been added following code 88332 to refer users to code 0842T when the digitization of glass microscope slides is performed.

Refer to the codebook and the Rationale for code 0842T for a full discussion of these changes.

88333 cytologic examination (eg, touch prep, squash prep), initial site

►(Use 0843T in conjunction with 88333, when the digitization of glass microscope slides is performed)◄

Rationale

In support of the establishment of code 0843T, a parenthetical note has been added following code 88333 to refer users to code 0843T when the digitization of glass microscope slides is performed.

Refer to the codebook and the Rationale for code 0843T for a full discussion of these changes.

+ 88334 cytologic examination (eg, touch prep, squash prep), each additional site (List separately in addition to code for primary procedure)

(Use 88334 in conjunction with 88331, 88333)

►(Use 0844T in conjunction with 88334, when the digitization of glass microscope slides is performed)◄

(For intraoperative consultation on a specimen requiring both frozen section and cytologic evaluation, use 88331 and 88334)

(For percutaneous needle biopsy requiring intraprocedural cytologic examination, use 88333)

(Do not report 88333 and 88334 for non-intraoperative cytologic examination, see 88160-88162)

(Do not report 88333 and 88334 for intraprocedural cytologic evaluation of fine needle aspirate, see 88172)

Rationale

In support of the establishment of code 0844T, a parenthetical note has been added following code 88334 to refer users to code 0844T when the digitization of glass microscope slides is performed.

Refer to the codebook and the Rationale for code 0844T for a full discussion of these changes.

88346   Immunofluorescence, per specimen; initial single antibody stain procedure

▶(Use 0845T in conjunction with 88346, when the digitization of glass microscope slides is performed)◀

Rationale

In support of the establishment of code 0845T, a parenthetical note has been added following code 88346 to refer users to code 0845T when the digitization of glass microscope slides is performed.

Refer to the codebook and the Rationale for code 0845T for a full discussion of these changes.

#+ 88350   each additional single antibody stain procedure (List separately in addition to code for primary procedure)

▶(Use 0846T in conjunction with 88350, when the digitization of glass microscope slides is performed)◀

(Report 88350 in conjunction with 88346)

(Do not report 88346 and 88350 for fluorescent in situ hybridization studies, see 88364, 88365, 88366, 88367, 88368, 88369, 88373, 88374, and 88377)

(Do not report 88346 and 88350 for multiplex immunofluorescence analysis, use 88399)

Rationale

In support of the establishment of code 0846T, a parenthetical note has been added following code 88350 to refer users to code 0846T when the digitization of glass microscope slides is performed.

Refer to the codebook and the Rationale for code 0846T for a full discussion of these changes.

88348   Electron microscopy, diagnostic

▶(Use 0856T in conjunction with 88348, when the digitization of glass microscope slides is performed)◀

Rationale

In support of the establishment of code 0856T, a parenthetical note has been added following code 88348 to refer users to code 0856T when the digitization of glass microscope slides is performed.

Refer to the codebook and the Rationale for code 0856T for a full discussion of these changes.

88363   Examination and selection of retrieved archival (ie, previously diagnosed) tissue(s) for molecular analysis (eg, KRAS mutational analysis)

▶(Use 0847T in conjunction with 88363, when the digitization of glass microscope slides is performed)◀

Rationale

In support of the establishment of code 0847T, a parenthetical note has been added following code 88363 to refer users to code 0847T when the digitization of glass microscope slides is performed.

Refer to the codebook and the Rationale for code 0847T for a full discussion of these changes.

88365   In situ hybridization (eg, FISH), per specimen; initial single probe stain procedure

▶(Use 0848T in conjunction with 88365, when the digitization of glass microscope slides is performed)◀

Rationale

In support of the establishment of code 0848T, a parenthetical note has been added following code 88365 to refer users to code 0848T when the digitization of glass microscope slides is performed.

Refer to the codebook and the Rationale for code 0848T for a full discussion of these changes.

#+ 88364   each additional single probe stain procedure (List separately in addition to code for primary procedure)

(Use 88364 in conjunction with 88365)

▶(Use 0849T in conjunction with 88364, when the digitization of glass microscope slides is performed)◀

Rationale

In support of the establishment of code 0849T, a parenthetical note has been added following code 88364 to refer users to code 0849T when the digitization of glass microscope slides is performed.

Refer to the codebook and the Rationale for code 0849T for a full discussion of these changes.

88366   each multiplex probe stain procedure

▶(Use 0850T in conjunction with 88366, when the digitization of glass microscope slides is performed)◀

(Do not report 88365, 88366 in conjunction with 88367, 88368, 88374, 88377 for the same probe)

Rationale

In support of the establishment of code 0850T, a parenthetical note has been added following code 88366 to refer users to code 0850T when the digitization of glass microscope slides is performed.

Refer to the codebook and the Rationale for code 0850T for a full discussion of these changes.

88367   Morphometric analysis, in situ hybridization (quantitative or semi-quantitative), using computer-assisted technology, per specimen; initial single probe stain procedure

#+ 88373   each additional single probe stain procedure (List separately in addition to code for primary procedure)

88368   Morphometric analysis, in situ hybridization (quantitative or semi-quantitative), manual, per specimen; initial single probe stain procedure

▶(Use 0851T in conjunction with 88368, when the digitization of glass microscope slides is performed)◀

Rationale

In support of the establishment of code 0851T, a parenthetical note has been added following code 88368 to refer users to code 0851T when the digitization of glass microscope slides is performed.

Refer to the codebook and the Rationale for code 0851T for a full discussion of these changes.

+ 88369   each additional single probe stain procedure (List separately in addition to code for primary procedure)

(Use 88369 in conjunction with 88368)

▶(Use 0852T in conjunction with 88369, when the digitization of glass microscope slides is performed)◀

Rationale

In support of the establishment of code 0852T, a parenthetical note has been added following code 88369 to refer users to code 0852T when the digitization of glass microscope slides is performed.

Refer to the codebook and the Rationale for code 0852T for a full discussion of these changes.

 # 88377   each multiplex probe stain procedure

▶(Use 0853T in conjunction with 88377, when the digitization of glass microscope slides is performed)◀

(Do not report 88368 or 88377 in conjunction with 88365, 88366, 88367, 88374 for the same probe)

(For morphometric in situ hybridization evaluation of urinary tract cytologic specimens, see 88120, 88121)

Rationale

In support of the establishment of code 0853T, a parenthetical note has been added following code 88377 to refer users to code 0853T when the digitization of glass microscope slides is performed.

Refer to the codebook and the Rationale for code 0853T for a full discussion of these changes.

Pathology and Laboratory   80047-89398, 0001U-0419U

In Vivo (eg, Transcutaneous) Laboratory Procedures

▶In vivo measurement procedures that are not specified in 88720, 88738, 88740, 88741 may be reported using the unlisted in vivo pathology procedure code 88749.◀

Rationale

In support of the changes for unlisted procedures and services, a new introductory guideline has been added in the In Vivo (eg, Transcutaneous) Laboratory Procedures subsection to provide instruction on how to report in vivo measurement procedures that are not specified in codes 88720, 88738, 88740, and 88741. The new guideline instructs that code 88749 may be reported when appropriate.

Refer to the codebook and the Rationale for the Unlisted Procedure or Service subsection of the Introduction section for a full discussion of these changes.

(For transdermal oxygen saturation, see 94760-94762)

Other Procedures

▶Other procedures that are not specified in 89049-89230 or in other subsections (Chemistry, Hematology and Coagulation, Immunology, Transfusion Medicine, Microbiology, Cytopathology) may be reported using the unlisted miscellaneous pathology test code 89240.◀

Rationale

In support of the changes for unlisted procedures and services, a new introductory guideline has been added in the Other Procedures subsection to provide instruction on how to report other procedures that are not specified in codes 89049-89230 or in the codes in the Chemistry, Hematology and Coagulation, Immunology, Transfusion Medicine, Microbiology, and Cytopathology subsections. The new guideline instructs that code 89240 may be reported when appropriate.

Refer to the codebook and the Rationale for the Unlisted Procedure or Service subsection of the Introduction section for a full discussion of these changes.

89049　Caffeine halothane contracture test (CHCT) for malignant hyperthermia susceptibility, including interpretation and report

Reproductive Medicine Procedures

▶Reproductive medicine procedures that are not specified in 89250-89356 may be reported using the unlisted reproductive medicine laboratory procedure code 89398.◀

Rationale

In support of the changes for unlisted procedures and services, a new introductory guideline has been added in the Reproductive Medicine Procedures subsection to provide instruction on how to report reproductive medicine procedures that are not specified in codes 89250-89356. The new guideline instructs that code 89398 may be reported when appropriate.

Refer to the codebook and the Rationale for the Unlisted Procedure or Service subsection of the Introduction section for a full discussion of these changes.

89250　Culture of oocyte(s)/embryo(s), less than 4 days;

89251　　with co-culture of oocyte(s)/embryos

(For extended culture of oocyte[s]/embryo[s], see 89272)

Proprietary Laboratory Analyses

▲ 0022U　Targeted genomic sequence analysis panel, non-small cell lung neoplasia, DNA and RNA analysis, 23 genes, interrogation for sequence variants and rearrangements, reported as presence or absence of variants and associated therapy(ies) to consider

▶(0053U has been deleted)◀

▶(0066U has been deleted)◀

▲ 0095U　Eosinophilic esophagitis (Eotaxin-3 *[CCL26 {C-C motif chemokine ligand 26}]* and major basic protein *[PRG2 {proteoglycan 2, pro eosinophil major basic protein}]*), enzyme-linked immunosorbent assays (ELISA), specimen obtained by esophageal string test device, algorithm reported as probability of active or inactive eosinophilic esophagitis

▶(0143U has been deleted)◀

▶(0144U has been deleted)◀

▶(0145U has been deleted)◀

▶(0146U has been deleted)◀

▶(0147U has been deleted)◀

▶(0148U has been deleted)◀

★ = Telemedicine　◀ = Audio-only　✚ = Add-on code　✗ = FDA approval pending　# = Resequenced code　⊘ = Modifier 51 exempt

▶(0149U has been deleted)◀

▶(0150U has been deleted)◀

▲ **0269U** Hematology (autosomal dominant congenital thrombocytopenia), genomic sequence analysis of 22 genes, blood, buccal swab, or amniotic fluid

▲ **0271U** Hematology (congenital neutropenia), genomic sequence analysis of 24 genes, blood, buccal swab, or amniotic fluid

▲ **0272U** Hematology (genetic bleeding disorders), genomic sequence analysis of 60 genes and duplication/deletion of *PLAU*, blood, buccal swab, or amniotic fluid, comprehensive

▲ **0274U** Hematology (genetic platelet disorders), genomic sequence analysis of 62 genes and duplication/deletion of *PLAU*, blood, buccal swab, or amniotic fluid

▲ **0277U** Hematology (genetic platelet function disorder), genomic sequence analysis of 40 genes and duplication/deletion of *PLAU*, blood, buccal swab, or amniotic fluid

▲ **0278U** Hematology (genetic thrombosis), genomic sequence analysis of 14 genes, blood, buccal swab, or amniotic fluid

▲ **0308U** Cardiology (coronary artery disease [CAD]), analysis of 3 proteins (high sensitivity [hs] troponin, adiponectin, and kidney injury molecule-1 [KIM-1]) with 3 clinical parameters (age, sex, history of cardiac intervention), plasma, algorithm reported as a risk score for obstructive CAD

▶(0324U has been deleted)◀

▶(0325U has been deleted)◀

✂ **0345U** Psychiatry (eg, depression, anxiety, attention deficit hyperactivity disorder [ADHD]), genomic analysis panel, variant analysis of 15 genes, including deletion/duplication analysis of *CYP2D6*

▶(For additional PLA code with identical clinical descriptor, see 0411U. See Appendix O to determine appropriate code assignment)◀

● **0355U** *APOL1 (apolipoprotein L1)* (eg, chronic kidney disease), risk variants (G1, G2)

● **0356U** Oncology (oropharyngeal), evaluation of 17 DNA biomarkers using droplet digital PCR (ddPCR), cell-free DNA, algorithm reported as a prognostic risk score for cancer recurrence

▶(0357U has been deleted)◀

● **0358U** Neurology (mild cognitive impairment), analysis of ß-amyloid 1-42 and 1-40, chemiluminescence enzyme immunoassay, cerebral spinal fluid, reported as positive, likely positive, or negative

● **0359U** Oncology (prostate cancer), analysis of all prostate-specific antigen (PSA) structural isoforms by phase separation and immunoassay, plasma, algorithm reports risk of cancer

● **0360U** Oncology (lung), enzyme-linked immunosorbent assay (ELISA) of 7 autoantibodies (p53, NY-ESO-1, CAGE, GBU4-5, SOX2, MAGE A4, and HuD), plasma, algorithm reported as a categorical result for risk of malignancy

● **0361U** Neurofilament light chain, digital immunoassay, plasma, quantitative

▲ **0362U** Oncology (papillary thyroid cancer), gene-expression profiling via targeted hybrid capture–enrichment RNA sequencing of 82 content genes and 10 housekeeping genes, fine needle aspirate or formalin-fixed paraffin-embedded (FFPE) tissue, algorithm reported as one of three molecular subtypes

● **0363U** Oncology (urothelial), mRNA, gene-expression profiling by real-time quantitative PCR of 5 genes *(MDK, HOXA13, CDC2 [CDK1], IGFBP5,* and *CXCR2)*, utilizing urine, algorithm incorporates age, sex, smoking history, and macrohematuria frequency, reported as a risk score for having urothelial carcinoma

● **0364U** Oncology (hematolymphoid neoplasm), genomic sequence analysis using multiplex (PCR) and next-generation sequencing with algorithm, quantification of dominant clonal sequence(s), reported as presence or absence of minimal residual disease (MRD) with quantitation of disease burden, when appropriate

● **0365U** Oncology (bladder), analysis of 10 protein biomarkers (A1AT, ANG, APOE, CA9, IL8, MMP9, MMP10, PAI1, SDC1, and VEGFA) by immunoassays, urine, algorithm reported as a probability of bladder cancer

● **0366U** Oncology (bladder), analysis of 10 protein biomarkers (A1AT, ANG, APOE, CA9, IL8, MMP9, MMP10, PAI1, SDC1, and VEGFA) by immunoassays, urine, algorithm reported as a probability of recurrent bladder cancer

● **0367U** Oncology (bladder), analysis of 10 protein biomarkers (A1AT, ANG, APOE, CA9, IL8, MMP9, MMP10, PAI1, SDC1, and VEGFA) by immunoassays, urine, diagnostic algorithm reported as a risk score for probability of rapid recurrence of recurrent or persistent cancer following transurethral resection

● **0368U** Oncology (colorectal cancer), evaluation for mutations of *APC, BRAF, CTNNB1, KRAS, NRAS, PIK3CA, SMAD4,* and *TP53,* and methylation markers (MYO1G, KCNQ5, C9ORF50, FLI1, CLIP4, ZNF132, and TWIST1), multiplex quantitative polymerase chain reaction (qPCR), circulating cell-free DNA (cfDNA), plasma, report of risk score for advanced adenoma or colorectal cancer

Pathology and Laboratory 80047-89398, 0001U-0419U

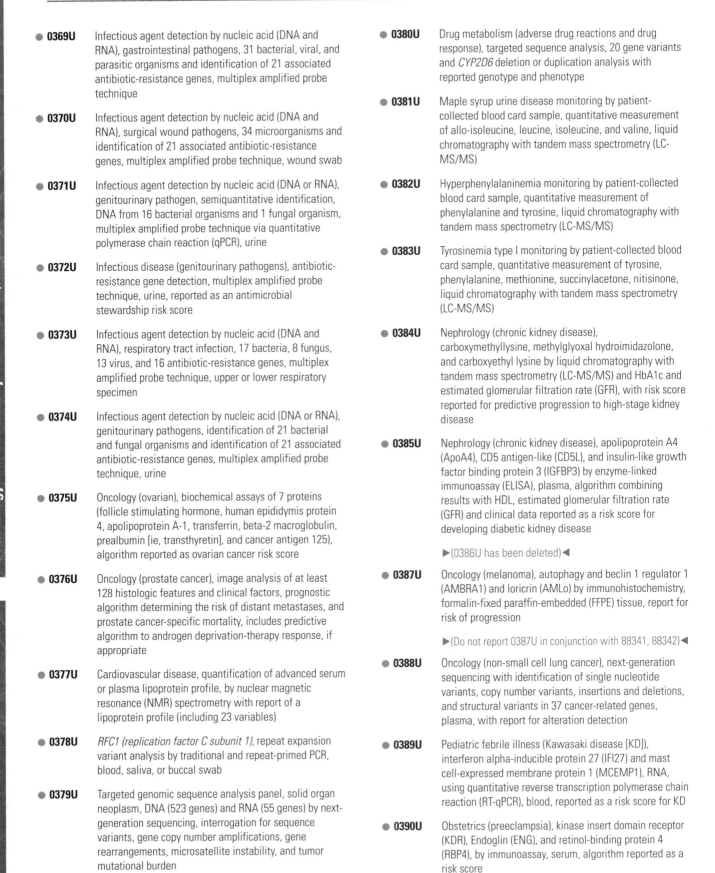

● **0369U** Infectious agent detection by nucleic acid (DNA and RNA), gastrointestinal pathogens, 31 bacterial, viral, and parasitic organisms and identification of 21 associated antibiotic-resistance genes, multiplex amplified probe technique

● **0370U** Infectious agent detection by nucleic acid (DNA and RNA), surgical wound pathogens, 34 microorganisms and identification of 21 associated antibiotic-resistance genes, multiplex amplified probe technique, wound swab

● **0371U** Infectious agent detection by nucleic acid (DNA or RNA), genitourinary pathogen, semiquantitative identification, DNA from 16 bacterial organisms and 1 fungal organism, multiplex amplified probe technique via quantitative polymerase chain reaction (qPCR), urine

● **0372U** Infectious disease (genitourinary pathogens), antibiotic-resistance gene detection, multiplex amplified probe technique, urine, reported as an antimicrobial stewardship risk score

● **0373U** Infectious agent detection by nucleic acid (DNA and RNA), respiratory tract infection, 17 bacteria, 8 fungus, 13 virus, and 16 antibiotic-resistance genes, multiplex amplified probe technique, upper or lower respiratory specimen

● **0374U** Infectious agent detection by nucleic acid (DNA or RNA), genitourinary pathogens, identification of 21 bacterial and fungal organisms and identification of 21 associated antibiotic-resistance genes, multiplex amplified probe technique, urine

● **0375U** Oncology (ovarian), biochemical assays of 7 proteins (follicle stimulating hormone, human epididymis protein 4, apolipoprotein A-1, transferrin, beta-2 macroglobulin, prealbumin [ie, transthyretin], and cancer antigen 125), algorithm reported as ovarian cancer risk score

● **0376U** Oncology (prostate cancer), image analysis of at least 128 histologic features and clinical factors, prognostic algorithm determining the risk of distant metastases, and prostate cancer-specific mortality, includes predictive algorithm to androgen deprivation-therapy response, if appropriate

● **0377U** Cardiovascular disease, quantification of advanced serum or plasma lipoprotein profile, by nuclear magnetic resonance (NMR) spectrometry with report of a lipoprotein profile (including 23 variables)

● **0378U** *RFC1 (replication factor C subunit 1),* repeat expansion variant analysis by traditional and repeat-primed PCR, blood, saliva, or buccal swab

● **0379U** Targeted genomic sequence analysis panel, solid organ neoplasm, DNA (523 genes) and RNA (55 genes) by next-generation sequencing, interrogation for sequence variants, gene copy number amplifications, gene rearrangements, microsatellite instability, and tumor mutational burden

● **0380U** Drug metabolism (adverse drug reactions and drug response), targeted sequence analysis, 20 gene variants and *CYP2D6* deletion or duplication analysis with reported genotype and phenotype

● **0381U** Maple syrup urine disease monitoring by patient-collected blood card sample, quantitative measurement of allo-isoleucine, leucine, isoleucine, and valine, liquid chromatography with tandem mass spectrometry (LC-MS/MS)

● **0382U** Hyperphenylalaninemia monitoring by patient-collected blood card sample, quantitative measurement of phenylalanine and tyrosine, liquid chromatography with tandem mass spectrometry (LC-MS/MS)

● **0383U** Tyrosinemia type I monitoring by patient-collected blood card sample, quantitative measurement of tyrosine, phenylalanine, methionine, succinylacetone, nitisinone, liquid chromatography with tandem mass spectrometry (LC-MS/MS)

● **0384U** Nephrology (chronic kidney disease), carboxymethyllysine, methylglyoxal hydroimidazolone, and carboxyethyl lysine by liquid chromatography with tandem mass spectrometry (LC-MS/MS) and HbA1c and estimated glomerular filtration rate (GFR), with risk score reported for predictive progression to high-stage kidney disease

● **0385U** Nephrology (chronic kidney disease), apolipoprotein A4 (ApoA4), CD5 antigen-like (CD5L), and insulin-like growth factor binding protein 3 (IGFBP3) by enzyme-linked immunoassay (ELISA), plasma, algorithm combining results with HDL, estimated glomerular filtration rate (GFR) and clinical data reported as a risk score for developing diabetic kidney disease

▶(0386U has been deleted)◀

● **0387U** Oncology (melanoma), autophagy and beclin 1 regulator 1 (AMBRA1) and loricrin (AMLo) by immunohistochemistry, formalin-fixed paraffin-embedded (FFPE) tissue, report for risk of progression

▶(Do not report 0387U in conjunction with 88341, 88342)◀

● **0388U** Oncology (non-small cell lung cancer), next-generation sequencing with identification of single nucleotide variants, copy number variants, insertions and deletions, and structural variants in 37 cancer-related genes, plasma, with report for alteration detection

● **0389U** Pediatric febrile illness (Kawasaki disease [KD]), interferon alpha-inducible protein 27 (IFI27) and mast cell-expressed membrane protein 1 (MCEMP1), RNA, using quantitative reverse transcription polymerase chain reaction (RT-qPCR), blood, reported as a risk score for KD

● **0390U** Obstetrics (preeclampsia), kinase insert domain receptor (KDR), Endoglin (ENG), and retinol-binding protein 4 (RBP4), by immunoassay, serum, algorithm reported as a risk score

★ = Telemedicine ◀ = Audio-only ✚ = Add-on code ✎ = FDA approval pending # = Resequenced code ⊘ = Modifier 51 exempt

● **0391U** Oncology (solid tumor), DNA and RNA by next-generation sequencing, utilizing formalin-fixed paraffin-embedded (FFPE) tissue, 437 genes, interpretive report for single nucleotide variants, splice-site variants, insertions/deletions, copy number alterations, gene fusions, tumor mutational burden, and microsatellite instability, with algorithm quantifying immunotherapy response score

● **0392U** Drug metabolism (depression, anxiety, attention deficit hyperactivity disorder [ADHD]), gene-drug interactions, variant analysis of 16 genes, including deletion/duplication analysis of *CYP2D6*, reported as impact of gene-drug interaction for each drug

● **0393U** Neurology (eg, Parkinson disease, dementia with Lewy bodies), cerebrospinal fluid (CSF), detection of misfolded α-synuclein protein by seed amplification assay, qualitative

● **0394U** Perfluoroalkyl substances (PFAS) (eg, perfluorooctanoic acid, perfluorooctane sulfonic acid), 16 PFAS compounds by liquid chromatography with tandem mass spectrometry (LC-MS/MS), plasma or serum, quantitative

● **0395U** Oncology (lung), multi-omics (microbial DNA by shotgun next-generation sequencing and carcinoembryonic antigen and osteopontin by immunoassay), plasma, algorithm reported as malignancy risk for lung nodules in early-stage disease

● **0396U** Obstetrics (pre-implantation genetic testing), evaluation of 300000 DNA single-nucleotide polymorphisms (SNPs) by microarray, embryonic tissue, algorithm reported as a probability for single-gene germline conditions

▶(0397U has been deleted)◀

● **0398U** Gastroenterology (Barrett's esophagus), *P16, RUNX3, HPP1,* and *FBN1* DNA methylation analysis using PCR, formalin-fixed paraffin-embedded (FFPE) tissue, algorithm reported as risk score for progression to high-grade dysplasia or cancer

● **0399U** Neurology (cerebral folate deficiency), serum, detection of anti-human folate receptor IgG-binding antibody and blocking autoantibodies by enzyme-linked immunoassay (ELISA), qualitative, and blocking autoantibodies, using a functional blocking assay for IgG or IgM, quantitative, reported as positive or not detected

● **0400U** Obstetrics (expanded carrier screening), 145 genes by next-generation sequencing, fragment analysis and multiplex ligation-dependent probe amplification, DNA, reported as carrier positive or negative

● **0401U** Cardiology (coronary heart disease [CHD]), 9 genes (12 variants), targeted variant genotyping, blood, saliva, or buccal swab, algorithm reported as a genetic risk score for a coronary event

● **0402U** Infectious agent (sexually transmitted infection), Chlamydia trachomatis, Neisseria gonorrhoeae, Trichomonas vaginalis, Mycoplasma genitalium, multiplex amplified probe technique, vaginal, endocervical, or male urine, each pathogen reported as detected or not detected

● **0403U** Oncology (prostate), mRNA, gene expression profiling of 18 genes, first-catch post-digital rectal examination urine (or processed first-catch urine), algorithm reported as percentage of likelihood of detecting clinically significant prostate cancer

● **0404U** Oncology (breast), semiquantitative measurement of thymidine kinase activity by immunoassay, serum, results reported as risk of disease progression

● **0405U** Oncology (pancreatic), 59 methylation haplotype block markers, next-generation sequencing, plasma, reported as cancer signal detected or not detected

● **0406U** Oncology (lung), flow cytometry, sputum, 5 markers (meso-tetra [4-carboxyphenyl] porphyrin [TCPP], CD206, CD66b, CD3, CD19), algorithm reported as likelihood of lung cancer

● **0407U** Nephrology (diabetic chronic kidney disease [CKD]), multiplex electrochemiluminescent immunoassay (ECLIA) of soluble tumor necrosis factor receptor 1 (sTNFR1), soluble tumor necrosis receptor 2 (sTNFR2), and kidney injury molecule 1 (KIM-1) combined with clinical data, plasma, algorithm reported as risk for progressive decline in kidney function

● **0408U** Infectious agent antigen detection by bulk acoustic wave biosensor immunoassay, severe acute respiratory syndrome coronavirus 2 (SARS-CoV-2) (coronavirus disease [COVID-19])

● **0409U** Oncology (solid tumor), DNA (80 genes) and RNA (36 genes), by next-generation sequencing from plasma, including single nucleotide variants, insertions/deletions, copy number alterations, microsatellite instability, and fusions, report showing identified mutations with clinical actionability

● **0410U** Oncology (pancreatic), DNA, whole genome sequencing with 5-hydroxymethylcytosine enrichment, whole blood or plasma, algorithm reported as cancer detected or not detected

✚● **0411U** Psychiatry (eg, depression, anxiety, attention deficit hyperactivity disorder [ADHD]), genomic analysis panel, variant analysis of 15 genes, including deletion/duplication analysis of *CYP2D6*

▶(For additional PLA code with identical clinical descriptor, see 0345U. See Appendix O to determine appropriate code assignment)◀

● **0412U** Beta amyloid, Aß42/40 ratio, immunoprecipitation with quantitation by liquid chromatography with tandem mass spectrometry (LC-MS/MS) and qualitative ApoE isoform-specific proteotyping, plasma combined with age, algorithm reported as presence or absence of brain amyloid pathology

● **0413U** Oncology (hematolymphoid neoplasm), optical genome mapping for copy number alterations, aneuploidy, and balanced/complex structural rearrangements, DNA from blood or bone marrow, report of clinically significant alterations

● **0414U** Oncology (lung), augmentative algorithmic analysis of digitized whole slide imaging for 8 genes (ALK, BRAF, EGFR, ERBB2, MET, NTRK1-3, RET, ROS1), and KRAS G12C and PD-L1, if performed, formalin-fixed paraffin-embedded (FFPE) tissue, reported as positive or negative for each biomarker

● **0415U** Cardiovascular disease (acute coronary syndrome [ACS]), IL-16, FAS, FASLigand, HGF, CTACK, EOTAXIN, and MCP-3 by immunoassay combined with age, sex, family history, and personal history of diabetes, blood, algorithm reported as a 5-year (deleted risk) score for ACS

● **0416U** Infectious agent detection by nucleic acid (DNA), genitourinary pathogens, identification of 20 bacterial and fungal organisms, including identification of 20 associated antibiotic-resistance genes, if performed, multiplex amplified probe technique, urine

● **0417U** Rare diseases (constitutional/heritable disorders), whole mitochondrial genome sequence with heteroplasmy detection and deletion analysis, nuclear-encoded mitochondrial gene analysis of 335 nuclear genes, including sequence changes, deletions, insertions, and copy number variants analysis, blood or saliva, identification and categorization of mitochondrial disorder–associated genetic variants

● **0418U** Oncology (breast), augmentative algorithmic analysis of digitized whole slide imaging of 8 histologic and immunohistochemical features, reported as a recurrence score

● **0419U** Neuropsychiatry (eg, depression, anxiety), genomic sequence analysis panel, variant analysis of 13 genes, saliva or buccal swab, report of each gene phenotype

---

Rationale

A total of 61 new proprietary laboratory analyses (PLA) codes have been established for the CPT 2024 code set. PLA test codes are released and posted online at https://www.ama-assn.org/practice-management/cpt/cpt-pla-codes on a quarterly basis (fall, winter, spring, and summer). New codes are effective the quarter following their publication online. Other changes include the deletion of 15 codes (0053U, 0066U, 0143U-0150U, 0324U, 0325U, 0357U, 0386U, 0397U); the revision of 10 codes (0022U, 0095U, 0269U, 0271U, 0272U, 0274U 0277U, 0278U, 0308U, 0362U); the revision of three test names (0308U-0310U); and the revision of the test name, laboratory name, and manufacturer name for code 0113U.

Clinical Example (0022U)

A 58-year-old female was recently diagnosed with stage IV adenocarcinoma of the lung, based on biopsy. The oncologist requests broad molecular profiling to inform first-line therapy options, including Food and Drug Administration (FDA)-approved therapies.

Description of Procedure (0022U)

Isolate and subject DNA from formalin-fixed paraffin-embedded (FFPE) tissue from a non-small cell lung cancer specimen to undergo targeted high-throughput, parallel sequencing to detect single nucleotide variants and deletions from 23 genes from DNA and fusions in ROS1 and RET genes from isolated RNA.

Clinical Example (0095U)

A 17-year-old male with eosinophilic esophagitis presents after 12 weeks of treatment with dietary exclusion of candidate food allergens. His symptoms have resolved. An esophageal string test is performed, and the esophageal sample is submitted.

Description of Procedure (0095U)

Elute supernatant from string test sample and subject to enzyme-linked immunosorbent assay (ELISA) for two eosinophil-associated protein biomarkers, Eotaxin-3 and major basic protein-1. An eosinophilic esophagitis score based on their concentrations is reported as the probability of having active disease. Issue the report to the ordering provider.

Clinical Example (0269U)

A 14-year-old healthy male with a personal and family history of mild chronic thrombocytopenia is evaluated by a hematologist. Genetic testing is ordered for possible inherited thrombocytopenia with autosomal dominant inheritance.

Description of Procedure (0269U)

Isolate and subject high-quality genomic DNA from the submitted specimen to NGS of 22 genes (ACTB, ACTN1, ANKRD26, CDC42, CYCS, DIAPH1, ETV6, FLI1, GFI1B, GP1BA, GP1BB, GP9, HOXA11, ITGA2B, ITGB3, MECOM, MYH9, RUNX1, SLFN14, SRC, STIM1, TUBB1). A qualified laboratory professional analyzes the data and composes a report.

Clinical Example (0271U)

A 14-year-old female with short stature, skin hypopigmentation, and nail dyskeratosis has lifelong mild to moderate isolated neutropenia. A younger brother has similar skin findings. A congenital neutropenia panel is ordered.

★ = Telemedicine   ◀ = Audio-only   ✚ = Add-on code   ✗ = FDA approval pending   # = Resequenced code   ⊘ = Modifier 51 exempt

Description of Procedure (0271U)

Isolate and subject high-quality genomic DNA from the submitted specimen whole blood to NGS of 24 genes (AP3B1, AP3D1, CSF3R, CXCR4, ELANE, G6PC3, GATA1, GATA2, GFI1, HAX1, JAGN1, LAMTOR2, LYST, RAB27A, RAC2, SBDS, SLC37A4, TAZ, TCIRG1, USB1, VPS13B, VPS45, WAS, WIPF1). A qualified laboratory professional analyzes the data and composes a report.

Clinical Example (0272U)

A 45-year-old female presents with lifelong bleeding and impaired wound healing. A combined coagulation factor deficiency and platelet function disorder is suspected. A comprehensive bleeding disorder panel is ordered.

Description of Procedure (0272U)

Isolate and subject high-quality gDNA to NGS of 60 genes (ANO6, AP3B1, AP3D1, ARPC1B, BLOC1S3, BLOC1S6, DTNBP1, F10, F11, F13A1, F13B, F2, F5, F7, F8, F9, FERMT3, FGA, FGB, FGG, FLI1, FLNA, FYB1, GATA1, GFI1B, GGCX, GP1BA, GP1BB, GP6, GP9, HPS1, HPS3, HPS4, HPS5, HPS6, ITGA2B, ITGB3, KDSR, LMAN1, LYST, MCFD2, NBEA, NBEAL2, P2RY12, PLA2G4A, PRKACG, RASGRP2, RUNX1, SERPINA1, SERPINE1, SERPINF2, SLFN14, SRC, STIM1, TBXA2R, TBXAS1, VIPAS39, VKORC1, VPS33B, VWF) and PLAU by aCGH. A qualified laboratory professional analyzes the data and composes a report.

Clinical Example (0274U)

A 9-year-old male presents with recurrent epistaxis and thrombocytopenia since birth. The bleeding is out of proportion to the degree of thrombocytopenia. A comprehensive genetic platelet disorder panel is ordered.

Description of Procedure (0274U)

Isolate and subject high-quality gDNA to NGS of 62 genes (ABCG5, ABCG8, ACTB, ACTN1, ANKRD26, ANO6, AP3B1, AP3D1, ARPC1B, BLOC1S3, BLOC1S6, CDC42, CYCS, DIAPH1, DTNBP1, ETV6, FERMT3, FLI1, FLNA, FYB1, GATA1, GFI1B, GNE, GP1BA, GP1BB, GP6, GP9, HOXA11, HPS1, HPS3, HPS4, HPS5, HPS6, ITGA2B, ITGB3, KDSR, LYST, MECOM, MPIG6B, MPL, MYH9, NBEA, NBEAL2, P2RY12, PLA2G4A, PRKACG, RASGRP2, RBM8A, RNU4ATAC, RUNX1, SLFN14, SRC, STIM1, STXBP2, TBXA2R, TBXAS1, THPO, TUBB1, VIPAS39, VPS33B, WAS, WIPF1) and PLAU by aCGH. A qualified laboratory professional reviews the data and reports the results to the ordering provider.

Clinical Example (0277U)

A 3-year-old male has recurrent bleeding leading to anemia. Platelet aggregation is abnormal with adenosine diphosphate and arachidonic acid. An inherited platelet dysfunction is suspected. Genetic testing is ordered.

Description of Procedure (0277U)

Isolate and subject high-quality genomic DNA from the specimen to NGS of 40 genes (ANO6, AP31B, AP3D1, ARPC1B, BLOC1S3, BLOC1S6, DTNBP1, FERMT3, FLI1, FLNA, FYB1, GATA1, GFI1B, GP6, GP9, GPIBA, GPIBB, HPS1, HPS3, HPS4, HPS5, HPS6, ITGA2B, ITGB3, KDSR, LYST, NBEA, NBEAL2, P2RY12, PLA2G4A, PRKACG, RASGRP2, RUNX1, SLFN14, SRC, STIM1, TBXA2R, TBXAS1, VIPAS39, VPS33B) and PLAU by aCGH. A qualified laboratory professional analyzes the data and composes a report.

Clinical Example (0278U)

A 32-year-old male presents with an unprovoked pulmonary embolus and bilateral deep venous thromboses. An inherited hypercoagulopathy panel is ordered.

Description of Procedure (0278U)

Isolate and subject high-quality genomic DNA from the submitted specimen to NGS of 14 genes (ADAMTS13, F2, F5, FGA, FGB, FGG, HRG, KNG1, PLG, PROC, PROS1, SERPINC1, SERPIND1, THPD). A qualified laboratory professional analyzes the data and composes a report.

Clinical Example (0356U)

A 52-year-old male presents to his radiation oncologist for surveillance of a previously treated human papillomavirus (HPV)-driven oropharyngeal cancer. Whole blood is sent for circulating tumor tissue modified HPV DNA testing.

Description of Procedure (0356U)

Isolate and subject cell-free DNA (cfDNA) from plasma to droplet digital PCR to profile the fragmentation pattern of HPV DNA using 17 DNA biomarkers. An algorithm generates a tumor tissue modified viral prognostic risk score for cancer recurrence. A qualified laboratory professional prepares a report and sends it to the ordering provider.

Clinical Example (0358U)

A 65-year-old male is evaluated and found to have mild cognitive impairment. Cerebrospinal fluid (CSF) is submitted to evaluate the risk for Alzheimer's disease pathology.

Description of Procedure (0358U)

Use CSF after a lumbar puncture to assess ß-amyloid 1-40 and ß-amyloid 1-42 using immunoassay reagents and to quantitatively measure ß-amyloid 1-42 in human CSF specimens based on chemiluminescence enzyme immunoassay technology using a two-step sandwich immunoassay method. A qualified laboratory professional reviews the findings and reports them to the ordering provider.

Clinical Example (0359U)

A 55-year-old male is referred to a urologist with a prostate-specific antigen (PSA) of 4.5 ng/mL and a free fraction of 25%. Physical shows no abnormalities. Plasma is submitted to determine the patient's risk for prostate cancer.

Description of Procedure (0359U)

The laboratory performs a PSA test to confirm that PSA is greater than 4.0 ng/mL. Analyze plasma for PSA isoforms. Measure the total and free PSA concentrations in the pre-processed sample and native plasma. Calculate a risk index. A qualified laboratory professional composes a report for the ordering provider, specifying the patient's risk for high-grade prostate cancer.

Clinical Example (0360U)

A 67-year-old female presents with a 10-year smoking history and cough. Computed tomography (CT) evaluation shows an 8-mm spiculated nodule in the right upper lobe of the lung. Plasma is submitted to determine the nodule's malignancy risk.

Description of Procedure (0360U)

Analyze plasma using an enzyme-linked immunosorbent assay to measure seven lung-cancer associated autoantibodies (p53, NY-ESO-1, CAGE, GBU4-5, SOX2, MAGE A4, and HuD). Integrate autoantibody levels using an algorithm to yield the risk of malignancy.

Clinical Example (0361U)

A 60-year-old male presents for neurologic evaluation of gradual cognitive decline. Measurement of neurofilament light chain (NfL) is requested to assess if his cognitive decline is due to neurodegeneration.

Description of Procedure (0361U)

Analyze plasma for NfL by immunoassay using monoclonal anti-NfL antibody–coated paramagnetic-capture beads and labeled biotinylated detector antibody. Determine NfL concentration using a proprietary software and algorithm to report a quantitative NfL result.

Clinical Example (0362U)

A 36-year-old female presents with a 2-cm thyroid nodule. A fine-needle aspiration confirms papillary thyroid cancer. The specimen is submitted to determine the molecular subtype.

Description of Procedure (0362U)

Isolate RNA from a fine-needle aspirate biopsy and conduct targeted hybrid-capture enrichment sequencing of 82 prognostic genes and 10 housekeeping genes. Proprietary software identifies the molecular subtypes and determines high- or low-recurrence risk. A qualified laboratory professional reviews the findings and reports the results to the ordering provider.

Clinical Example (0363U)

A 47-year-old female is referred to her urologist with a history of microscopic hematuria. She has a negative history of gross hematuria and a positive smoking history. A urine sample is submitted to assess the patient's risk for urothelial carcinoma.

Description of Procedure (0363U)

Subject mRNA isolated from urine to RT-qPCR of five genes (MDK, HOXA13, CDC2 [CDK1], IGFBP5, and CXCR2). Incorporate mRNA levels into an algorithm, along with risk factors of age, sex, smoking history, and macrohematuria frequency, to calculate a risk score for urothelial carcinoma. A qualified laboratory professional prepares a report specifying the risk status and communicates to the ordering provider.

Clinical Example (0364U)

A 45-year-old male with acute lymphoblastic leukemia received induction chemotherapy. Bone marrow is submitted to evaluate the patient for therapeutic response.

Description of Procedure (0364U)

Extract genomic DNA from bone marrow, lymph node, skin, or peripheral blood and subjected to multiplex PCR. Prepare libraries from barcoded amplified DNA and sequence by NGS. Analyze sequence data and process using a proprietary algorithm. The pathologist or other qualified laboratory professional reviews the report that quantifies residual disease, if present. Communicate the results to the ordering provider.

★ = Telemedicine ◀ = Audio-only ✚ = Add-on code ✒ = FDA approval pending # = Resequenced code ⊘ = Modifier 51 exempt

Clinical Example (0365U)

A 66-year-old female presents to her physician with hematuria, initially diagnosed as a urinary tract infection (UTI) that has recurred in 2 months. A voided urine sample is submitted to determine the probability of bladder cancer.

Description of Procedure (0365U)

Analzye urine using a multiplexed immunoassay for A1AT, ANG, APOE, CA9, IL8, MMP9, MMP10, PAI1, SDC1, and VEGFA. Quantify each protein and using a bladder cancer proprietary algorithm, which includes age, race, and gender, provide a risk score for the likelihood of bladder cancer.

Clinical Example (0366U)

A 66-year-old female with a history of tumor (T)1 (T1) high-grade bladder cancer diagnosed a year ago is seen in follow-up. A voided urine sample is submitted to determine the probability of recurrent bladder cancer.

Description of Procedure (0366U)

Analyze urine using a multiplexed immunoassay for A1AT, ANG, APOE, CA9, IL8, MMP9, MMP10, PAI1, SDC1, and VEGFA. Quantify each protein and using a bladder cancer proprietary algorithm provide a risk score for the likelihood of recurrent bladder cancer.

Clinical Example (0367U)

A 76-year-old male underwent bladder resection for urothelial carcinoma. Metastatic workup was negative. Voided urine is submitted to determine the risk of tumor recurrence if treated with Bacillus Calmette–Guérin therapy.

Description of Procedure (0367U)

Analyze urine using a multiplexed immunoassay for A1AT, ANG, APOE, CA9, IL8, MMP9, MMP10, PAI1, SDC1, and VEGFA. Quantify each protein and using a bladder cancer proprietary algorithm, which includes tumor stage and grade, provide a risk score for the likelihood of rapid failure following transurethral resection.

Clinical Example (0368U)

A 50-year-old male presents with rectal bleeding and abdominal pain. Blood is submitted to evaluate the patient's risk for harboring advanced adenoma and/or colorectal cancer.

Description of Procedure (0368U)

Subject cfDNA from blood to PCR-based xeno nucleic acid technology to detect APC, BRAF, CTNNB1, KRAS, NRAS, PIK3CA, SMAD4, and TP53 mutations, and methylation markers for MYO1G, KCNQ5, C9ORF50, FLI1, CLIP4, ZNF132, and TWIST1. Determine the presence or absence of gene mutations and methylation associated with colorectal cancer and its precursors and generate a report using an algorithm to determine risk for harboring advanced adenoma and/or colorectal cancer.

Clinical Example (0369U)

A 35-year-old healthy female presents with abdominal pain and diarrhea for 4 days; CT scan shows abdominal inflammation. A fecal swab is submitted for analysis.

Description of Procedure (0369U)

Isolate and subject DNA and RNA from a fecal swab to amplification and load on predesigned open array for gene expression. A qualified laboratory professional reviews data and prepares a report and sends it to the ordering provider.

Clinical Example (0370U)

A 68-year-old male with a chronic wound infection presents to his physician. A swab is submitted to characterize the bacteria responsible for the wound and possible resistance.

Description of Procedure (0370U)

Isolate and treat DNA and RNA from a wound sample with primers for multiple bacteria and place on predesigned open array gene expression panel. Obtain data and analyze for each microbial target. A qualified laboratory professional interprets and reports the results to the ordering provider.

Clinical Example (0371U)

An 80-year-old male presents with a history of recurrent UTIs that have been unresponsive to several courses of antibiotics. His physician orders an infectious disease panel.

Description of Procedure (0371U)

Extract and subject DNA from urine to a multiplex amplified probe technique via RT-PCR for 17 pathogens (Acinetobacter baumannii, Citrobacter freundii, Enterobacter aerogenes, Enterobacter cloacae, Enterococcus faecalis, Enterococcus faecium, Escherichia coli, Klebsiella oxytoca, Klebsiella pneumoniae, Morganella morganii, Proteus mirabilis, Proteus vulgaris, Providencia stuartii, Pseudomonas aeruginosa, Staphylococcus saprophyticus, Streptococcus agalactiae, Candida albicans). Analyze results, which are reported as negative or positive, semi-quantitated.

Clinical Example (0372U)

An 80-year-old male presents with a history of recurrent UTIs that have been unresponsive to several courses of antibiotics. His physician orders an infectious disease panel, which is positive, and reflexes to antibiotic-resistance panel.

Description of Procedure (0372U)

Extract and subject DNA from urine to a multiplex amplified probe technique via RT-PCR for 23 antibiotic-resistance genes: APH(3')-VI, AAC(6')-lb, AAC(6')-lb-cr, blaMOX/blaCMY, blaCTX-M (subset 1), dfrA, gyrA, mcr-1/mcr-2, sul1/sul2, MecA/MecC, Mef(A)/Ere(B), VanA/VanB, blaKPC, blaIMP, blaNDM, blaVIM, blaOXA, blaFOX, blaTEM, erm(B), cfr, blaPER, blaCTX-M (subset 2). Analyze results and report using the Arkstone Antibiotic Stewardship score.

Clinical Example (0373U)

A 53-year-old female presents with flu-like symptoms and a negative coronavirus disease 2019 (COVID-19) test. A throat swab is submitted to identify the possible source of infection.

Description of Procedure (0373U)

Isolate and treat DNA and RNA from a respiratory specimen with primers for multiple pathogens and place on predesigned open array gene expression panel. Obtain data and analyze for each microbial target. A qualified laboratory professional interprets and reports results to the ordering provider.

Clinical Example (0374U)

A 45-year-old female with recurring UTIs returned with burning and frequency. A midstream urine sample is submitted to determine pathogens present and resistance patterns.

Description of Procedure (0374U)

Isolate and subject microbial nucleic acids from urine to undergo RT-PCR. A clinical laboratory scientist analyzes the data and prepares a report to show any organisms present and resistance. Send the information to the ordering provider.

Clinical Example (0375U)

A 45-year-old female presents with mild pelvic pain, and transvaginal ultrasound showed an adnexal mass, which

was considered indeterminate by the clinician. Serum is submitted to determine the risk for ovarian cancer.

Description of Procedure (0375U)

Analyze serum using electrochemiluminescence technology to determine the concentration of seven biomarker values. The proprietary algorithm produces a risk score for ovarian cancer, which is communicated to the ordering physician.

Clinical Example (0376U)

A 75-year-old male with intermediate risk prostate cancer (by National Comprehensive Cancer Network [NCCN] criteria) had histologic slides evaluated by augmentative algorithmic analysis to determine prognosis.

Description of Procedure (0376U)

Digitize FFPE prostate cancer specimens from the patient that have been stained with hematoxylin and eosin (H&E) using a whole-slide scanner for analysis. Combine clinical data and digitized images and analyze with algorithms using multilayer neural networks. Algorithms report prognostic scores and/or drug response classification as indicated based on the patient's NCCN-risk grouping.

Clinical Example (0377U)

A 51-year-old male presents with uncontrolled type 2 diabetes. Serum is submitted for an advanced lipoprotein profile to assess the patient's risk for cardiovascular disease.

Description of Procedure (0377U)

Analyze serum or plasma using two-dimensional nuclear magnetic resonance spectrometry. Process results using an algorithm to obtain quantitative data for advanced lipoprotein parameters. A qualified laboratory professional reviews the results and sends them to the ordering provider.

Clinical Example (0378U)

A 55-year-old female presents to her physician with ataxia, mild speech impairment, and a chronic cough. She has nystagmus and sensory neuropathy. She has two similarly affected siblings with balance issues. Blood is submitted for RFC1 repeat–expansion analysis.

Description of Procedure (0378U)

Isolate and subject DNA to PCR analysis across the repeat region of the RFC1 gene and repeat-prime PCR-specific for the normal and pathogenic repeat motifs within the RFC1 gene. A qualified laboratory professional analyzes the data and issues a report to the ordering provider.

Clinical Example (0379U)

A 53-year-old female with metastatic stage 4 lung cancer desires to maximize therapeutic options, including targeted therapy, immune/oncology-based therapy, and clinical trial enrollment. Her physician orders the solid tumor expanded panel.

Description of Procedure (0379U)

Extract genomic DNA and RNA from an FFPE-embedded sample. Interrogate PCR and NGS for 523 DNA and 55 RNA genes (for fusion detection only) for variant types, microsatellite instability (MSI), and TMB. A qualified laboratory professional reviews the data and issues a report to the physician.

Clinical Example (0380U)

A 23-year-old female with poor response to antidepressant therapy has a buccal swab sent for genetic testing to determine alternate antidepressant drug options.

Description of Procedure (0380U)

Isolate and analyze DNA from buccal smears on mass array spectra chip for 20 genes, including ABCB1, ANKK1/DRD2, APOE, COMT, CYP1A2, CYP2B6, CYP2C19, CYP2C9, CYP2D6, CYP3A4, CYP3A5, F2, F5, GLP1R, MTHFR, OPRM1, PNPLA5, SLCO1B1, SULT4A1, and VKORC1, and characterized by bioinformatics software. A qualified laboratory professional reviews the data, finalizes the report, and communicates it to the ordering provider.

Clinical Example (0381U)

An asymptomatic newborn male with maple syrup urine disease was identified via newborn screening. To prevent onset of symptoms, dietary restriction of branched chain amino acids was initiated. A dried blood spot (DBS) card is submitted to monitor clinical status and treatment efficacy.

Description of Procedure (0381U)

Send a collection kit to the patient's parent to self-collect a DBS card. Send the DBS to the laboratory for testing. Punch a 3-mm disk from the DBS onto a 96-well plate. Measure analytes by liquid chromatography-tandem mass spectrometry (LC-MS/MS). Report results to the ordering physician.

Clinical Example (0382U)

An asymptomatic newborn female with hyperphenylalaninemia was identified via newborn screening. To prevent onset of symptoms, dietary restriction of phenylalanine (Phe) was initiated. A DBS card is submitted to monitor clinical status and treatment efficacy.

Description of Procedure (0382U)

Send a collection kit to the patient's parent to self-collect a DBS card. Send the DBS to the laboratory for testing. Punch a 3-mm disk from the DBS onto a 96-well plate. Measure analytes by LC-MS/MS. Report results to the ordering physician.

Clinical Example (0383U)

An asymptomatic newborn male with tyrosinemia type I (hepatorenal tyrosinemia) was identified via newborn screening. To prevent onset of symptoms, dietary restriction of Phe and tyrosine was initiated in conjunction with nitisinone therapy. A DBS card is submitted to monitor ongoing clinical status and treatment efficacy.

Description of Procedure (0383U)

Send a collection kit to the patient's parent to self-collect a DBS card. Send the DBS card to the laboratory for testing. Punch a 3-mm disk from the DBS onto a 96-well plate. Measure analytes by LC-MS/MS. Report results to the ordering physician.

Clinical Example (0384U)

A 62-year-old female with type 2 diabetes, elevated hemoglobin A1c (HbA1c), and no clinical evidence of diabetic kidney disease presents to her physician. A fasting-blood specimen is submitted to predict her risk of developing diabetic kidney disease.

Description of Procedure (0384U)

Analyze advanced glycation end products (carboxymethyllysine, methylglyoxal hydroimidazolone, and carboxyethyl lysine) from a fasting-blood sample by LC-MS/MS. Combine those measurements in a proprietary algorithm with HbA1c and estimated glomerular rate (eGFR) results to calculate a predictive risk score for developing diabetic kidney disease.

Clinical Example (0385U)

A 74-year-old male with type 2 diabetes and other risk factors presents to his physician. He is asymptomatic for diabetic kidney disease. His compliance with medications and blood sugar control is subpar. Plasma is submitted to predict his risk for progression of kidney disease in the next 4 years.

Description of Procedure (0385U)

Analyze plasma from patient for ApoA4, CD5L, and IGFBP3 by ELISA. Measure high-density lipoprotein and eGFR (derived from creatinine) on a chemistry analyzer. A qualified laboratory professional inputs data for algorithmic analysis that returns risk scores for future disease. Review and send the report to the ordering provider.

Clinical Example (0387U)

A 57-year-old female has been diagnosed with early-stage primary cutaneous melanoma. To guidepost excision management, her oncologist requests that biopsy specimen be evaluated to assess the risk of progression.

Description of Procedure (0387U)

FFPE tissue sections from a non-ulcerated cutaneous melanoma specimen undergo immunohistochemistry staining for AMBRA1 and Loricrin. A trained laboratory professional analyzes the immunohistochemistry stains in conjunction with an H&E-stained slide of the same tissue and then scores results as "At-Risk" or "Low-Risk" for melanoma progression.

Clinical Example (0388U)

A 66-year-old male smoker presents with recent diagnosis of lung adenocarcinoma. Blood is submitted to identify targeted-therapy options.

Description of Procedure (0388U)

Extract and sequence cfDNA from plasma to detect the presence of single nucleotide variants, insertion deletions (Indels), copy number variations, and structural variants in 37 cancer-related genes. A qualified laboratory professional reviews the report that indicates the patient's mutation status and communicates the results to the ordering provider.

Clinical Example (0389U)

A 3-year-old male presents with a fever persisting for 5 days with redness of the lips and oral mucosa, a polymorphous exanthema, and non-purulent cervical lymphadenopathy. Whole blood is submitted to determine the risk for Kawasaki disease (KD).

Description of Procedure (0389U)

Subject RNA extracted from whole blood to reverse transcription PCR for IFI27 and MCEMP1. Examine quantified RNA values to determine a KD risk score. A qualified laboratory professional reviews the report specifying the risk for KD and communicates to the ordering provider.

Clinical Example (0390U)

A 25-year-old pregnant female presents with a history of pre-eclampsia before 20 weeks of pregnancy. Serum is submitted to assess the patient's serum protein biomarker levels to determine the risk of developing pre-eclampsia.

Description of Procedure (0390U)

Analyze serum for kinase insert domain receptor, endoglin, and retinol binding protein 4 by immunoassay. Evaluate concentrations of these biomarkers algorithmically to provide a pre-eclampsia risk-assessment score. A qualified laboratory professional reviews findings and issues a report specifying the risk to the ordering provider.

Clinical Example (0391U)

A 66-year-old female presents with stage IV estrogen receptors/progesterone receptors (ER/PR+) human epidermal growth factor receptor 2 (HER2)-negative breast cancer that has progressed on first-line therapy. Her physician submits tissue from the tumor to identify potential immunotherapy response.

Description of Procedure (0391U)

Isolate DNA and RNA from a solid tumor to undergo NGS by multiplex PCR. Assess select genes for RNA expression. Generate a report that includes genomic alterations and genomic signatures, including MSI and TMB, with an immunotherapy response score and associated therapies. A qualified laboratory professional reviews the report and communicates the results to the ordering physician.

Clinical Example (0392U)

A 35-year-old male on antidepressants started to experience bouts of drowsiness, insomnia, anxiety, and other reactions after unsuccessful multiple selective serotonin reuptake inhibitors (SSRI) medications. A buccal swab is submitted for genomic testing to assess the patient's gene/variant mutation status.

Description of Procedure (0392U)

Isolate and analyze DNA from a buccal swab for ADRA2A, COMT, CYP1A2, CYP2B6, DRD2, GRIK4, HTR2A, HTR2C, OPRM1, SLC6A4, CYP2C9, CYP2C19, CYP2D6, CYP3A4, CYP3A5, MTHFR by RT-PCR/fluorescence to detect clinically relevant genes with variant psychiatric mutations from wild type. A qualified laboratory professional provides results; a pharmacist reviews and prepares a report that communicates a pharmacogenomic analysis to the ordering provider.

★=Telemedicine ◀=Audio-only ✚=Add-on code ✐=FDA approval pending #=Resequenced code ⊘=Modifier 51 exempt

Clinical Example (0393U)

A 65-year-old female presents with findings of a possible parkinsonian neurodegenerative disorder. The ordering physician submits a CSF specimen to differentiate, confirm, or exclude the diagnosis.

Description of Procedure (0393U)

Subject CSF to qualitative seed amplification assay to detect misfolded aggregates of α-synuclein protein. A qualified laboratory professional reviews the fluorescence signals produced and applies an algorithm to classify the result as "Detected" or "Not Detected." Provide the report to the ordering physician.

Clinical Example (0394U)

A 51-year-old male with suspected exposure to per- and polyfluorinated substances (PFAS) presents to his physician. A plasma sample is submitted to determine exposure.

Description of Procedure (0394U)

Analyze plasma or serum by high-performance liquid chromatography/tandem mass spectrometry (HPLC-MS/MS) for 16 PFAS compounds and report quantitatively with a calculated National Academies of Science, Engineering and Medicine (NASEM) summation value (NASEM guidance value).

Clinical Example (0395U)

A 65-year-old female smoker has an indeterminant 1.5-cm lesion found on low-dose CT. Plasma is submitted to assist in determining the risk category of malignancy.

Description of Procedure (0395U)

Subject plasma to shotgun NGS to detect microbial DNA and immunoassay to determine carcinoembryonic antigen and osteopontin. A qualified laboratory professional combines results with patient data (eg, gender and age) and lung nodule characteristics to determine a lung cancer malignancy risk category for lung cancer. Communicate results to the ordering provider.

Clinical Example (0396U)

A couple, each with a deletion in the SMN1 gene, present to the obstetrician. Because there is a 25% chance with each pregnancy for a child with spinal muscular atrophy, they decide to pursue in-vitro fertilization with preimplantation genetic testing. Embryo biopsy samples are submitted for evaluation.

Description of Procedure (0396U)

Individually analyze embryonic samples using whole genome amplification. Analysis includes an algorithm that references parental genotypes to the result. The report states which embryos are affected or unaffected and aneuploid or euploid.

Clinical Example (0398U)

A 50-year-old male with gastrointestinal reflux undergoes upper endoscopy and is found to have non-dysplastic Barrett's esophagus. Tissue is submitted to determine the risk for future advanced disease.

Description of Procedure (0398U)

Extract DNA from FFPE tissue. Analyze purified DNA for P16, HPP1, RUNX3, and FBN1 plus beta-actin (internal control) using methylation-specific PCR. Add normalized methylation values into a multigene algorithm to develop a risk score. A qualified laboratory professional reviews findings and sends report to the ordering provider.

Clinical Example (0399U)

A 2-year-old female presents with developmental delay. The physician orders a blood test for the analysis of folate receptor alpha autoantibodies.

Description of Procedure (0399U)

Subject serum to enzyme-linked immunoassays for autoantibodies against folate receptors and/or binding affinity studies. Analyze results and issue a report to health care provider.

Clinical Example (0400U)

A 28-year-old pregnant female presents to her obstetrician for routine prenatal care who orders an expanded carrier screening to rule out the risk for the child having a genetic disorder.

Description of Procedure (0400U)

Isolate and subject high-quality genomic DNA from whole blood to NGS, PCR with fragment analysis, and multiplex ligation probe-dependent amplification of 145 genes. A laboratory professional analyzes the data and composes a report.

Clinical Example (0401U)

A 45-year-old male presents to his physician with cardiovascular risk factors. Blood, saliva, or buccal swab is submitted to determine polygenic risk of coronary artery disease.

Description of Procedure (0401U)

Isolate and subject high-quality genomic DNA from blood, saliva, or buccal swab to hydrolysis probe analysis for genetic variants (AL0X5AP, CDKN2A/B, SLC5A3/KCNE2, LPA, TAF1A, MRAS, PHACTR1, WDR12, CXCL12). The algorithm generates a risk score from the data. A qualified laboratory professional reviews the findings and composes a report.

Clinical Example (0402U)

A 24-year-old female presents with vaginal discharge and dysuria. A vaginal swab is collected in viral transport media and is sent to the laboratory for Chlamydia trachomatis, Neisseria gonorrhoeae, Trichomonas vaginalis, and Mycoplasma genitalium.

Description of Procedure (0402U)

Extract and rehydrate nucleic acid and perform target nucleic acid amplification using PCR probes for Chlamydia trachomatis, Neisseria gonorrhoeae, Trichomonas vaginalis, and Mycoplasma genitalium. A laboratory professional reviews the findings and issues a report to the ordering provider.

Clinical Example (0403U)

A 65-year-old male presents with an elevated prostate-specific antigen level of 9.3 ng/mL. A urologist performs a digital rectal examination and obtains the first-catch urine sample.

Description of Procedure (0403U)

Subject a first post-digital rectal examination urine collection to qPCR to analyze 18 biomarkers. Calculate score using a proprietary algorithm that reports as a percentage risk for clinically significant prostate cancer.

Clinical Example (0404U)

A 60-year-old female presents to her oncologist with metastatic hormone receptor positive, HER2-negative breast cancer. Serum is submitted to determine thymidine kinase activity.

Description of Procedure (0404U)

Subject serum to a multistep end-point ELISA. Use supplied calibrators to generate a standard curve by which the optical density (OD) readings from the patient are converted to thymidine kinase activity. A qualified laboratory professional reviews the results and reports them to the ordering provider.

Clinical Example (0405U)

A 50-year-old female presents with a family history of pancreatic cancer and upper gastrointestinal pain. Blood is submitted to assess if the patient has developed pancreatic cancer.

Description of Procedure (0405U)

Isolate cfDNA from plasma and subject to bisulfite treatment NGS. Compare the methylation haplotype blocks signals from NGS data to a proprietary model. A qualified laboratory professional reviews the findings and issues a report to the ordering provider.

Clinical Example (0406U)

A 66-year-old male smoker with a 6-mm lung nodule found on CT scan submits a sputum sample to determine the likelihood of malignancy.

Description of Procedure (0406U)

Process sputum to create a single-cell suspension and stain with TCPP, CD206, CD66b, CD3, CD19, and FVS510 markers. Use flow cytometry to quantify these markers and use a proprietary algorithm to evaluate data combined with the patient's age to produce a score reflecting the likelihood of lung cancer. A qualified laboratory professional reviews the findings and issues a report to the ordering provider.

Clinical Example (0407U)

A 60-year-old female presents with hypertension and type 2 diabetes, eGFR 65 mL/min/1.73 m2, and a urine albumin/creatinine ratio of 50 mg/g. Plasma is submitted to determine the risk for progressive decline in renal function.

Description of Procedure (0407U)

Analyze plasma isolated from peripheral blood using an electrochemiluminescence immunoassay to quantify soluble tumor necrosis factor receptor 1 and 2 and the kidney injury molecule 1. Evaluate results combined with clinical data using an algorithm to predict risk of progressive decline in kidney function over 5 years for a patient with type 2 diabetes. A qualified laboratory professional reviews the results and reports them to the ordering provider.

Clinical Example (0408U)

A 40-year-old male presents with slight respiratory distress and an infrequent cough. An anterior nasal swab is submitted for rapid antigen-based detection.

★ = Telemedicine   ◀ = Audio-only   ✚ = Add-on code   ✗ = FDA approval pending   # = Resequenced code   ⊘ = Modifier 51 exempt

Description of Procedure (0408U)

Extract nasal secretions using lysis buffer and add to the cartridge chamber. Through an enzymatically enhanced reaction, the sample is bound to the bulk acoustic wave (BAW) biosensor and undergoes immunohistochemical analysis of the frequency shift within the BAW. A QHP reviews the results and communicates them directly to the patient.

Clinical Example (0409U)

A 76-year-old male presents with recently diagnosed lung cancer. Blood is submitted to identify biomarkers to guide treatment selection.

Description of Procedure (0409U)

Whole blood undergoes plasma extraction, nucleic acid extraction, and library preparation and sequencing to identify DNA and RNA mutations, including single-nucleotide variants, insertions/deletions, copy number alterations, microsatellite instability, and fusions. A qualified laboratory professional reviews the variant cells and issues a report to the treating physician.

Clinical Example (0410U)

A 65-year-old male presents with recent onset of type 2 diabetes, poor glycemic control, and weight loss. Blood is submitted to evaluate for the presence or absence of pancreatic ductal adenocarcinoma.

Description of Procedure (0410U)

Extract cfDNA from the plasma to undergo library preparation involving enrichment of genome-wide 5-hydroxymethylation and a parallel low-coverage whole genome sequencing (1x). Enter sequencing data into an algorithm for classification. A qualified laboratory professional reviews the findings and provides a report to the ordering provider showing the presence or absence of pancreatic cancer.

Clinical Example (0411U)

A 72-year-old female is diagnosed with major depressive disorder and prescribed an SSRI. She reports skipping doses due to side effects and asks her physician about other treatment options. A buccal swab is submitted for pharmacogenetic analysis to help guide treatment decision making.

Description of Procedure (0411U)

Isolate and subject high-quality genomic DNA from a buccal swab to hydrolysis probe and capillary electrophoresis techniques for variants in 15 genes

(ABCB1, ADRA2A, COMT, CYP1A2, CYP2C19, CYP2C9, CYP2D6, CYP3A4, CYP3A5, HTR2A, HTR2C, MTHFR, NAT2, OPRM1, and SLC6A4) and CYP2D6 copy number. Compose a report based on patient-specific drug-gene, drug-drug interactions, and lifestyle factors. A qualified laboratory professional evaluates the findings and provides the results to the ordering provider.

Clinical Example (0412U)

A 72-year-old female presents with progressive cognitive decline. Blood is submitted to assess the presence or absence of brain amyloid pathology.

Description of Procedure (0412U)

Process plasma using LC-MS/MS and Aß42/Aß40 ratio. Combine APOE isoform results with the patient's age to generate an amyloid probability score. A qualified laboratory professional reviews the report and communicates the findings to the ordering physician.

Clinical Example (0413U)

A 54-year-old male presents with AML. Blood is submitted for cytogenomic analysis.

Extract megabase-sized genomic DNA to undergo optical genome mapping to detect structural and copy number variants. The pathologist or other QHP analyzes the data and composes a report.

Description of Procedure (0413U)

Extract megabase-sized genomic DNA to undergo optical genome mapping to detect structural and copy number variants. The pathologist or other QHP analyzes the data and composes a report.

Clinical Example (0414U)

A 67-year-old male presents with shortness of breath and hemoptysis. Biopsy confirms early-stage on-small cell lung cancer. Tissue is submitted to help guide patient management.

Description of Procedure (0414U)

Evaluate FFPE lung tumor slides using artificial intelligence of H&E–stained slides for 8 genes (ALK, BRAF, EGFR, ERBB2, MET, NTRK1-3, RET, ROS1), and KRAS G12C and PD-L1, if ordered. A proprietary algorithm detects variants and/or rearrangements. A qualified laboratory professional review results for each gene and report to the ordering provider.

Clinical Example (0415U)

A 66-year-old male presents with fatigue and shortness of breath. The physician submits a blood sample to determine the presence of vascular inflammation.

Description of Procedure (0415U)

Analyze serum for IL-16, FAS, FASLigand, HGF, CTACK, EOTAXIN, and MCP-3 using a multiplexed chemiluminescence sandwich immunoassay. Combine results in an algorithm to produce an absolute probability score. A qualified laboratory professional reviews the findings and reports them to the ordering provider.

Clinical Example (0416U)

A 75-year-old female presents with recurrent and resistant UTIs. Urine is sent to the laboratory to assess for infectious pathogens and antibiotic resistance, if needed.

Description of Procedure (0416U)

Extract cellular DNA from urine via magnetic bead separation and nucleotide purification, followed by DNA amplification using RT-PCR to identify 15 bacterial and five fungal pathogens. A positive bacterial infection triggers a reflex to antibiotic-resistance gene reporting. A qualified laboratory professional analyzes the data and reports findings to the ordering provider.

Clinical Example (0417U)

A 15-year-old male presents with migraines, seizures, tremor, weight loss, poor appetite, hyperuricosuria, electroencephalogram changes, and other neurologic findings. Blood is submitted to identify if a genetic variant known to cause mitochondrial disorder(s) is responsible for the patient's clinical presentation.

Description of Procedure (0417U)

Isolate and sequence high-quality genomic DNA from blood or saliva. Perform whole mitochondrial genome sequencing, including heteroplasmy detection and deletion analysis. Evaluate a total of 335 nuclear-encoded mitochondrial genes for sequence changes, deletions, insertions, and copy number variants analysis. A qualified laboratory professional examines genetic variants and correlates them with the patient's phenotype, matching the phenotype and observed variants for pathogenicity based on American College of Medical Genetics and Genomics guidelines. A report specifying the findings is issued to the ordering provider.

Clinical Example (0418U)

A 51-year-old postmenopausal female was recently diagnosed with invasive breast cancer with two positive lymph nodes. The biopsy is submitted for further evaluation to determine the risk of recurrence.

Description of Procedure (0418U)

Interrogate H&E digital whole-slide scanned images from an invasive breast cancer biopsy with image analysis software. Evaluate eight features and combine morphometric features with clinical data using an algorithm to produce a risk of recurrence. A qualified laboratory professional prepares and sends the report to the ordering provider.

Clinical Example (0419U)

A 23-year-old male on treatment for depression presents with agitation and increased appetite. Symptoms persisted despite a medication change. Saliva is submitted to assess genetic alterations and metabolism status.

Description of Procedure (0419U)

Isolate DNA from saliva or buccal swab for genomic sequence analysis by matrix-assisted laser desorption ionization–time-of-flight for nine pharmacokinetic genes (CYP1A2, CYP2B6, CYP2C19, CYP2C9, CYP2D6, CYP3A4, CYP3A5, UGT1A4, UGT2B15); two pharmacodynamic genes (HTR2A, SLC6A4); and two immunological genes (HLA-A, HLA-B). Use capillary electrophoresis for CYP2D6 deletion/duplication analysis. A qualified laboratory professional reviews and reports the genetic results, metabolism status, and gene–drug interactions to the ordering provider.

★ = Telemedicine ◀ = Audio-only ✚ = Add-on code ⅄ = FDA approval pending # = Resequenced code ⊘ = Modifier 51 exempt

Medicine

Summary of Additions, Deletions, and Revisions

The summary of changes shows the actual changes that have been made to the code descriptors.

New codes appear with a bullet (●) and are indicated as "Code added." Revised codes are preceded with a triangle (▲). Within revised codes, or if a code symbol has been deleted, the deleted language and code symbol appear with a ~~strikethrough~~, while new text appears <u>underlined</u>.

The ✔ symbol is used to identify codes for vaccines that are pending FDA approval. The # symbol is used to identify codes that have been resequenced. CPT add-on codes are annotated by the ✚ symbol. The ⊘ symbol is used to identify codes that are exempt from the use of modifier 51. The ★ symbol is used to identify codes that may be used for reporting telemedicine services. The ✗ is used to identify proprietary laboratory analyses (PLA) test that has an identical descriptor as another PLA test. A PLA code that satisfies Category I code criteria and has been accepted by the CPT Editorial Panel is annotated with the ↕ symbol. The ◀ symbol is used to identify codes that may be used to report audio-only telemedicine services when appended by modifier 93 **(see Appendix T)**.

Code	Description
●**90380**	Code added
●**90381**	Code added
#●**0121A**	Code added
#▲**0124A**	~~Immunization administration by intramuscular injection of severe acute respiratory syndrome coronavirus 2 (SARS-CoV-2) (coronavirus disease [COVID-19]) vaccine, mRNA-LNP, bivalent spike protein, preservative free, 30 mcg/0.3 mL dosage, tris-sucrose formulation,; booster~~<u>additional</u> dose
#●**0151A**	Code added
#▲**0154A**	~~Immunization administration by intramuscular injection of severe acute respiratory syndrome coronavirus 2 (SARS-CoV-2) (coronavirus disease [COVID-19]) vaccine, mRNA-LNP, bivalent spike protein, preservative free, 10 mcg/0.2 mL dosage, diluent reconstituted, tris-sucrose formulation,; booster~~<u>additional</u> dose
#●**0171A**	Code added
#●**0172A**	Code added
#▲**0173A**	~~Immunization administration by intramuscular injection of severe acute respiratory syndrome coronavirus 2 (SARS-CoV-2) (coronavirus disease [COVID-19]) vaccine, mRNA-LNP, bivalent spike protein, preservative free, 3 mcg/0.2 mL dosage, diluent reconstituted, tris-sucrose formulation, third dose;~~ <u>third dose</u>
#▲**0174A**	~~booster~~<u>additional</u> dose
#▲**0134A**	Immunization administration by intramuscular injection of severe acute respiratory syndrome coronavirus 2 (SARS-CoV-2) (coronavirus disease [COVID-19]) vaccine, mRNA-LNP, spike protein, bivalent, preservative free, 50 mcg/0.5 mL dosage, ~~booster~~<u>additional</u> dose
#●**0141A**	Code added
#●**0142A**	Code added

▲ = Revised code ● = New code ▶ ◀ = Contains new or revised text ✗ = Duplicate PLA test ↕ = Category I PLA American Medical Association **109**

Medicine 90281-99607

Code	Description
#▲0144A	~~Immunization administration by intramuscular injection of severe acute respiratory syndrome coronavirus 2 (SARS-CoV-2) (coronavirus disease [COVID-19]) vaccine, mRNA-LNP, spike protein, bivalent, preservative free, 25 mcg/0.25 mL dosage,; booster~~additional dose
#●0091A	Code added
#●0092A	Code added
#●0093A	Code added
#▲0094A	~~Immunization administration by intramuscular injection of severe acute respiratory syndrome coronavirus 2 (SARS-CoV-2) (coronavirus disease [COVID-19]) vaccine, mRNA-LNP, spike protein, preservative free, 50 mcg/0.5 mL dosage,;~~ booster dose, when administered to individuals 18 years and older
●0044A	Code added
●0113A	Code added
▲0164A	Immunization administration by intramuscular injection of severe acute respiratory syndrome coronavirus 2 (SARS-CoV-2) (coronavirus disease [COVID-19]) vaccine, mRNA-LNP, spike protein, bivalent, preservative free, 10 mcg/0.2 mL dosage, ~~booster~~additional dose
#●91312	Code added
#●91315	Code added
#●91317	Code added
#●91313	Code added
#●91314	Code added
#●91316	Code added
#✎●90589	Code added
●90679	Code added
#✎●90683	Code added
#●90611	Code added
#●90622	Code added
#✎●90623	Code added
●92622	Code added
✛●92623	Code added
#✛●92972	Code added
#●93150	Code added
#●93151	Code added
#●93152	Code added
#●93153	Code added
#✛●93584	Code added

★ =Telemedicine   ◀ =Audio-only   ✛ =Add-on code   ✎ =FDA approval pending   # =Resequenced code   ⊘ =Modifier 51 exempt

Code	Description
#+●93585	Code added
#+●93586	Code added
#+●93587	Code added
#+●93588	Code added
▲96446	Chemotherapy administration into the peritoneal cavity via ~~indwelling~~ implanted port or catheter
+●96547	Code added
+●96548	Code added
▲96920	Excimer ~~L~~laser treatment for ~~inflammatory skin disease~~ (psoriasis); total area less than 250 sq cm
▲96921	250 sq cm to 500 sq cm
▲96922	over 500 sq cm
#●97037	Code added
●97550	Code added
+●97551	Code added
●97552	Code added

Medicine

Immune Globulins, Serum or Recombinant Products

Codes 90281-90399 identify the serum globulins, extracted from human blood; or recombinant immune globulin products created in a laboratory through genetic modification of human and/or animal proteins. Both are reported in addition to the administration codes 96365, 96366, 96367, 96368, 96369, 96370, 96371, 96372, 96374, 96375, as appropriate. Modifier 51 should not be reported with this section of products codes when performed with another procedure. The serum or recombinant globulin products listed here include broad-spectrum anti-infective immune globulins, antitoxins, various isoantibodies, and monoclonal antibodies. See the Introduction section of the CPT code set for a complete list of the dates of release and implementation.

▶To assist users in reporting the most recent new or revised immune globulin product codes, the American Medical Association (AMA) currently uses the CPT website (ama-assn.org/cpt-cat-i-immunization-codes) to feature updates from the CPT Editorial Panel actions regarding these products. See the Introduction section of the CPT code set for a complete list of the dates of release and implementation.

In recognition of public health interest in immune globulin products, the CPT Editorial Panel has chosen to publish new immune globulin product codes prior to approval by the US Food and Drug Administration (FDA). These codes are indicated with the ∕ symbol and will be tracked by the AMA to monitor FDA approval status. Once the FDA status changes to approved, the ∕ symbol will be removed. CPT code users should refer to the AMA CPT website (ama-assn.org/cpt-cat-i-immunization-codes) for the most up-to-date information on codes with the ∕ symbol.◀

Rationale

Guidelines in the Medicine/Immune Globulins, Serum or Recombinant Products subsection have been revised to amend the intended use of the US Food and Drug Administration (FDA) approval in recognition of public health interests. Therefore, these codes will carry the FDA approval-pending symbol (∕) similar to vaccine products that are awaiting such approval.

Previously, the FDA approval-pending symbol was intended to be reported for vaccine/toxoids products only. However, by adding immune globulin products in the guidelines and immune globulin product codes with the

FDA approval-pending symbol in the CPT 2024 code set, technological advancements in medicine and the growth in use of immune globulins to provide patients with immunity against infection for diseases, including the use of passive immunity (ie, short-term immunity that results from the introduction of antibodies from another person or animal) to treat patients, the importance of public health interest is taken into consideration and enabled in the CPT code set.

In addition, the use of the FDA approval-pending symbol (∕) also indicates that evidence substantiating completion of Phase III clinical trials and review of unblinded data has been provided although the product has not received the FDA's approval.

To support these revisions, the introduction for Appendix K (Product Pending FDA Approval) has been revised as well.

The change will also be reflected within appropriate locations of the code change application to provide initial instruction to users regarding the new intent for use of the symbol and criteria for assignment/usage and code development.

Because immune globulin products will be part of the CPT codes with the FDA approval-pending symbol (∕), interim updates on the FDA status of these codes will be reflected on the American Medical Association (AMA) CPT website at https://www.ama-assn.org/system/files/vaccine-long-descriptors.pdf, under the CPT Category I Vaccine Codes.

90378 Respiratory syncytial virus, monoclonal antibody, recombinant, for intramuscular use, 50 mg, each

● **90380** Respiratory syncytial virus, monoclonal antibody, seasonal dose; 0.5 mL dosage, for intramuscular use

● **90381** 1 mL dosage, for intramuscular use

Rationale

Immune globulin product codes 90380 and 90381 have been established in the Immune Globulins, Serum or Recombinant Products subsection to report respiratory syncytial monoclonal antibody used for immunization against respiratory syncytial virus (RSV) infection. In addition, guidelines and parenthetical notes have been added, revised, or deleted to accommodate the changes, to direct users to the appropriate codes to report immune globulin product used for RSV immunization, and to provide instruction regarding appropriate coding for immune globulin administration.

Immune globulin product codes 90380 and 90381 are intended to be used for reporting seasonal immunization against respiratory disease caused by RSV. Specifically,

★ = Telemedicine   ◀ = Audio-only   ✚ = Add-on code   ∕ = FDA approval pending   # = Resequenced code   ⦵ = Modifier 51 exempt use of this product affords patients passive immunity (ie, short-term immunity that results from the introduction of antibodies from another person or animal) for the prevention of lower respiratory tract infection caused by RSV. Administration of the immune globulin is reported separately using immune globulin and monoclonal antibodies administration codes (96365-96372, 96374, 96375).

The Centers for Disease Control and Prevention (CDC) Advisory Committee on Immunization Practices (ACIP) has not assigned a US vaccine/immune globulin abbreviation for this product. Visit the AMA CPT website for updates on the US vaccine/immune abbreviation status for this immunization product.

Clinical Example (90380)

A parent or guardian of a child seeks protection for their child against the respiratory syncytial virus (RSV) infection to decrease the risk of contracting this disease. The physician or other qualified health care professional (QHP) determines that the child is an appropriate candidate for RSV immunization and orders its administration.

Description of Procedure (90380)

The physician or other QHP selects the appropriate RSV immunization dosage, obtains informed consent from the child's parent or guardian, and dispenses a dose of the RSV immunoglobulin. Report the administration of the immunoglobulin separately.

Clinical Example (90381)

A parent or guardian of a child seeks protection for their child against RSV infection to decrease the risk of contracting this disease. The physician or other QHP determines that the child is an appropriate candidate for RSV immunization and orders its administration.

Description of Procedure (90381)

The physician or other QHP selects the appropriate RSV immunization dosage, obtains informed consent from the child's parent or guardian, and dispenses the dose of the RSV immunoglobulin. Report the administration of the immunoglobulin separately.

Immunization Administration for Vaccines/Toxoids

▶Report vaccine immunization administration codes (90460, 90461, 90471-90474, 0001A, 0002A, 0003A, 0004A, 0011A, 0012A, 0013A, 0021A, 0022A, 0031A, 0034A, 0041A, 0042A, 0044A, 0051A, 0052A, 0053A, 0054A, 0064A, 0071A, 0072A, 0073A, 0074A, 0081A, 0082A, 0083A, 0091A, 0092A, 0093A, 0094A, 0104A, 0111A, 0112A, 0113A, 0121A, 0124A, 0134A, 0141A, 0142A, 0144A, 0151A, 0154A, 0164A, 0171A, 0172A, 0173A, 0174A) in addition to the vaccine and toxoid code(s) (90476-90759, 91300-91317).◀

Report codes 90460 and 90461 only when the physician or other qualified health care professional provides face-to-face counseling of the patient/family during the administration of a vaccine other than when performed for severe acute respiratory syndrome coronavirus 2 (SARS-CoV-2) (coronavirus disease [COVID-19]) vaccines. For immunization administration of any vaccine, other than SARS-CoV-2 (coronavirus disease [COVID-19]) vaccines, that is not accompanied by face-to-face physician or other qualified health care professional counseling to the patient/family/guardian or for administration of vaccines to patients over 18 years of age, report codes 90471-90474. (See also **Instructions for Use of the CPT Codebook** for definition of reporting qualifications.)

▶Report 0001A, 0002A, 0003A, 0004A, 0011A, 0012A, 0013A, 0021A, 0022A, 0031A, 0034A, 0041A, 0042A, 0044A, 0051A, 0052A, 0053A, 0054A, 0064A, 0071A, 0072A, 0073A, 0074A, 0081A, 0082A, 0083A, 0091A, 0092A, 0093A, 0094A, 0104A, 0111A, 0112A, 0113A, 0121A, 0124A, 0134A, 0141A, 0142A, 0144A, 0151A, 0154A, 0164A, 0171A, 0172A, 0173A, 0174A for immunization administration of SARS-CoV-2 (coronavirus disease [COVID-19]) vaccines only. Each administration code is specific to each individual vaccine product (eg, 91300-91317), the dosage schedule (eg, first dose, second dose), and counseling, when performed. The appropriate administration code is chosen based on the type of vaccine and the specific dose number the patient receives in the schedule. For example, 0012A is reported for the second dose of vaccine 91301. Do not report 90460-90474 for the administration of SARS-CoV-2 (coronavirus disease [COVID-19]) vaccines. Codes related to SARS-CoV-2 (coronavirus disease [COVID-19]) vaccine administration are listed in Appendix Q, with their associated vaccine code descriptors, vaccine administration codes, patient age, vaccine manufacturer, vaccine name(s), National Drug Code (NDC) Labeler Product ID, and interval between doses. In order to report these codes, the vaccine must fulfill the code descriptor and must be the vaccine represented by the manufacturer and vaccine name listed in Appendix Q.◀

Medicine 90281-99607

Rationale

The codes listed in the Immunization Administration for Vaccines/Toxoids guidelines have been updated to reflect the ranges and codes added for reporting coronavirus disease 2019 (COVID-19) vaccinations.

Refer to the codebook and the Rationale for COVID-19 administration codes for a full discussion of these changes.

If a significant separately identifiable evaluation and management service (eg, new or established patient office or other outpatient services [99202-99215], office or other outpatient consultations [99242, 99243, 99244, 99245], emergency department services [99281-99285], preventive medicine services [99381-99429]) is performed, the appropriate E/M service code should be reported in addition to the vaccine and toxoid administration codes.

▶For immune globulins and monoclonal antibodies immunizations, see 90281-90399. For administration of immune globulins and monoclonal antibodies immunizations, see 96365, 96366, 96367, 96368, 96369, 96370, 96371, 96372, 96374.◄

Rationale

To accommodate the addition of immune globulin product codes 90380 and 90381, guidelines have been added within the Immunization Administration for Vaccines/Toxoids subsection to direct users to the appropriate codes to report immune globulins and monoclonal antibodies immunizations and their administration. In addition, a parenthetical note following code 90472 with this same information has been removed because this language is now located in the guidelines.

Refer to the codebook and the Rationale for the Immune Globulins, Serum, or Recombinant Products guidelines for a full discussion of these changes.

90460   Immunization administration through 18 years of age via any route of administration, with counseling by physician or other qualified health care professional; first or only component of each vaccine or toxoid administered

+ 90461   each additional vaccine or toxoid component administered (List separately in addition to code for primary procedure)

(Use 90460 for each vaccine administered. For vaccines with multiple components [combination vaccines], report 90460 in conjunction with 90461 for each additional component in a given vaccine)

▶(Do not report 90460, 90461 in conjunction with 91300-91317, unless both a severe acute respiratory syndrome coronavirus 2 [SARS-CoV-2] [coronavirus disease {COVID-19}] vaccine/toxoid product and at least one vaccine/toxoid product from 90476-90759 are administered at the same encounter)◄

90471   Immunization administration (includes percutaneous, intradermal, subcutaneous, or intramuscular injections); 1 vaccine (single or combination vaccine/toxoid)

(Do not report 90471 in conjunction with 90473)

+ 90472   each additional vaccine (single or combination vaccine/toxoid) (List separately in addition to code for primary procedure)

(Use 90472 in conjunction with 90460, 90471, 90473)

▶(Do not report 90471, 90472 in conjunction with 91300-91317, unless both a severe acute respiratory syndrome coronavirus 2 [SARS-CoV-2] [coronavirus disease {COVID-19}] vaccine/toxoid product and at least one vaccine/toxoid product from 90476-90759 are administered at the same encounter)◄

(For intravesical administration of BCG vaccine, see 51720, 90586)

90473   Immunization administration by intranasal or oral route; 1 vaccine (single or combination vaccine/toxoid)

(Do not report 90473 in conjunction with 90471)

+ 90474   each additional vaccine (single or combination vaccine/toxoid) (List separately in addition to code for primary procedure)

(Use 90474 in conjunction with 90460, 90471, 90473)

▶(Do not report 90473, 90474 in conjunction with 91300-91317, unless both a severe acute respiratory syndrome coronavirus 2 [SARS-CoV-2] [coronavirus disease {COVID-19}] vaccine/toxoid product and at least one vaccine/toxoid product from 90476-90759 are administered at the same encounter)◄

0001A   Immunization administration by intramuscular injection of severe acute respiratory syndrome coronavirus 2 (SARS-CoV-2) (coronavirus disease [COVID-19]) vaccine, mRNA-LNP, spike protein, preservative free, 30 mcg/0.3 mL dosage, diluent reconstituted; first dose

0002A   second dose

0003A   third dose

0004A   booster dose

(Report 0001A, 0002A, 0003A, 0004A for the administration of vaccine 91300)

▶(Do not report 0001A, 0002A, 0003A, 0004A in conjunction with 91305, 91307, 91308, 91312, 91315, 91317)◄

0051A   Immunization administration by intramuscular injection of severe acute respiratory syndrome coronavirus 2 (SARS-CoV-2) (coronavirus disease [COVID-19]) vaccine, mRNA-LNP, spike protein, preservative free, 30 mcg/0.3 mL dosage, tris-sucrose formulation; first dose

0052A   second dose

0053A   third dose

0054A   booster dose

(Report 0051A, 0052A, 0053A, 0054A for the administration of vaccine 91305)

►(Do not report 0051A, 0052A, 0053A, 0054A in conjunction with 91300, 91307, 91308, 91312, 91315, 91317)◄

#● 0121A   Immunization administration by intramuscular injection of severe acute respiratory syndrome coronavirus 2 (SARS-CoV-2) (coronavirus disease [COVID-19]) vaccine, mRNA-LNP, bivalent spike protein, preservative free, 30 mcg/0.3 mL dosage, tris-sucrose formulation; single dose

#▲ 0124A   additional dose

►(Report 0121A, 0124A for the administration of vaccine 91312)◄

►(Do not report 0121A, 0124A in conjunction with 91300, 91305, 91307, 91308, 91315, 91317)◄

0071A   Immunization administration by intramuscular injection of severe acute respiratory syndrome coronavirus 2 (SARS-CoV-2) (coronavirus disease [COVID-19]) vaccine, mRNA-LNP, spike protein, preservative free, 10 mcg/0.2 mL dosage, diluent reconstituted, tris-sucrose formulation; first dose

0072A   second dose

0073A   third dose

0074A   booster dose

(Report 0071A, 0072A, 0073A, 0074A for the administration of vaccine 91307)

►(Do not report 0071A, 0072A, 0073A, 0074A in conjunction with 91300, 91305, 91308, 91312, 91315, 91317)◄

#● 0151A   Immunization administration by intramuscular injection of severe acute respiratory syndrome coronavirus 2 (SARS-CoV-2) (coronavirus disease [COVID-19]) vaccine, mRNA-LNP, bivalent spike protein, preservative free, 10 mcg/0.2 mL dosage, diluent reconstituted, tris-sucrose formulation; single dose

#▲ 0154A   additional dose

►(Report 0151A, 0154A for the administration of vaccine 91315)◄

►(Do not report 0151A, 0154A in conjunction with 91300, 91305, 91307, 91308, 91312, 91317)◄

0081A   Immunization administration by intramuscular injection of severe acute respiratory syndrome coronavirus 2 (SARS-CoV-2) (coronavirus disease [COVID-19]) vaccine, mRNA-LNP, spike protein, preservative free, 3 mcg/0.2 mL dosage, diluent reconstituted, tris-sucrose formulation; first dose

0082A   second dose

0083A   third dose

(Report 0081A, 0082A, 0083A for the administration of vaccine 91308)

►(Do not report 0081A, 0082A, 0083A in conjunction with 91300, 91305, 91307, 91312, 91315, 91317)◄

#● 0171A   Immunization administration by intramuscular injection of severe acute respiratory syndrome coronavirus 2 (SARS-CoV-2) (coronavirus disease [COVID-19]) vaccine, mRNA-LNP, bivalent spike protein, preservative free, 3 mcg/0.2 mL dosage, diluent reconstituted, tris-sucrose formulation; first dose

#● 0172A   second dose

#▲ 0173A   third dose

#▲ 0174A   additional dose

►(Report 0171A, 0172A, 0173A, 0174A for the administration of vaccine 91317)◄

►(Use 0174A in conjunction with 91317 when used as an additional dose administration of primary series for 91308, [ie, following administration of 0081A, 0082A, 0083A])◄

►(Do not report 0171A, 0172A, 0173A, 0174A in conjunction with 91300, 91305, 91307, 91308, 91312, 91315)◄

0011A   Immunization administration by intramuscular injection of severe acute respiratory syndrome coronavirus 2 (SARS-CoV-2) (coronavirus disease [COVID-19]) vaccine, mRNA-LNP, spike protein, preservative free, 100 mcg/0.5 mL dosage; first dose

0012A   second dose

0013A   third dose

(Report 0011A, 0012A, 0013A for the administration of vaccine 91301)

►(Do not report 0011A, 0012A, 0013A in conjunction with 91306, 91309, 91311, 91313, 91314, 91316)◄

0064A   Immunization administration by intramuscular injection of severe acute respiratory syndrome coronavirus 2 (SARS-CoV-2) (coronavirus disease [COVID-19]) vaccine, mRNA-LNP, spike protein, preservative free, 50 mcg/0.25 mL dosage, booster dose

(Report 0064A for the administration of vaccine 91306)

►(Do not report 0064A in conjunction with 91301, 91309, 91311, 91313, 91314, 91316)◄

#▲ **0134A** Immunization administration by intramuscular injection of severe acute respiratory syndrome coronavirus 2 (SARS-CoV-2) (coronavirus disease [COVID-19]) vaccine, mRNA-LNP, spike protein, bivalent, preservative free, 50 mcg/0.5 mL dosage, additional dose

▶(Report 0134A for the administration of vaccine 91313)◀

▶(Do not report 0134A in conjunction with 91301, 91306, 91309, 91311, 91314, 91316)◀

#● **0141A** Immunization administration by intramuscular injection of severe acute respiratory syndrome coronavirus 2 (SARS-CoV-2) (coronavirus disease [COVID-19]) vaccine, mRNA-LNP, spike protein, bivalent, preservative free, 25 mcg/0.25 mL dosage; first dose

#● **0142A** second dose

#▲ **0144A** additional dose

▶(Report 0141A, 0142A, 0144A for the administration of vaccine 91314)◀

▶(Do not report 0141A, 0142A, 0144A in conjunction with 91301, 91306, 91309, 91311, 91313, 91316)◀

#● **0091A** Immunization administration by intramuscular injection of severe acute respiratory syndrome coronavirus 2 (SARS-CoV-2) (coronavirus disease [COVID-19]) vaccine, mRNA-LNP, spike protein, preservative free, 50 mcg/0.5 mL dosage; first dose, when administered to individuals 6 through 11 years

#● **0092A** second dose, when administered to individuals 6 through 11 years

#● **0093A** third dose, when administered to individuals 6 through 11 years

#▲ **0094A** booster dose, when administered to individuals 18 years and older

▶(Report 0091A, 0092A, 0093A, 0094A for the administration of vaccine 91309)◀

▶(Do not report 0091A, 0092A, 0093A, 0094A in conjunction with 91301, 91306, 91311, 91313, 91314, 91316)◀

0041A Immunization administration by intramuscular injection of severe acute respiratory syndrome coronavirus 2 (SARS-CoV-2) (coronavirus disease [COVID-19]) vaccine, recombinant spike protein nanoparticle, saponin-based adjuvant, preservative free, 5 mcg/0.5 mL dosage; first dose

0042A second dose

● **0044A** booster dose

▶(Report 0041A, 0042A, 0044A for the administration of vaccine 91304)◀

0091A Code is out of numerical sequence. See 0003A-0022A

0092A Code is out of numerical sequence. See 0003A-0022A

0093A Code is out of numerical sequence. See 0003A-0022A

0111A Immunization administration by intramuscular injection of severe acute respiratory syndrome coronavirus 2 (SARS-CoV-2) (coronavirus disease [COVID-19]) vaccine, mRNA-LNP, spike protein, preservative free, 25 mcg/0.25 mL dosage; first dose

0112A second dose

● **0113A** third dose

▶(Report 0111A, 0112A, 0113A for the administration of vaccine 91311)◀

▶(Do not report 0111A, 0112A, 0113A in conjunction with 91301, 91306, 91309, 91313, 91314, 91316)◀

0121A Code is out of numerical sequence. See 0003A-0022A

0124A Code is out of numerical sequence. See 0003A-0022A

0134A Code is out of numerical sequence. See 0003A-0022A

0141A Code is out of numerical sequence. See 0003A-0022A

0142A Code is out of numerical sequence. See 0003A-0022A

0144A Code is out of numerical sequence. See 0003A-0022A

0151A Code is out of numerical sequence. See 0003A-0022A

0154A Code is out of numerical sequence. See 0003A-0022A

▲ **0164A** Immunization administration by intramuscular injection of severe acute respiratory syndrome coronavirus 2 (SARS-CoV-2) (coronavirus disease [COVID-19]) vaccine, mRNA-LNP, spike protein, bivalent, preservative free, 10 mcg/0.2 mL dosage, additional dose

▶(Report 0164A for the administration of vaccine 91316)◀

▶(Do not report 0164A in conjunction with 91301, 91306, 91309, 91311, 91313, 91314)◀

0171A Code is out of numerical sequence. See 0003A-0022A

0172A Code is out of numerical sequence. See 0003A-0022A

0173A Code is out of numerical sequence. See 0003A-0022A

0174A Code is out of numerical sequence. See 0003A-0022A

Rationale

It is important to note that subsequent to the printing of the CPT codebook, the CPT Editorial Panel approved five new COVID-19 vaccine product codes and one administration code in August 2023. These new COVID-19 codes replaced all previously approved, specific COVID-19 product and administration codes, with the exception of vaccine product code 91304. In addition, Appendix Q has been deleted from the CPT code set effective November 1,

★ = Telemedicine   ◀ = Audio-only   ✚ = Add-on code   � = FDA approval pending   # = Resequenced code   ⊘ = Modifier 51 exempt

2023. To view the most current CPT codes to report for COVID-19 administration and products, refer to the AMA CPT public website at ama-assn.org/cpt-cat-i-immunization-codes. Because the decision to delete these codes took place after the *CPT 2024* codebook has been finalized, these deleted codes and Appendix Q are included in the *CPT 2024* codebook and *CPT Changes 2024*. Therefore, the following rationale only discusses the content that have been included in the *CPT 2024* codebook, which was finalized before the August 2023 revisions.

New vaccine product (91312-91317) and administration (0044A, 0091A-0093A, 0113A, 0121A, 0124A, 0134A, 0141A, 0142A, 0144A, 0151A, 0154A, 0164A, 0171A-0174A) codes have been established for reporting new severe acute respiratory syndrome coronavirus 2 (SARS-CoV-2) (coronavirus disease 2019 [COVID-19]) vaccine products and administration. In addition, new parenthetical notes have been added and changes have been made to Appendix Q and to existing guidelines and parenthetical notes throughout the CPT code set to accommodate the new code additions. This includes updates that conform to decisions made by government agencies regarding future reporting for COVID-19 vaccinations.

To address urgent health care needs and in continuation of the ongoing efforts to control the spread of the COVID-19 virus throughout the US, the FDA continued the emergency use authorization (EUA) for the development of new vaccine products and their administration. The EUA was continued to allow more rapid development of vaccine codes requested from multiple manufacturers and to make COVID-19 vaccine products available earlier for code development.

Recent decisions resulted in midyear updates for reporting of certain vaccines. The CDC has made midyear determinations that simplify reporting for Pfizer and Moderna vaccines. As has been conducted during previous EUA, with the development of better and more complete vaccines, the CDC has decided that the use of available bivalent vaccines should supersede the use of monovalent COVID-19 vaccine products from Pfizer and Moderna that may still be available for use. This is because the bivalent vaccines provide immunity against more COVID-19 viral strains that are currently in circulation within the population. This includes transition to using the bivalent vaccine for primary administrations for initial immunity for patients who may not have received any COVID-19 vaccination, as well as use of bivalent vaccine for patients who may have received monovalent administrations for their initial or booster immunity.

As a result, the CDC has authorized and instructed providers (ie, physicians and other qualified health care professionals) to switch immunization administration from monovalent Pfizer and Moderna products to their bivalent products for vaccinations and administration, where available.

The new codes that have been included in the Vaccine, Toxoids subsection reflect the addition of codes before and after the CDC's decision. These codes allow (1) reporting of separate COVID-19 vaccine product codes according to the vaccine product manufacturer and (2) reporting of specific administration codes that are unique to the various COVID-19 vaccine products. This is exemplified by the inclusion of six new codes for COVID-19 vaccine products (91312-91317) and 18 COVID-19 vaccine administration codes (0044A, 0091A-0093A, 0113A, 0121A, 0124A, 0134A, 0141A, 0142A, 0144A, 0151A, 0154A, 0164A, 0171A-0174A) that are reported according to the COVID-19 vaccine product administered.

The changes to this specific section of the code set include:

- Addition of a booster administration code (0044A) for code 91304 (product).

- Addition of new bivalent single-dose product and administration codes to report tris-sucrose (91312, 0121A) and the diluent reconstituted tris-sucrose (91315, 0151A) formulations of COVID-19 vaccine.

- Revisions to codes 0124A and 0154A, which have been indented as child codes of new codes 0121A and 0151A, to reinforce their use as *additional* doses for these newly created codes. The term "booster" has been replaced with "additional" to demonstrate the intent for administration as an added dose as opposed to a booster dose (in compliance with the CDC's new instructions regarding the use of bivalent products).

- Addition of codes 0171A/0172A and 0141A/0142A for use as the administration of the first and second dose of vaccine products described by codes 91317 and 91314, respectively (in compliance with the new CDC instruction for its preference of using the new bivalent products for future immunizations).

- Revision of codes 0144A and 0173A as child codes (for code 0173A, it indicates its use for the third dose of the new bivalent primary series).

- Revision of codes 0134A, 0144A, 0164A, and 0174A to reflect their use as additional doses, instead of booster doses.

- Addition of monovalent primary administration codes 0091A-0093A for reporting administration of the vaccine product represented by code 91309.

Medicine 90281-99607

Medicine 90281-99607

- Revision of the age specification noted within administration code 0094A for the booster dose described by code 91309 and its status as a child code for inclusion within the family of administration codes for code 91309.

- Addition of a third-dose administration code (0113A) for the product described in code 91311.

- Addition of bivalent product codes 91312-91317 with accompanying parenthetical reporting instructions.

- Update of guidelines and parenthetical notes (including additions or deletions as necessary) to reflect addition of the new codes and to provide guidance regarding the appropriate reporting between the product and the administration codes (ie, codes that may or may not be used together for reporting).

Several changes have also been included within the Appendix Q table to reflect (1) updates to ages for which the codes are intended to be used; (2) updates regarding instructions for dosing schedules; and (3) addition of the new administration and product codes previously noted.

Finally, on the AMA's COVID-19 CPT Coding and Guidance website (https://www.ama-assn.org/find-covid-19-vaccine-codes), a built-in tool has also been included to assist vaccine product code and administration code selection. The AMA COVID-19 website should be consulted for frequent updates to CPT codes for COVID-19 vaccines and services.

Clinical Example (0044A)

A 33-year-old individual who was previously immunized with a primary series seeks booster immunization against SARS-CoV-2 to decrease the risk of contracting this disease, consistent with evidence-supported guidelines. The individual is offered and accepts an intramuscular injection of SARS-CoV-2 vaccine for this purpose.

Description of Procedure (0044A)

The physician or other QHP reviews the patient's chart to confirm that vaccination to decrease the risk of COVID-19 is indicated. Counsel the patient on the benefits and risks of vaccination to decrease the risk of COVID-19 and obtain consent. Administer the booster dose of the COVID-19 vaccine by intramuscular injection in the upper arm. Monitor the patient for any adverse reaction. Update the patient's immunization record (and registry when applicable) to reflect the vaccine administered.

Clinical Example (0091A)

A parent or guardian of a 7-year-old child seeks immunization against SARS-CoV-2 to decrease the risk of contracting this disease, consistent with evidence-supported guidelines. The parent or guardian is offered and agrees to an intramuscular injection of SARS-CoV-2 vaccine for the child for this purpose.

Description of Procedure (0091A)

The physician or other QHP reviews the patient's chart to confirm that vaccination to decrease the risk of COVID-19 is indicated. Counsel the parent or guardian on the benefits and risks of vaccination to decrease the risk of COVID-19 and obtain consent. Administer the first dose of the COVID-19 vaccine by intramuscular injection. Monitor the patient for any adverse reaction. Update the patient's immunization record (and registry when applicable) to reflect the vaccine administered.

Clinical Example (0092A)

A parent or guardian of a 7-year-old child seeks immunization against SARS-CoV-2 to decrease the risk of contracting this disease, consistent with evidence-supported guidelines. The parent or guardian is offered and agrees to an intramuscular injection of SARS-CoV-2 vaccine for the child for this purpose.

Description of Procedure (0092A)

The physician or other QHP reviews the patient's chart to confirm that vaccination to decrease the risk of COVID-19 is indicated. Counsel the parent or guardian on the benefits and risks of vaccination to decrease the risk of COVID-19 and obtain consent. Administer the second dose of the COVID-19 vaccine by intramuscular injection. Monitor the patient for any adverse reaction. Update the patient's immunization record (and registry when applicable) to reflect the vaccine administered.

Clinical Example (0093A)

A parent or guardian of a 7-year-old child seeks immunization against SARS-CoV-2 to decrease the risk of contracting this disease, consistent with evidence-supported guidelines. The parent or guardian is offered and agrees to an intramuscular injection of SARS-CoV-2 vaccine for the child for this purpose.

Description of Procedure (0093A)

The physician or other QHP reviews the patient's chart to confirm that vaccination to decrease the risk of COVID-19 is indicated. Counsel the parent or guardian on the benefits and risks of vaccination to decrease the risk of COVID-19 and obtain consent. Administer the third dose of the COVID-19 vaccine by intramuscular injection. Monitor the patient for any adverse reaction. Update the patient's immunization record (and registry when applicable) to reflect the vaccine administered.

Clinical Example (0094A)

A 33-year-old individual who was previously immunized with a primary series seeks booster immunization against SARS-CoV-2 to decrease the risk of contracting this disease, consistent with evidence-supported guidelines. The individual is offered and accepts an intramuscular injection of SARS-CoV-2 vaccine for this purpose.

Description of Procedure (0094A)

The physician or other QHP reviews the patient's chart to confirm that vaccination to decrease the risk of COVID-19 is indicated. Counsel the patient on the benefits and risks of vaccination to decrease the risk of COVID-19 and obtain consent. Administer the booster dose of the COVID-19 vaccine by intramuscular injection in the upper arm. Monitor the patient for any adverse reaction. Update the patient's immunization record (and registry when applicable) to reflect the vaccine administered.

Clinical Example (0113A)

A parent or guardian of a 1-year-old child seeks immunization against SARS-CoV-2 to decrease the risk of contracting this disease, consistent with evidence-supported guidelines. The parent or guardian is offered and agrees to an intramuscular injection of SARS-CoV-2 vaccine for the child for this purpose.

Description of Procedure (0113A)

The physician or other QHP reviews the patient's chart to confirm that vaccination to decrease the risk of COVID-19 is indicated. Counsel the parent or guardian on the benefits and risks of vaccination to decrease the risk of COVID-19 and obtain consent. Administer the third dose of the COVID-19 vaccine by intramuscular injection. Monitor the patient for any adverse reaction. Update the patient's immunization record (and registry when applicable) to reflect the vaccine administered.

Clinical Example (0121A)

A 33-year-old individual seeks immunization against SARS-CoV-2 to decrease the risk of contracting this disease, consistent with evidence-supported guidelines. The individual is offered and accepts an intramuscular injection of SARS-CoV-2 vaccine for this purpose.

Description of Procedure (0121A)

The physician or other QHP reviews the patient's chart to confirm that vaccination to decrease the risk of

COVID-19 is indicated. Counsel the patient on the benefits and risks of vaccination to decrease the risk of COVID-19 and obtain consent. Administer the bivalent first dose of the COVID-19 vaccine by intramuscular injection. Monitor the patient for any adverse reaction. Update the patient's immunization record (and registry when applicable) to reflect the vaccine administered.

Clinical Example (0124A)

A 33-year-old individual who was previously immunized with a primary series seeks booster immunization against SARS-CoV-2 to decrease the risk of contracting this disease, consistent with evidence-supported guidelines. The individual is offered and accepts an intramuscular injection of SARS-CoV-2 vaccine for this purpose.

Description of Procedure (0124A)

The physician or other QHP reviews the patient's chart to confirm that vaccination to decrease the risk of COVID-19 is indicated. Counsel the patient on the benefits and risks of vaccination to decrease the risk of COVID-19 and obtain consent. Administer the booster dose of the COVID-19 vaccine by intramuscular injection in the upper arm. Monitor the patient for any adverse reaction. Update the patient's immunization record (and registry when applicable) to reflect the vaccine administered.

Clinical Example (0134A)

A 33-year-old individual who was previously immunized with a primary series seeks booster immunization against SARS-CoV-2 to decrease the risk of contracting this disease, consistent with evidence-supported guidelines. The individual is offered and accepts an intramuscular injection of SARS-CoV-2 vaccine for this purpose.

Description of Procedure (0134A)

The physician or other QHP reviews the patient's chart to confirm that vaccination to decrease the risk of COVID-19 is indicated. Counsel the patient on the benefits and risks of vaccination to decrease the risk of COVID-19 and obtain consent. Administer the booster dose of the COVID-19 vaccine by intramuscular injection in the upper arm. Monitor the patient for any adverse reaction. Update the patient's immunization record (and registry when applicable) to reflect the vaccine administered.

Clinical Example (0141A)

A parent or guardian of a 7-year-old child seeks a bivalent first dose immunization against SARS-CoV-2 to decrease the risk of contracting this disease, consistent with evidence-supported guidelines. The parent or guardian is offered and agrees to an intramuscular injection of SARS-CoV-2 vaccine for the child for this purpose.

Description of Procedure (0141A)

The physician or other QHP reviews the patient's chart to confirm that vaccination to decrease the risk of COVID-19 is indicated. Counsel the parent or guardian on the benefits and risks of vaccination to decrease the risk of COVID-19 and obtain consent. Administer the bivalent first dose of the bivalent COVID-19 vaccine by intramuscular injection. Monitor the patient for any adverse reaction. Update the patient's immunization record (and registry when applicable) to reflect the vaccine administered.

Clinical Example (0142A)

A parent or guardian of a 7-year-old child seeks a bivalent second dose immunization against SARS-CoV-2 to decrease the risk of contracting this disease, consistent with evidence-supported guidelines. The parent or guardian is offered and agrees to an intramuscular injection of SARS-CoV-2 vaccine for the child for this purpose.

Description of Procedure (0142A)

The physician or other QHP reviews the patient's chart to confirm that vaccination to decrease the risk of COVID-19 is indicated. Counsel the parent or guardian on the benefits and risks of vaccination to decrease the risk of COVID-19 and obtain consent. Administer the bivalent second dose of the bivalent COVID-19 vaccine by intramuscular injection. Monitor the patient for any adverse reaction. Update the patient's immunization record (and registry when applicable) to reflect the vaccine administered.

Clinical Example (0144A)

A parent or guardian of a 7-year-old child who was previously immunized with a primary series seeks booster immunization against SARS-CoV-2 to decrease the risk of contracting this disease, consistent with evidence-supported guidelines. The individual is offered and accepts an intramuscular injection of SARS-CoV-2 vaccine for this purpose.

Description of Procedure (0144A)

The physician or other QHP reviews the patient's chart to confirm that vaccination to decrease the risk of COVID-19 is indicated. Counsel the patient on the benefits and risks of vaccination to decrease the risk of COVID-19 and obtain consent. Administer the booster dose of the COVID-19 vaccine by intramuscular injection in the upper arm. Monitor the patient for any adverse reaction. Update the patient's immunization record (and registry when applicable) to reflect the vaccine administered.

Clinical Example (0151A)

A parent or guardian of a 7-year-old child seeks a bivalent first dose immunization against SARS-CoV-2 to decrease the risk of contracting this disease, consistent with evidence-supported guidelines. The parent or guardian is offered and agrees to an intramuscular injection of SARS-CoV-2 vaccine for the child for this purpose.

Description of Procedure (0151A)

The physician or other QHP reviews the patient's chart to confirm that vaccination to decrease the risk of COVID-19 is indicated. Counsel the parent or guardian on the benefits and risks of vaccination to decrease the risk of COVID-19 and obtain consent. Administer the bivalent first dose of the bivalent COVID-19 vaccine by intramuscular injection. Monitor the patient for any adverse reaction. Update the patient's immunization record (and registry when applicable) to reflect the vaccine administered.

Clinical Example (0154A)

A parent or guardian of a 7-year-old child who was previously immunized with a primary series seeks booster immunization against SARS-CoV-2 to decrease the risk of contracting this disease, consistent with evidence-supported guidelines. The individual is offered and accepts an intramuscular injection of SARS-CoV-2 vaccine for this purpose.

Description of Procedure (0154A)

The physician or other QHP reviews the patient's chart to confirm that vaccination to decrease the risk of COVID-19 is indicated. Counsel the patient on the benefits and risks of vaccination to decrease the risk of COVID-19 and obtain consent. Administer the booster dose of the COVID-19 vaccine by intramuscular injection in the upper arm. Monitor the patient for any adverse reaction. Update the patient's immunization record (and registry when applicable) to reflect the vaccine administered.

Clinical Example (0164A)

A parent or guardian of a 1-year-old child who was previously immunized with a primary series seeks a bivalent booster immunization against SARS-CoV-2 to decrease the risk of contracting this disease, consistent with evidence-supported guidelines. The parent or guardian is offered and agrees to an intramuscular injection of SARS-CoV-2 vaccine for the child for this purpose.

Description of Procedure (0164A)

The physician or other QHP reviews the patient's chart to confirm that vaccination to decrease the risk of COVID-19 is indicated. Counsel the parent or guardian on the benefits and risks of vaccination to decrease the risk of COVID-19 and obtain consent. Administer the bivalent booster dose of the COVID-19 vaccine by intramuscular injection in the upper arm. Monitor the patient for any adverse reaction. Update the patient's immunization record (and registry when applicable) to reflect the vaccine administered.

Clinical Example (0171A)

A parent or guardian of a 1-year-old child seeks bivalent immunization against SARS-CoV-2 to decrease the risk of contracting this disease, consistent with evidence-supported guidelines. The parent or guardian is offered and agrees to an intramuscular injection of SARS-CoV-2 vaccine for the child for this purpose.

Description of Procedure (0171A)

The physician or other QHP reviews the patient's chart to confirm that vaccination to decrease the risk of COVID-19 is indicated. Counsel the parent or guardian on the benefits and risks of vaccination to decrease the risk of COVID-19 and obtain consent. Administer the first dose of the bivalent COVID-19 vaccine by intramuscular injection. Monitor the patient for any adverse reaction. Update the patient's immunization record (and registry when applicable) to reflect the vaccine administered.

Clinical Example (0172A)

A parent or guardian of a 1-year-old child seeks bivalent immunization against SARS-CoV-2 to decrease the risk of contracting this disease, consistent with evidence-supported guidelines. The parent or guardian is offered and agrees to an intramuscular injection of SARS-CoV-2 vaccine for the child for this purpose.

Description of Procedure (0172A)

The physician or other QHP reviews the patient's chart to confirm that vaccination to decrease the risk of COVID-19 is indicated. Counsel the parent or guardian on the benefits and risks of vaccination to decrease the risk of COVID-19 and obtain consent. Administer the second dose of the bivalent COVID-19 vaccine by intramuscular injection. Monitor the patient for any adverse reaction. Update the patient's immunization record (and registry when applicable) to reflect the vaccine administered.

Clinical Example (0173A)

A parent or guardian of a 1-year-old child seeks a bivalent third dose immunization against SARS-CoV-2 to decrease the risk of contracting this disease, consistent with evidence-supported guidelines. The parent or guardian is offered and agrees to an intramuscular injection of SARS-CoV-2 vaccine for the child for this purpose.

Description of Procedure (0173A)

The physician or other QHP reviews the patient's chart to confirm that vaccination to decrease the risk of COVID-19 is indicated. Counsel the parent or guardian on the benefits and risks of vaccination to decrease the risk of COVID-19 and obtain consent. Administer the bivalent third dose of the bivalent COVID-19 vaccine by intramuscular injection. Monitor the patient for any adverse reaction. Update the patient's immunization record (and registry when applicable) to reflect the vaccine administered.

Clinical Example (0174A)

A parent or guardian of a 1-year-old child who was previously immunized with a primary series seeks bivalent booster immunization against SARS-CoV-2 to decrease the risk of contracting this disease, consistent with evidence-supported guidelines. The parent or guardian is offered and agrees to an intramuscular injection of SARS-CoV-2 vaccine for the child for this purpose.

Description of Procedure (0174A)

The physician or other QHP reviews the patient's chart to confirm that vaccination to decrease the risk of COVID-19 is indicated. Counsel the parent or guardian on the benefits and risks of vaccination to decrease the risk of COVID-19 and obtain consent. Administer the booster dose of the primary series of the bivalent COVID-19 vaccine by intramuscular injection. Monitor the patient for any adverse reaction. Update the patient's immunization record (and registry when applicable) to reflect the vaccine administered.

Vaccines, Toxoids

▶Codes 90476-90759, 91300-91317 identify the vaccine product **only**. To report the administration of a vaccine/toxoid other than SARS-CoV-2 (coronavirus disease [COVID-19]), the vaccine/toxoid product codes (90476-90759) must be used in addition to an immunization administration code(s) (90460, 90461, 90471, 90472, 90473, 90474). To report the administration of a SARS-CoV-2 (coronavirus disease [COVID-19]) vaccine, the vaccine/toxoid product codes (91300-91317) should be reported with the corresponding immunization administration codes (0001A, 0002A, 0003A, 0004A, 0011A, 0012A, 0013A, 0021A, 0022A, 0031A, 0034A, 0041A, 0042A, 0044A, 0051A, 0052A, 0053A, 0054A, 0064A, 0071A, 0072A, 0073A, 0074A, 0081A, 0082A, 0083A, 0091A, 0092A, 0093A, 0094A, 0104A, 0111A, 0112A, 0113A, 0121A, 0124A, 0134A, 0141A, 0142A, 0144A, 0151A, 0154A, 0164A, 0171A, 0172A, 0173A, 0174A). All SARS-CoV-2 (coronavirus disease [COVID-19]) vaccine codes in this section are listed in Appendix Q with their associated vaccine code descriptors, vaccine administration codes, patient age, vaccine manufacturer, vaccine name(s), NDC Labeler Product ID, and interval between doses. In order to report these codes, the vaccine must fulfill the code descriptor and must be the vaccine represented by the manufacturer and vaccine name listed in Appendix Q.

Do not report 90476-90759 in conjunction with the SARS-CoV-2 (coronavirus disease [COVID-19]) immunization administration codes 0001A, 0002A, 0003A, 0004A, 0011A, 0012A, 0013A, 0021A, 0022A, 0031A, 0034A, 0041A, 0042A, 0044A, 0051A, 0052A, 0053A, 0054A, 0064A, 0071A, 0072A, 0073A, 0074A, 0081A, 0082A, 0083A, 0091A, 0092A, 0093A, 0094A, 0104A, 0111A, 0112A, 0113A, 0121A, 0124A, 0134A, 0141A, 0142A, 0144A, 0151A, 0154A, 0164A, 0171A, 0172A, 0173A, 0174A, unless both a SARS-CoV-2 (coronavirus disease [COVID-19]) vaccine/toxoid product and at least one vaccine/toxoid product from 90476-90759 are administered at the same encounter.

Modifier 51 should not be reported with vaccine/toxoid codes 90476-90759, 91300-91317, when reported in conjunction with administration codes 90460, 90461, 90471, 90472, 90473, 90474, 0001A, 0002A, 0003A, 0004A, 0011A, 0012A, 0013A, 0021A, 0022A, 0031A, 0034A, 0041A, 0042A, 0044A, 0051A, 0052A, 0053A, 0054A, 0064A, 0071A, 0072A, 0073A, 0074A, 0081A, 0082A, 0083A, 0091A, 0092A, 0093A, 0094A, 0104A, 0111A, 0112A, 0113A, 0121A, 0124A, 0134A, 0141A, 0142A, 0144A, 0151A, 0154A, 0164A, 0171A, 0172A, 0173A, 0174A.◄

If a significantly separately identifiable Evaluation and Management (E/M) service (eg, office or other outpatient services, preventive medicine services) is performed, the appropriate E/M service code should be reported in addition to the vaccine and toxoid administration codes.

To meet the reporting requirements of immunization registries, vaccine distribution programs, and reporting systems (eg, Vaccine Adverse Event Reporting System) the exact vaccine product administered needs to be reported. Multiple codes for a particular vaccine are provided in the CPT codebook when the schedule (number of doses or timing) differs for two or more products of the same vaccine type (eg, hepatitis A, Hib) or the vaccine product is available in more than one chemical formulation, dosage, or route of administration.

The "when administered to" age descriptions included in CPT vaccine codes are not intended to identify a product's licensed age indication. The term "preservative free" includes use for vaccines that contain no preservative and vaccines that contain trace amounts of preservative agents that are not present in a sufficient concentration for the purpose of preserving the final vaccine formulation. The absence of a designation regarding a preservative does not necessarily indicate the presence or absence of preservative in the vaccine. Refer to the product's prescribing information (PI) for the licensed age indication before administering vaccine to a patient.

Separate codes are available for combination vaccines (eg, Hib-HepB, DTap-IPV/Hib). It is inappropriate to code each component of a combination vaccine separately. If a specific vaccine code is not available, the unlisted procedure code should be reported, until a new code becomes available.

►The vaccine/toxoid abbreviations listed in codes 90476-90759, 91300-91317 reflect the most recent US vaccine abbreviation references used in the Advisory Committee on Immunization Practices (ACIP) recommendations at the time of CPT code set publication. Interim updates to vaccine code descriptors will be made following abbreviation approval by the ACIP on a timely basis via the AMA CPT website (ama-assn.org/cpt-cat-i-immunization-codes). The accuracy of the ACIP vaccine abbreviation designations in the CPT code set does not affect the validity of the vaccine code and its reporting function.

For the purposes of severe acute respiratory syndrome coronavirus 2 (SARS-CoV-2) (coronavirus disease [COVID-19]) vaccinations, codes 0003A, 0013A, 0053A, 0073A, 0083A, 0093A, 0113A, and 0173A represent the administration of a third dose in the primary series (eg, patient with immunocompromising condition or patient age 6 months through 4 years). In contrast, the booster or additional dose codes 0004A, 0034A, 0044A, 0054A, 0064A, 0074A, 0094A, 0104A, 0124A, 0134A, 0144A, 0154A, 0164A, and 0174A represent the administration of a dose of vaccine when the initial immune response to a primary vaccine series was sufficient, but has likely waned over time.◄

►(For immune globulins and monoclonal antibodies immunizations, see 90281-90399. For administration of immune globulins and monoclonal antibodies immunizations, see 96365-96375)◄

\# **91300**   Severe acute respiratory syndrome coronavirus 2 (SARS-CoV-2) (coronavirus disease [COVID-19]) vaccine, mRNA-LNP, spike protein, preservative free, 30 mcg/0.3 mL dosage, diluent reconstituted, for intramuscular use

(Report 91300 with administration codes 0001A, 0002A, 0003A, 0004A)

★=Telemedicine   ◄=Audio-only   +=Add-on code   ✗=FDA approval pending   #=Resequenced code   ⦸=Modifier 51 exempt

▶(Do not report 91300 in conjunction with administration codes 0051A, 0052A, 0053A, 0054A, 0071A, 0072A, 0073A, 0074A, 0081A, 0082A, 0083A, 0121A, 0124A, 0151A, 0154A, 0171A, 0172A, 0173A, 0174A)◀

91305 Severe acute respiratory syndrome coronavirus 2 (SARS-CoV-2) (coronavirus disease [COVID-19]) vaccine, mRNA-LNP, spike protein, preservative free, 30 mcg/0.3 mL dosage, tris-sucrose formulation, for intramuscular use

(Report 91305 with administration codes 0051A, 0052A, 0053A, 0054A)

▶(Do not report 91305 in conjunction with administration codes 0001A, 0002A, 0003A, 0004A, 0071A, 0072A, 0073A, 0074A, 0081A, 0082A, 0083A, 0121A, 0124A, 0151A, 0154A, 0171A, 0172A, 0173A, 0174A)◀

#● 91312 Severe acute respiratory syndrome coronavirus 2 (SARS-CoV-2) (coronavirus disease [COVID-19]) vaccine, mRNA-LNP, bivalent spike protein, preservative free, 30 mcg/0.3 mL dosage, tris-sucrose formulation, for intramuscular use

▶(Report 91312 with administration codes 0121A, 0124A)◀

▶(Do not report 91312 in conjunction with administration codes 0001A, 0002A, 0003A, 0004A, 0051A, 0052A, 0053A, 0054A, 0071A, 0072A, 0073A, 0074A, 0081A, 0082A, 0083A, 0151A, 0154A, 0171A, 0172A, 0173A, 0174A)◀

91307 Severe acute respiratory syndrome coronavirus 2 (SARS-CoV-2) (coronavirus disease [COVID-19]) vaccine, mRNA-LNP, spike protein, preservative free, 10 mcg/0.2 mL dosage, diluent reconstituted, tris-sucrose formulation, for intramuscular use

(Report 91307 with administration codes 0071A, 0072A, 0073A, 0074A)

▶(Do not report 91307 in conjunction with administration codes 0001A, 0002A, 0003A, 0004A, 0051A, 0052A, 0053A, 0054A, 0081A, 0082A, 0083A, 0121A, 0124A, 0151A, 0154A, 0171A, 0172A, 0173A, 0174A)◀

#● 91315 Severe acute respiratory syndrome coronavirus 2 (SARS-CoV-2) (coronavirus disease [COVID-19]) vaccine, mRNA-LNP, bivalent spike protein, preservative free, 10 mcg/0.2 mL dosage, diluent reconstituted, tris-sucrose formulation, for intramuscular use

▶(Report 91315 with administration codes 0151A, 0154A)◀

▶(Do not report 91315 in conjunction with administration codes 0001A, 0002A, 0003A, 0004A, 0051A, 0052A, 0053A, 0054A, 0071A, 0072A, 0073A, 0074A, 0081A, 0082A, 0083A, 0121A, 0124A, 0171A, 0172A, 0173A, 0174A)◀

91308 Severe acute respiratory syndrome coronavirus 2 (SARS-CoV-2) (coronavirus disease [COVID-19]) vaccine, mRNA-LNP, spike protein, preservative free, 3 mcg/0.2 mL dosage, diluent reconstituted, tris-sucrose formulation, for intramuscular use

(Report 91308 with administration codes 0081A, 0082A, 0083A)

▶(Do not report 91308 in conjunction with administration codes 0001A, 0002A, 0003A, 0004A, 0051A, 0052A, 0053A, 0054A, 0071A, 0072A, 0073A, 0074A, 0121A, 0124A, 0151A, 0154A, 0171A, 0172A, 0173A, 0174A)◀

#● 91317 Severe acute respiratory syndrome coronavirus 2 (SARS-CoV-2) (coronavirus disease [COVID-19]) vaccine, mRNA-LNP, bivalent spike protein, preservative free, 3 mcg/0.2 mL dosage, diluent reconstituted, tris-sucrose formulation, for intramuscular use

▶(Report 91317 with administration codes 0171A, 0172A, 0173A, 0174A)◀

▶(Use 91317 as the third dose in the primary series, with the first two doses reported using 91308, 0081A, 0082A)◀

▶(Use 91317 as the additional dose in the primary series, with the first three doses reported using 91308, 0081A, 0082A, 0083A)◀

▶(Do not report 91317 in conjunction with administration codes 0001A, 0002A, 0003A, 0004A, 0051A, 0052A, 0053A, 0054A, 0071A, 0072A, 0073A, 0074A, 0081A, 0082A, 0083A, 0121A, 0124A, 0151A, 0154A)◀

91301 Severe acute respiratory syndrome coronavirus 2 (SARS-CoV-2) (coronavirus disease [COVID-19]) vaccine, mRNA-LNP, spike protein, preservative free, 100 mcg/0.5 mL dosage, for intramuscular use

(Report 91301 with administration codes 0011A, 0012A, 0013A)

▶(Do not report 91301 in conjunction with administration codes 0064A, 0091A, 0092A, 0093A, 0094A, 0111A, 0112A, 0113A, 0134A, 0141A, 0142A, 0144A, 0164A)◀

91306 Severe acute respiratory syndrome coronavirus 2 (SARS-CoV-2) (coronavirus disease [COVID-19]) vaccine, mRNA-LNP, spike protein, preservative free, 50 mcg/0.25 mL dosage, for intramuscular use

(Report 91306 with administration code 0064A)

▶(Do not report 91306 in conjunction with administration codes 0011A, 0012A, 0013A, 0091A, 0092A, 0093A, 0094A, 0111A, 0112A, 0113A, 0134A, 0141A, 0142A, 0144A, 0164A)◀

#● 91313 Severe acute respiratory syndrome coronavirus 2 (SARS-CoV-2) (coronavirus disease [COVID-19]) vaccine, mRNA-LNP, spike protein, bivalent, preservative free, 50 mcg/0.5 mL dosage, for intramuscular use

▶(Report 91313 with administration code 0134A)◀

▶(Do not report 91313 in conjunction with administration codes 0011A, 0012A, 0013A, 0064A, 0091A, 0092A, 0093A, 0094A, 0111A, 0112A, 0113A, 0141A, 0142A, 0144A, 0164A)◀

#● **91314** Severe acute respiratory syndrome coronavirus 2 (SARS-CoV-2) (coronavirus disease [COVID-19]) vaccine, mRNA-LNP, spike protein, bivalent, preservative free, 25 mcg/0.25 mL dosage, for intramuscular use

▶(Report 91314 with administration codes 0141A, 0142A, 0144A)◀

▶(Do not report 91314 in conjunction with administration codes 0011A, 0012A, 0013A, 0064A, 0091A, 0092A, 0093A, 0094A, 0111A, 0112A, 0113A, 0134A, 0164A)◀

91311 Severe acute respiratory syndrome coronavirus 2 (SARS-CoV-2) (coronavirus disease [COVID-19]) vaccine, mRNA-LNP, spike protein, preservative free, 25 mcg/0.25 mL dosage, for intramuscular use

▶(Report 91311 with administration codes 0111A, 0112A, 0113A)◀

▶(Do not report 91311 in conjunction with administration codes 0011A, 0012A, 0013A, 0064A, 0091A, 0092A, 0093A, 0094A, 0134A, 0141A, 0142A, 0144A, 0164A)◀

#● **91316** Severe acute respiratory syndrome coronavirus 2 (SARS-CoV-2) (coronavirus disease [COVID-19]) vaccine, mRNA-LNP, spike protein, bivalent, preservative free, 10 mcg/0.2 mL dosage, for intramuscular use

▶(Report 91316 with administration code 0164A)◀

▶(Do not report 91316 in conjunction with administration codes 0011A, 0012A, 0013A, 0064A, 0091A, 0092A, 0093A, 0094A, 0111A, 0112A, 0113A, 0134A, 0141A, 0142A, 0144A)◀

91309 Severe acute respiratory syndrome coronavirus 2 (SARS-CoV-2) (coronavirus disease [COVID-19]) vaccine, mRNA-LNP, spike protein, preservative free, 50 mcg/0.5 mL dosage, for intramuscular use

▶(Report 91309 with administration codes 0091A, 0092A, 0093A, 0094A)◀

▶(Do not report 91309 in conjunction with administration codes 0011A, 0012A, 0013A, 0064A, 0111A, 0112A, 0113A, 0134A, 0141A, 0142A, 0144A, 0164A)◀

91304 Severe acute respiratory syndrome coronavirus 2 (SARS-CoV-2) (coronavirus disease [COVID-19]) vaccine, recombinant spike protein nanoparticle, saponin-based adjuvant, preservative free, 5 mcg/0.5 mL dosage, for intramuscular use

▶(Report 91304 with administration codes 0041A, 0042A, 0044A)◀

#✗ **91310** Severe acute respiratory syndrome coronavirus 2 (SARS-CoV-2) (coronavirus disease [COVID-19]) vaccine, monovalent, preservative free, 5 mcg/0.5 mL dosage, adjuvant AS03 emulsion, for intramuscular use

(Report 91310 with administration code 0104A)

90476 Adenovirus vaccine, type 4, live, for oral use

Rationale

To accommodate the addition of new codes for reporting COVID-19 vaccine products, codes 91312-91317 and associated parenthetical notes have been added, and the existing Vaccines, Toxoids subsection guidelines and related parenthetical notes have been revised.

Refer to the codebook and the Rationale for COVID-19 product administration codes 0044A-0174A for a full discussion of these changes.

Also, to accommodate the addition of immune globulin product codes 90380 and 90381, the parenthetical note following the Vaccines, Toxoids guidelines has been revised to include consistent language for immune globulin and monoclonal antibody immunizations.

Refer to the codebook and the Rationale for the Immune Globulins, Serum, or Recombinant Products guidelines for a full discussion of these changes.

Clinical Example (91312)

A 33-year-old individual seeks immunization against SARS-CoV-2 to decrease the risk of contracting this disease, consistent with evidence-supported guidelines. The individual is offered and accepts an intramuscular injection of SARS-CoV-2 vaccine for this purpose.

Description of Procedure (91312)

The physician or other QHP determines that the SARS-CoV-2 vaccine is appropriate for this patient and dispenses the vaccine according to the dose scheduled in the administration code for the SARS-CoV-2 vaccine.

Clinical Example (91313)

A 33-year-old individual seeks immunization against SARS-CoV-2 to decrease the risk of contracting this disease, consistent with evidence-supported guidelines. The individual is offered and accepts an intramuscular injection of SARS-CoV-2 vaccine for this purpose.

Description of Procedure (91313)

The physician or other QHP determines that the SARS-CoV-2 vaccine is appropriate for this patient and dispenses the vaccine according to the dose scheduled in the administration code for the SARS-CoV-2 vaccine.

Clinical Example (91314)

A parent or guardian of a 7-year-old child seeks immunization against SARS-CoV-2 to decrease the risk of contracting this disease, consistent with evidence-supported guidelines. The individual is offered and accepts an intramuscular injection of SARS-CoV-2 vaccine for this purpose.

Description of Procedure (91314)

The physician or other QHP determines that the SARS-CoV-2 vaccine is appropriate for this patient and dispenses the vaccine according to the dose scheduled in the administration code for the SARS-CoV-2 vaccine.

Clinical Example (91315)

A parent or guardian of a 7-year-old child seeks immunization against SARS-CoV-2 to decrease the risk of contracting this disease, consistent with evidence-supported guidelines. The individual is offered and accepts an intramuscular injection of SARS-CoV-2 vaccine for this purpose.

Description of Procedure (91315)

The physician or other QHP determines that the SARS-CoV-2 vaccine is appropriate for this patient and dispenses the vaccine according to the dose scheduled in the administration code for the SARS-CoV-2 vaccine.

Clinical Example (91316)

A parent or guardian of a 1-year-old child who was previously immunized with a primary series seeks a bivalent booster immunization against SARS-CoV-2 to decrease the risk of contracting this disease, consistent with evidence-supported guidelines. The parent or guardian is offered and accepts an intramuscular injection of SARS-CoV-2 vaccine for the child for this purpose.

Description of Procedure (91316)

The physician or other QHP determines that the bivalent SARS-CoV-2 vaccine is appropriate for this patient and dispenses the vaccine according to the dose scheduled in the administration code for the SARS-CoV-2 vaccine.

Clinical Example (91317)

A parent or guardian of a 1-year-old child seeks bivalent immunization against SARS-CoV-2 to decrease the risk of contracting this disease, consistent with evidence-supported guidelines. The parent or guardian is offered and agrees to an intramuscular injection of SARS-CoV-2 vaccine for the child for this purpose.

Description of Procedure (91317)

The physician or other QHP determines that the bivalent SARS-CoV-2 vaccine is appropriate for this patient and dispenses the vaccine according to the dose scheduled in the administration code for the SARS-CoV-2 vaccine.

| 90586 | Bacillus Calmette-Guerin vaccine (BCG) for bladder cancer, live, for intravesical use |
| #✎● 90589 | Chikungunya virus vaccine, live attenuated, for intramuscular use |

Rationale

New vaccine product code 90589 has been established in the Vaccines, Toxoids subsection to report chikungunya virus vaccine. Code 90589 describes a live, attenuated vaccine administered intramuscularly for the prevention of disease caused by the chikungunya virus. Administration of the vaccine is reported separately using codes 90460-90474 (immunization administration for vaccines/toxoids). Code 90589 carries the FDA approval pending symbol (✎); therefore, interim updates on the FDA status of this code will be reflected on the AMA CPT website at https://www.ama-assn.org/system/files/vaccine-long-descriptors.pdf under the CPT Category I Vaccine Codes.

The CDC ACIP has not assigned a US vaccine abbreviation for this vaccine. Visit the AMA CPT website for updates on the US vaccine abbreviation status for this vaccine.

Clinical Example (90589)

A 45-year-old female visits her physician or other QHP because she will be traveling to Africa on business. After assessing her itinerary and risk of exposure to mosquitos, the physician or other QHP recommends immunization against chikungunya virus and orders administration of the vaccine.

Description of Procedure (90589)

The physician or other QHP confirms the need for vaccination against chikungunya virus. After counseling and obtaining informed consent, reconstitute the vaccine and administer intramuscularly. Record the vaccination and report the vaccination administration separately.

Medicine 90281-99607

#✗ **90584** Dengue vaccine, quadrivalent, live, 2 dose schedule, for subcutaneous use

90589 Code is out of numerical sequence. See 90585-90632

90611 Code is out of numerical sequence. See 90710-90715

90622 Code is out of numerical sequence. See 90714-90717

90623 Code is out of numerical sequence. See 90717-90739

● **90679** Respiratory syncytial virus vaccine, preF, recombinant, subunit, adjuvanted, for intramuscular use

Rationale

New vaccine product code 90679 has been established in the Vaccines, Toxoids subsection to report RSV vaccine. Code 90679 describes a recombinant, adjuvanted, preF, subunit RSV vaccine administered intramuscularly for the prevention of disease caused by the RSV virus. Administration of the vaccine is reported separately using codes 90460-90474 (immunization administration for vaccines/toxoids).

The CDC ACIP has not assigned a US vaccine abbreviation for this vaccine. Visit the AMA CPT website for updates on the US vaccine abbreviation status for this vaccine.

Clinical Example (90679)

A 67-year-old male presents for evaluation, and the physician or other QHP determines that he should receive the RSV vaccine and orders its administration.

Description of Procedure (90679)

The physician or other QHP selects the appropriate RSV vaccine. After counseling and obtaining informed consent, administer the immunization intramuscularly. Report the vaccine administration separately from the vaccine product.

#✗● **90683** Respiratory syncytial virus vaccine, mRNA lipid nanoparticles, for intramuscular use

▶(For seasonal respiratory syncytial virus [RSV] monoclonal antibodies immunization codes, see 90380, 90381. For administration of seasonal RSV monoclonal antibodies immunizations, use 96372)◀

Rationale

New vaccine product code 90683 has been established in the Vaccines, Toxoids subsection to report RSV vaccine that uses mRNA lipid nanoparticles. This differentiates the use of this vaccine product from the recombinant, adjuvanted, preF, subunit RSV vaccine administered intramuscularly for the prevention of disease caused by

the RSV virus (90679). Administration of the vaccine is reported separately using codes 90460-90474 (immunization administration for vaccines/toxoids). Code 90683 carries the FDA approval pending symbol (✗); therefore, interim updates on the FDA status of this code will be reflected on the AMA CPT website at https://www.ama-assn.org/system/files/vaccine-long-descriptors.pdf under the CPT Category I Vaccine Codes.

The CDC ACIP has not assigned a US vaccine abbreviation for this vaccine. Visit the AMA CPT website for updates on the US vaccine abbreviation status for this vaccine.

To accommodate the addition of immune globulin product codes 90380 and 90381, a parenthetical note following code 90683 has been added to direct users to the appropriate codes to report seasonal RSV monoclonal antibodies immunizations (90380, 90381) and their administration (96372).

Refer to the codebook and the Rationale for codes 90380 and 90381 for a full discussion of these changes.

Clinical Example (90683)

A 60-year-old female is seen for a preventive medicine visit. In accordance with the national recommendations for immunizations, the physician determines that a vaccine to prevent RSV-associated lower respiratory tract disease (LRTD) is recommended for the patient. The patient is offered and agrees to an intramuscular injection of an RSV vaccine for this purpose.

Description of Procedure (90683)

The physician or other QHP reviews the patient's chart to confirm that vaccination to prevent RSV-associated LRTD is indicated. Obtain informed consent and dispense a dose of the RSV vaccine.

90683 Code is out of numerical sequence. See 90678-90681

90713 Poliovirus vaccine, inactivated (IPV), for subcutaneous or intramuscular use

#● **90611** Smallpox and monkeypox vaccine, attenuated vaccinia virus, live, non-replicating, preservative free, 0.5 mL dosage, suspension, for subcutaneous use

Rationale

New vaccine product code 90611 has been established in the Vaccines, Toxoids subsection to report attenuated vaccinia virus vaccine for immunization against contracting smallpox and monkeypox. This vaccine product uses live, nonreplicating virus that is preservative-free and administered subcutaneously. Administration of the

★ = Telemedicine   ◀ = Audio-only   ✚ = Add-on code   ✗ = FDA approval pending   # = Resequenced code   ⊘ = Modifier 51 exempt

vaccine is reported separately using codes 90460-90474 (immunization administration for vaccines/toxoids).

The CDC ACIP has not assigned a US vaccine abbreviation for this vaccine. Visit the AMA CPT website for updates on the US vaccine abbreviation status for this vaccine.

Clinical Example (90611)

A 36-year-old male who is at risk for exposure to an orthopoxvirus (ie, monkeypox virus) presents for vaccination.

Description of Procedure (90611)

The physician or other QHP determines that the orthopoxvirus (ie, monkeypox virus) vaccine is appropriate for him and dispenses the vaccine according to the dose scheduled for the orthopoxvirus (ie, monkeypox virus) vaccine.

#● **90622**   Vaccinia (smallpox) virus vaccine, live, lyophilized, 0.3 mL dosage, for percutaneous use

Rationale

New vaccine product code 90622 has been established in the Vaccines, Toxoids subsection to report lyophilized, vaccinia virus vaccine for immunization against contracting smallpox. This vaccine product uses lyophilized (ie, freeze-dried) vaccine product, and it is administered percutaneously. Administration of the vaccine is reported separately using codes 90460-90474 (immunization administration for vaccines/toxoids).

The CDC ACIP has not assigned a US vaccine abbreviation for this vaccine. Visit the AMA CPT website for updates on the US vaccine abbreviation status for this vaccine.

Clinical Example (90622)

A 36-year-old male who is at risk for exposure to an orthopoxvirus (ie, smallpox virus) presents for vaccination.

Description of Procedure (90622)

The physician or other QHP determines that the orthopoxvirus (ie, smallpox virus) vaccine is appropriate for him and dispenses the vaccine according to the dose scheduled for the orthopoxvirus (ie, smallpox virus) vaccine.

90734   Meningococcal conjugate vaccine, serogroups A, C, W, Y, quadrivalent, diphtheria toxoid carrier (MenACWY-D) or CRM197 carrier (MenACWY-CRM), for intramuscular use

90619   Meningococcal conjugate vaccine, serogroups A, C, W, Y, quadrivalent, tetanus toxoid carrier (MenACWY-TT), for intramuscular use

#⚡● **90623**   Meningococcal pentavalent vaccine, conjugated Men A, C, W, Y- tetanus toxoid carrier, and Men B-FHbp, for intramuscular use

Rationale

New vaccine product code 90623 has been established in the Vaccines, Toxoids subsection to report meningococcal pentavalent vaccine. Code 90623 describes use of a pentavalent meningococcal vaccine that uses bacterial meningococcal serogroup antigens A, C, W, and Y conjugated with tetanus toxoid carrier along with meningococcal serogroup B using the factor H-binding protein (FHbp) antigen as the carrier to elicit an immune response from the patient. It is administered intramuscularly for the prevention of disease caused by the meningococcal pentavalent bacteria. Administration of the vaccine is reported separately using codes 90460-90474 (immunization administration for vaccines/toxoids). Code 90623 carries the FDA approval-pending symbol (⚡); therefore, interim updates on the FDA status of this code will be reflected on the AMA CPT website at https://www.ama-assn.org/system/files/vaccine-long-descriptors.pdf under the CPT Category I Vaccine Codes.

The CDC ACIP has not assigned a US vaccine abbreviation for this vaccine. Visit the AMA CPT website for updates on the US vaccine abbreviation status for this vaccine.

Clinical Example (90623)

A parent or guardian of a child seeks immunization for the child against meningococcal infection to decrease the risk of contracting the disease. The physician or other QHP determines that the child is an appropriate candidate for the pentavalent meningococcal vaccine and orders its administration.

Description of Procedure (90623)

A physician or other QHP determines that the pentavalent meningococcal vaccine is appropriate for this patient. After counseling and obtaining informed consent, administer the immunization intramuscularly. Report the vaccination administration separately from the vaccine product.

▲ = Revised code   ● = New code   ▶◀ = Contains new or revised text   ✖ = Duplicate PLA test   ↑↓ = Category I PLA   American Medical Association   **127**

Medicine 90281-99607

Psychiatry

Psychiatric Diagnostic Procedures

Other Psychiatric Services or Procedures

90867 Therapeutic repetitive transcranial magnetic stimulation (TMS) treatment; initial, including cortical mapping, motor threshold determination, delivery and management

(Report only once per course of treatment)

(Do not report 90867 in conjunction with 90868, 90869, 95860, 95870, 95928, 95929, 95939)

▶(For peripheral nerve transcutaneous magnetic stimulation, see 0766T, 0767T)◀

Rationale

In accordance with the deletion of codes 0768T and 0769T, a parenthetical note following code 90867 has been revised to reflect the deleted codes and to direct users to the appropriate codes for reporting transcutaneous magnetic stimulation.

Refer to the codebook and the Rationale for codes 0766T-0769T for a full discussion of these changes.

Gastroenterology

Other Procedures

91299 Unlisted diagnostic gastroenterology procedure

91312 Code is out of numerical sequence. See 90473-90477

91313 Code is out of numerical sequence. See 90473-90477

91314 Code is out of numerical sequence. See 90473-90477

91315 Code is out of numerical sequence. See 90473-90477

91316 Code is out of numerical sequence. See 90473-90477

91317 Code is out of numerical sequence. See 90473-90477

Special Otorhinolaryngologic Services

Evaluative and Therapeutic Services

Codes 92601 and 92603 describe post-operative analysis and fitting of previously placed external devices, connection to the cochlear implant, and programming of the stimulator. Codes 92602 and 92604 describe subsequent sessions for measurements and adjustment of the external transmitter and re-programming of the internal stimulator.

(For placement of cochlear implant, use 69930)

▶Codes 92622, 92623 describe the analysis, programming, and verification of an auditory osseointegrated sound processor, any type. These services include evaluating the attachment of the processor, device feedback calibration, device programming, and verification of the processor performance. These codes should be used for subsequent reprogramming, when performed.◀

Rationale

In accordance with the establishment of codes 92622 and 92623, new guidelines have been added in the Evaluative and Therapeutic Services subsection. The guidelines explain the various components described in the codes and the work included in codes 92622 and 92623.

Refer to the codebook and the Rationale for codes 92622 and 92623 for a full discussion of these changes.

★ **92601** Diagnostic analysis of cochlear implant, patient younger than 7 years of age; with programming

★ **92602** subsequent reprogramming

(Do not report 92602 in addition to 92601)

★ **92603** Diagnostic analysis of cochlear implant, age 7 years or older; with programming

★ **92604** subsequent reprogramming

(Do not report 92604 in addition to 92603)

▶(For diagnostic analysis, programming, and verification of an auditory osseointegrated sound processor, use 92622)◀

▶(For evaluation of auditory function for surgically implanted device[s] candidacy or postoperative status of a surgically implanted device[s], use 92626)◀

▶(For aural rehabilitation services following auditory osseointegrated implant, see 92630, 92633)◀

(For initial and subsequent diagnostic analysis and programming of vestibular implant, see 0728T, 0729T)

92620 Evaluation of central auditory function, with report; initial 60 minutes

+ **92621** each additional 15 minutes (List separately in addition to code for primary procedure)

(Use 92621 in conjunction with 92620)

★ = Telemedicine ◀ = Audio-only + = Add-on code ⊘ = FDA approval pending # = Resequenced code ⊘ = Modifier 51 exempt

(Do not report 92620, 92621 in conjunction with 92521, 92522, 92523, 92524)

● **92622** Diagnostic analysis, programming, and verification of an auditory osseointegrated sound processor, any type; first 60 minutes

+● **92623** each additional 15 minutes (List separately in addition to code for primary procedure)

►(Use 92623 in conjunction with 92622)◄

►(Do not report 92622, 92623 in conjunction with 92626, 92627)◄

►(For diagnostic analysis of cochlear implant, with programming or subsequent reprogramming, see 92601, 92602, 92603, 92604)◄

►(For evaluation of auditory function for surgically implanted device[s] candidacy or postoperative status of a surgically implanted device[s], use 92626)◄

►(For aural rehabilitation services following auditory osseointegrated implant, see 92630, 92633)◄

Rationale

To provide specificity and capture the service provided to patients for disorders such as conductive or mixed-hearing disorders or single-sided deafness, code 92622 and add-on code 92623 have been established.

In addition, several changes have been made to the Medicine/Special Otorhinolaryngologic Services/Evaluative and Therapeutic Services and the Surgery/Auditory System/Middle Ear/Osseointegrated Implants subsections, including the addition of new guidelines and parenthetical notes for reporting analysis, programming, and verification of an auditory osseointegrated sound processor.

The services reflected in code 92626 and add-on code 92627 are separate and distinct from the services described in codes 92622 and 92623. The services reflected in codes 92622 and 92623 use different procedures, equipment, and supplies than those in codes 92626 and 92627. Code 92622 and add-on code 92623 describe the work of programming and configuring the auditory osseointegrated device to customize and optimize the device's performance for the patient. Variable time is required depending on the service or procedure performed. Specifically, code 92622 is intended to describe the first 60 minutes, and add-on code 92623 describes each additional 15 minutes of the service.

Code 92626 and add-on code 92627 reflect various diagnostic assessments that evaluate and measure a patient's auditory function (ie, their functional hearing performance).

These assessments, which are performed in the sound room, are used both:

1. Preoperatively to determine candidacy for a surgically implanted device and

2. Post-surgical implantation to assess the patient's functional hearing performance with the hearing implant.

The introductory guidelines included in the Evaluative and Therapeutic Services subsection have been revised to note that codes 92622 and 92623 describe analysis, programming, and verification of an auditory osseointegrated sound processor. Codes 92622 and 92623 should be reported for subsequent reprogramming, when performed. In addition, clarifying parenthetical notes and cross-reference parenthetical notes have been added following codes 92604, 92623, and 92627.

Clinical Example (92622)

A 56-year-old male presents with chronic otitis media resulting in otorrhea and mixed-hearing loss, and the former symptom prevents him from using traditional air-conduction hearing aids. An osseointegrated implant for an auditory osseointegrated device was placed to allow for bone-conducted sound delivery. Patient has returned for device activation, programming, and verification of the sound processor.

Description of Procedure (92622)

The QHP inspects the surgical site for skin irritation or overgrowth and performs an otoscopic examination. Affix the external sound processor to patient's head and adjust for a secure fit. Assess and calibrate the magnetic connection between the sound processor and implant as necessary. The QHP connects the external sound processor to computer programming software and performs a feedback calibration as appropriate. Adjust processor settings to prevent acoustic feedback. With the sound processor still connected to the programming software, measure patient's in situ bone-conduction responses using appropriate audiometric techniques. Responses are used for programming the device to optimize patient's auditory performance. Perform verification of the device to validate effective programming. Add or adjust additional sound processor settings and repeat verification as indicated. The QHP confirms connectivity to hearing-assistive technology, as needed, and confirms function. Export the finalized settings to the external processor. The QHP demonstrates and instructs patient and/or family/caregiver regarding sound processor attachment, retention, and microphone orientation for optimal hearing performance. The QHP prepares a report of the analysis, programming, and verification.

Clinical Example (92623)

A 56-year-old male who has just undergone 60 minutes of service requires and receives an additional 15 minutes of service beyond the first hour, during auditory osseointegrated sound processor diagnostic analysis, programming, and verification. [**Note:** This is an add-on code. Only consider the additional work related to the primary service.]

Description of Procedure (92623)

The QHP continues to make necessary adjustments to the processor settings to prevent auditory feedback. With the sound processor still connected to the programming software, measure patient's in situ bone-conduction responses using appropriate audiometric techniques. Responses are used for programming the device to optimize patient's auditory performance. Verification of the device is then performed to validate effective programming. Additional sound processor settings are added or adjusted, and verification is repeated, as indicated. The QHP confirms connectivity to hearing-assistive technology, as needed, and confirms function. The finalized settings are exported to the external processor. The QHP demonstrates and instructs patient and/or family/caregiver regarding sound processor attachment, retention, and microphone orientation for optimal hearing performance.

92625	Assessment of tinnitus (includes pitch, loudness matching, and masking)

(Do not report 92625 in conjunction with 92562)

(For unilateral assessment, use modifier 52)

92626	Evaluation of auditory function for surgically implanted device(s) candidacy or postoperative status of a surgically implanted device(s); first hour
+ 92627	each additional 15 minutes (List separately in addition to code for primary procedure)

(Use 92627 in conjunction with 92626)

(When reporting 92626, 92627, use the face-to-face time with the patient or family)

(Do not report 92626, 92627 in conjunction with 92590, 92591, 92592, 92593, 92594, 92595 for hearing aid evaluation, fitting, follow-up, or selection)

▶(Do not report 92626, 92627 in conjunction with 92622, 92623)◀

▶(For diagnostic analysis of cochlear implant, with programming or subsequent reprogramming, see 92601, 92602, 92603, 92604)◀

▶(For diagnostic analysis, programming, and verification of an auditory osseointegrated sound processor, use 92622)◀

Rationale

In accordance with the establishment of codes 92622 and 92623, three clarifying parenthetical notes have been added following code 92627 to accommodate these changes.

Refer to the codebook and the Rationale for codes 92622 and 92623 for a full discussion of these changes.

Cardiovascular

Therapeutic Services and Procedures

Other Therapeutic Services and Procedures

92970	Cardioassist-method of circulatory assist; internal
92971	external

(For balloon atrial septostomy, use 33741)

(For placement of catheters for use in circulatory assist devices such as intra-aortic balloon pump, use 33970)

92972	Code is out of numerical sequence. See 92997-93005

Coronary Therapeutic Services and Procedures

▶Codes 92920-92944 describe percutaneous revascularization services performed for occlusive disease of the coronary vessels (major coronary arteries, coronary artery branches, or coronary artery bypass grafts). These percutaneous coronary intervention (PCI) codes are built on progressive hierarchies with more intensive services inclusive of lesser intensive services. These PCI codes all include the work of accessing and selectively catheterizing the vessel, traversing the lesion, radiological supervision and interpretation directly related to the intervention(s) performed, closure of the arteriotomy when performed through the access sheath, and imaging performed to document completion of the intervention in addition to the intervention(s) performed. These codes include angioplasty (eg, balloon, cutting balloon, wired balloons, cryoplasty), atherectomy (eg, directional, rotational, laser), and stenting (eg, balloon expandable, self-expanding, bare metal, drug eluting, covered). Each code in this family includes balloon angioplasty, when performed. Diagnostic coronary angiography may be reported separately under specific circumstances. Percutaneous transluminal coronary lithotripsy may be reported using 92972 in conjunction with 92920, 92924, 92928, 92933, 92937, 92941, 92943, 92975, as appropriate. ◀

Diagnostic coronary angiography codes (93454-93461) and injection procedure codes (93563-93564) should not be used with percutaneous coronary revascularization services (92920-92944) to report:

1. Contrast injections, angiography, roadmapping, and/ or fluoroscopic guidance for the coronary intervention,

2. Vessel measurement for the coronary intervention, **or**

3. Post-coronary angioplasty/stent/atherectomy angiography, as this work is captured in the percutaneous coronary revascularization services codes (92920-92944).

Diagnostic angiography performed at the time of a coronary interventional procedure may be separately reportable if:

1. No prior catheter-based coronary angiography study is available, and a full diagnostic study is performed, and a decision to intervene is based on the diagnostic angiography, **or**

2. A prior study is available, but as documented in the medical record:

    a. The patient's condition with respect to the clinical indication has changed since the prior study, **or**

    b. There is inadequate visualization of the anatomy and/or pathology, **or**

    c. There is a clinical change during the procedure that requires new evaluation outside the target area of intervention.

Diagnostic coronary angiography performed at a separate session from an interventional procedure is separately reportable.

Major coronary arteries: The major coronary arteries are the left main, left anterior descending, left circumflex, right, and ramus intermedius arteries. All PCI procedures performed in all segments (proximal, mid, distal) of a single major coronary artery through the native coronary circulation are reported with one code. When one segment of a major coronary artery is treated through the native circulation and treatment of another segment of the same artery requires access through a coronary artery bypass graft, the intervention through the bypass graft is reported separately.

Coronary artery branches: Up to two coronary artery branches of the left anterior descending (diagonals), left circumflex (marginals), and right (posterior descending, posterolaterals) coronary arteries are recognized. The left main and ramus intermedius coronary arteries do not have recognized branches for reporting purposes. All PCI(s) performed in any segment (proximal, mid, distal) of a coronary artery branch is reported with one code. PCI is reported for up to two branches of a major coronary artery. Additional PCI in a third branch of the same major coronary artery is not separately reportable.

Coronary artery bypass grafts: Each coronary artery bypass graft represents a coronary vessel. A sequential bypass graft with more than one distal anastomosis represents only one graft. A branching bypass graft (eg, Y graft) represents a coronary vessel for the main graft, and each branch off the main graft constitutes an additional coronary vessel. PCI performed on major coronary arteries or coronary artery branches by access through a bypass graft is reported using the bypass graft PCI codes. All bypass graft PCI codes include the use of coronary artery embolic protection devices when performed.

Only one base code from this family may be reported for revascularization of a major coronary artery and its recognized branches. Only one base code should be reported for revascularization of a coronary artery bypass graft, its subtended coronary artery, and recognized branches of the subtended coronary artery. If one segment of a major coronary artery and its recognized branches is treated through the native circulation, and treatment of another segment of the same vessel requires access through a coronary artery bypass graft, an additional base code is reported to describe the intervention performed through the bypass graft. The PCI base codes are 92920, 92924, 92928, 92933, 92937, 92941, and 92943. The PCI base code that includes the most intensive service provided for the target vessel should be reported. The hierarchy of these services is built on an intensity of service ranked from highest to lowest as 92943 = 92941 = 92933 > 92924 > 92937 = 92928 > 92920.

PCI performed during the same session in additional recognized branches of the target vessel should be reported using the applicable add-on code(s). The add-on codes are 92921, 92925, 92928, 92934, 92938, and 92944 and follow the same principle in regard to reporting the most intensive service provided. The intensity of service is ranked from highest to lowest as 92944 = 92938 > 92934 > 92925 > 92929 > 92921.

PCI performed during the same session in additional major coronary or in additional coronary artery bypass grafts should be reported using the applicable additional base code(s). PCI performed during the same session in additional coronary artery branches should be reported using the applicable additional add-on code(s).

If a single lesion extends from one target vessel (major coronary artery, coronary artery bypass graft, or coronary artery branch) into another target vessel, but can be revascularized with a single intervention bridging the two vessels, this PCI should be reported with a single code despite treating more than one vessel. For example, if a left main coronary lesion extends into the proximal left circumflex coronary artery and a single stent is placed to treat the entire lesion, this PCI should be reported as a single vessel stent (92928). In this example, a code for additional vessel treatment (92929) would not be additionally reported.

When bifurcation lesions are treated, PCI is reported for both vessels treated. For example, when a bifurcation lesion involving the left anterior descending artery and the first diagonal artery is treated by stenting both vessels, 92928 and 92929 are both reported.

Target vessel PCI for acute myocardial infarction is inclusive of all balloon angioplasty, atherectomy, stenting, manual aspiration thrombectomy, distal protection, and intracoronary rheolytic agent administration performed. Mechanical thrombectomy is reported separately.

Chronic total occlusion of a coronary vessel is present when there is no antegrade flow through the true lumen, accompanied by suggestive angiographic and clinical criteria (eg, antegrade "bridging" collaterals present, calcification at the occlusion site, no current presentation with ST elevation or Q wave acute myocardial infarction attributable to the occluded target lesion). Current presentation with ST elevation or Q wave acute myocardial infarction attributable to the occluded target lesion, subtotal occlusion, and occlusion with dye staining at the site consistent with fresh thrombus are not considered chronic total occlusion.

▶Codes 92973 (percutaneous transluminal coronary thrombectomy, mechanical), 92974 (coronary brachytherapy), 92978 and 92979 (intravascular ultrasound/optical coherence tomography), 93571 and 93572 (intravascular Doppler velocity and/or pressure [fractional flow reserve {FFR} or coronary flow reserve {CFR}]), and 92972 (percutaneous transluminal coronary lithotripsy), are add-on codes for reporting procedures performed in addition to coronary and bypass graft diagnostic and interventional services, unless included in the base code. Non-mechanical, aspiration thrombectomy is not reported with 92973, and is included in the PCI code for acute myocardial infarction (92941), when performed.◀

(To report transcatheter placement of radiation delivery device for coronary intravascular brachytherapy, use 92974)

(For intravascular radioelement application, see 77770, 77771, 77772)

(For nonsurgical septal reduction therapy [eg, alcohol ablation], use 93799)

#+ **92934**   each additional branch of a major coronary artery (List separately in addition to code for primary procedure)

92943   Percutaneous transluminal revascularization of chronic total occlusion, coronary artery, coronary artery branch, or coronary artery bypass graft, any combination of intracoronary stent, atherectomy and angioplasty; single vessel

#+ **92944**   each additional coronary artery, coronary artery branch, or bypass graft (List separately in addition to code for primary procedure)

(Use 92944 in conjunction with 92924, 92928, 92933, 92937, 92941, 92943)

(To report transcatheter placement of radiation delivery device for coronary intravascular brachytherapy, use 92974)

(For intravascular radioelement application, see 77770, 77771, 77772)

#+● **92972**   Percutaneous transluminal coronary lithotripsy (List separately in addition to code for primary procedure)

▶(Use 92972 in conjunction with 92920, 92924, 92928, 92933, 92937, 92941, 92943, 92975)◀

Rationale

A new add-on code (92972) has been established for the CPT 2024 code set to describe percutaneous transluminal coronary lithotripsy procedure. This procedure may be used in the treatment of heavily calcified coronary arteries. This procedure is performed using pulsatile sonic pressure waves that pass through soft tissue and selectively interact strongly with high-density calcium, producing significant shear stresses that can fracture the calcium.

Percutaneous transluminal coronary lithotripsy code 92972 may be reported in conjunction with codes 92920, 92924, 92928, 92933, 92937, 92941, 92943, and 92975, as appropriate. Because code 92972 describes an add-on service, consider the additional work of performing percutaneous transluminal coronary lithotripsy and the resources related to percutaneous transluminal coronary lithotripsy when reporting the service.

In support of the establishment of code 92972, Category III code 0715T has been deleted for the CPT 2024 code set. A deletion parenthetical note and a cross-reference parenthetical note have been added to direct users to code 92972 in the Category III section.

In accordance with the deletion of Category III code 0715T and the establishment of add-on code 92972, the introductory guidelines in the Medicine Coronary Therapeutic Services and Procedures subsection have been revised to provide instruction on appropriate

Medicine 90281-99607

reporting of percutaneous transluminal coronary lithotripsy procedures. In addition, inclusionary and cross-reference parenthetical notes have been added and deleted in the code set to clarify the appropriate reporting of this new service.

Clinical Example (92972)

A 62-year-old male with a history of left anterior descending (LAD) coronary stent placement presents with exertional chest pain despite appropriate medical therapy. Coronary angiography (reported separately) reveals severe in-stent restenosis, and imaging shows a circumferential calcified ring in the distal portion of the stent. Patient is sent to an angioplasty center, and the lesion is treated with intravascular lithotripsy (IVL) to allow appropriate stent expansion with balloon dilation. [**Note:** This is an add-on code. Only consider the additional physician work related to percutaneous transluminal coronary lithotripsy.]

Description of Procedure (92972)

Based on separately reportable diagnostic coronary angiography, the presence of severe coronary artery calcium is observed. The appropriate diameter coronary IVL catheter is selected. The coronary IVL catheter is inserted over the standard guidewire and advanced to the target location using fluoroscopy and marker bands. Once the coronary IVL catheter is placed, the integrated balloon is inflated to 4 atmosphere (atm) or enough pressure to make contact with the vessel wall. The first lithotripsy cycle of pulses is then delivered. Once the cycle is complete, the integrated balloon is then inflated to its nominal pressure of 6 atm. The balloon is then deflated. The mid-LAD segment is also treated with the 3.0 mm x 20 mm balloon inflated at 8 atm for 50 seconds. Final angiogram shows good angiographic results in LAD with residual stenosis of 30%, no overt dissection, and thrombolysis in myocardial infarction (TIMI) 3 (TIMI 3) flow. No special patient care is needed postoperatively.

#✚ **92973**   Percutaneous transluminal coronary thrombectomy mechanical (List separately in addition to code for primary procedure)

(Use 92973 in conjunction with 92920, 92924, 92928, 92933, 92937, 92941, 92943, 92975, 93454-93461, 93563, 93564)

(Do not report 92973 for aspiration thrombectomy)

Cardiography

93050   Arterial pressure waveform analysis for assessment of central arterial pressures, includes obtaining waveform(s), digitization and application of nonlinear mathematical transformations to determine central arterial pressures and augmentation index, with interpretation and report, upper extremity artery, non-invasive

(Do not report 93050 in conjunction with diagnostic or interventional intra-arterial procedures)

93150   Code is out of numerical sequence. See 93297-93304

93151   Code is out of numerical sequence. See 93297-93304

93152   Code is out of numerical sequence. See 93297-93304

93153   Code is out of numerical sequence. See 93297-93304

▶Phrenic Nerve Stimulation System◀

▶Phrenic nerve stimulation system–therapy activation (93150) is performed once (after 30 days from implantation to allow for lead stabilization). Activation includes device evaluation and programming services: rate, pulse amplitude; pulse duration; configuration of waveform; battery status; electrode selection output modulation; cycling; impedance; and patient compliance measurements (eg, hours of therapy, sleeping position, and activity [sleep activity, awake activity, time in a sleep position]). Subsequent interrogation only (93153) or interrogation and programming (93151, 93152) may be performed to evaluate device function and to optimize performance incrementally. For patients that require programming during a polysomnogram, report 93152 once, regardless of how many programming changes are made over the course of the polysomnogram.◀

#● **93150**   Therapy activation of implanted phrenic nerve stimulator system, including all interrogation and programming

▶(Do not report 93150 in conjunction with 33276, 33277, 33278, 33279, 33280, 33281, 93151, 93152, 93153)◀

#● **93151**   Interrogation and programming (minimum one parameter) of implanted phrenic nerve stimulator system

▶(Do not report 93151 in conjunction with 93150, 93152, 93153)◀

▶(For interrogation without programming of implanted phrenic nerve stimulator system, use 93153)◀

#● **93152**   Interrogation and programming of implanted phrenic nerve stimulator system during polysomnography

▶(Do not report 93152 in conjunction with 33276, 93150, 93151, 93153)◀

▶(For polysomnography, see 95808, 95810, 95811, 95782, 95783)◀

Medicine 90281-99607

#● **93153**   Interrogation without programming of implanted phrenic nerve stimulator system

▶(Do not report 93153 in conjunction with 33276, 93150, 93151, 93152)◀

Rationale

Four new Category I codes (93150-93153) have been established to report programming for phrenic nerve stimulation system. In addition, new guidelines and parenthetical notes have also been included to provide instructions to users regarding appropriate reporting for these codes.

Codes 93150-93153 identify phrenic nerve stimulation system: therapy activation (93150), interrogation and programming (93151, 93152), and subsequent interrogation only (93153). These programming and interrogation codes are reported subsequent to phrenic nerve stimulation system services (33276-33281, 33287, 33288). As noted in the guidelines, these codes may be reported when separate programming or interrogation services are required (eg, evaluate device function, incremental performance optimization) and may not be reported for phrenic nerve stimulation system services performed on the same day. In addition, the guidelines include additional factors that are addressed as part of of the evaluation and programming.

New parenthetical notes have also been established to provide instruction on the appropriate reporting, which includes: (1) restriction for reporting interrogration and programming (93150) in conjunction with insertion (33276, 33277), removal (33278-33280), repositioning (33281), or individual interrogation and programming components (93151-93153); (2) two instructional parenthetical notes that direct reporting for interrogation without programming of implanted phrenic nerve stimulator system (93153), and reporting for polysomnography (95808, 95810, 95811, 95782, 95783).

To accommodate these changes, Category III codes 0424T-0436T and all related references have been deleted. New parenthetical notes have been established to direct users to the appropriate codes for these services.

Refer to the codebook and the Rationale for codes 33276-33288 for full discussion of these changes.

Clinical Example (93150)

A 66-year-old male, who had a phrenic nerve stimulator system implanted, recently returns to the clinic for initial activation of therapy.

Description of Procedure (93150)

Program the neurostimulator system for the first time after implanted to initiate therapy and to evaluate parameters of respiratory rate, pulse amplitude, pulse duration, selection of sensing vector, battery status, electrode selection, timing of stimulation impedance, and patient-compliance measurements for six leads. Historical data collected during monitoring mode before activation, query of patient-sleep patterns/habits in supine, left lateral and right lateral positions, and waveforms stored by neurostimulator are used to program initial settings. Educate patient about the system and how to optimally interact with the system. If patient has a concomitant device, testing for interaction is also performed during the visit prior to starting therapy. Evaluate all possible stimulation settings during the initial programming session. Utilize device data to determine the pacing configuration and stimulation frequency.

Clinical Example (93151)

A 68-year-old male, who has central sleep apnea and a previously implanted and activated phrenic nerve stimulator system, whose device programming needs to be adjusted due to recent new symptoms.

Description of Procedure (93151)

Patient had previously undergone implantation of a neurostimulator system, and the system has previously been programmed. From the supine, left lateral, and right lateral positions, the implantable pulse generator is interrogated to evaluate various parameters of rate, pulse amplitude, pulse duration, configuration of waveform, battery status, electrode selection, output modulation, impedance, timing of stimulation, and patient-compliance measurements. Patient is queried for input and feedback on personal perceptions about the system settings. At least one of these parameters is changed to provide optimal results. The device data are utilized to determine the pacing configuration and stimulation frequency.

Clinical Example (93152)

A 66-year-old male with a previously implanted phrenic nerve stimulation system requires evaluation while sleeping to confirm therapy efficacy and optimize programming during a polysomnogram.

Description of Procedure (93152)

Patient had previously undergone implantation of a neurostimulator system, and the system has previously been activated. During a sleep study, a programmer uses continuous evaluation to change parameters based on output during the attended-sleep study to optimize respiratory rate, pulse amplitude, pulse duration, and patient arousal threshold. Data captured after patient is awakened at set intervals to adjust settings in three positions (supine, left lateral, and right lateral) or based on the apnea hypopnea index. One programming adjustment is made based on the position in which the patient was still having events. Interpretation of neurostimulator data is performed at the same time the polysomnogram is interpreted. The device data are utilized to determine the pacing configuration and stimulation frequency that provide maximal physiologic diaphragm movement throughout the night in all sleeping positions.

Clinical Example (93153)

A 68-year-old male, who has central sleep apnea and an implantable phrenic nerve stimulator system, comes to clinic to check battery status and overall device function.

Description of Procedure (93153)

Patient had previously undergone implantation of a neurostimulator system, and the system has previously been programmed. The system is interrogated to evaluate parameters of rate, pulse amplitude, and pulse duration; configuration of waveform and battery status; and electrode selection, output modulation, impedance, and patient-compliance measurements. No changes are made to the previously programmed parameters.

Cardiac Catheterization

+ **93563**   Injection procedure during cardiac catheterization including imaging supervision, interpretation, and report; for selective coronary angiography during congenital heart catheterization (List separately in addition to code for primary procedure)

(Use 93563 in conjunction with 33741, 33745, 93582, 93593, 93594, 93595, 93596, 93597)

+ **93564**   for selective opacification of aortocoronary venous or arterial bypass graft(s) (eg, aortocoronary saphenous vein, free radial artery, or free mammary artery graft) to one or more coronary arteries and in situ arterial conduits (eg, internal mammary), whether native or used for bypass to one or more coronary arteries during congenital heart catheterization, when performed (List separately in addition to code for primary procedure)

(Use 93564 in conjunction with 93582, 93593, 93594, 93595, 93596, 93597)

(Do not report 93563, 93564 in conjunction with 33418, 0345T, 0483T, 0484T, 0544T, 0545T for coronary angiography intrinsic to the valve repair or annulus reconstruction procedure)

+ **93565**   for selective left ventricular or left atrial angiography (List separately in addition to code for primary procedure)

(Use 93565 in conjunction with 33741, 33745, 93582, 93593, 93594, 93595, 93596, 93597)

(Do not report 93563-93565 in conjunction with 93452-93461)

+ **93566**   for selective right ventricular or right atrial angiography (List separately in addition to code for primary procedure)

(Use 93566 in conjunction with 33741, 33745, 93451, 93453, 93456, 93457, 93460, 93461, 93582, 93593, 93594, 93595, 93596, 93597)

►(Do not report 93566 in conjunction with 33274, 0795T, 0796T, 0797T, 0801T, 0802T, 0803T, 0823T, 0824T, 0825T, for right ventriculography performed during leadless pacemaker insertion)◄

(Do not report 93566 in conjunction with 0545T for right ventricular or right atrial angiography procedures intrinsic to the annulus reconstruction procedure)

Rationale

In accordance with the establishment of codes 0795T-0803T, and 0823T-0825T, the exclusionary parenthetical note following code 93566 has been revised.

Refer to the codebook and the Rationale for codes 0795T-0803T and 0823T-0825T for a full discussion of these changes.

Repair of Structural Heart Defect

93583   Percutaneous transcatheter septal reduction therapy (eg, alcohol septal ablation) including temporary pacemaker insertion when performed

(93583 includes insertion of temporary pacemaker, when performed, and left heart catheterization)

(Do not report 93583 in conjunction with 33210, 93452, 93453, 93458, 93459, 93460, 93461, 93565, 93595, 93596, 93597)

(93583 includes left anterior descending coronary angiography for the purpose of roadmapping to guide the intervention. Do not report 93454, 93455, 93456, 93457, 93458, 93459, 93460, 93461, 93563 for coronary angiography performed during alcohol septal ablation for the purpose of roadmapping, guidance of the intervention, vessel measurement, and completion angiography)

▲=Revised code   ●=New code   ►◄=Contains new or revised text   ✕=Duplicate PLA test   ↕=Category I PLA   American Medical Association   **135**

Medicine 90281-99607

(Diagnostic cardiac catheterization procedures may be separately reportable when no prior catheter-based diagnostic study of the treatment zone is available, the prior diagnostic study is inadequate, or the patient's condition with respect to the clinical indication has changed since the prior study or during the intervention. Use the appropriate codes from 93451, 93454, 93455, 93456, 93457, 93563, 93564, 93566, 93567, 93568, 93593, 93594, 93598, 93569, 93573, 93574, 93575)

(Do not report 93583 in conjunction with 33210, 33211)

(Do not report 93463 for the injection of alcohol for this procedure)

(For intracardiac echocardiographic services performed at the time of alcohol septal ablation, use 93662)

(Other echocardiographic services provided by a separate physician are reported using the appropriate echocardiography services codes, 93312, 93313, 93314, 93315, 93316, 93317)

(For surgical ventriculomyotomy [-myectomy] for idiopathic hypertrophic subaortic stenosis, use 33416)

93584   Code is out of numerical sequence. See 93596-93598

93585   Code is out of numerical sequence. See 93596-93598

93586   Code is out of numerical sequence. See 93596-93598

93587   Code is out of numerical sequence. See 93596-93598

93588   Code is out of numerical sequence. See 93596-93598

Cardiac Catheterization for Congenital Heart Defects

Cardiac catheterization for the evaluation of congenital heart defect(s) is reported with 93593, 93594, 93595, 93596, 93597, 93598. Cardiac catheterization services for anomalous coronary arteries arising from the aorta or off of other coronary arteries, patent foramen ovale, mitral valve prolapse, and bicuspid aortic valve, in the absence of other congenital heart defects, are reported with 93451-93464, 93566, 93567, 93568. However, when these conditions exist in conjunction with other congenital heart defects, 93593, 93594, 93595, 93596, 93597 may be reported. Evaluation of anomalous coronary arteries arising from the pulmonary arterial system is reported with the cardiac catheterization for congenital heart defects codes.

For additional guidance on reporting cardiac catheterization services for congenital heart defects versus non-congenital indications, see Cardiac Catheterization guidelines.

Right heart catheterization for congenital heart defects (93593, 93594, 93596, 93597): includes catheter placement in one or more right-sided cardiac chamber(s) or structures (ie, the right atrium, right ventricle, pulmonary artery, pulmonary wedge), obtaining blood

samples for measurement of blood gases, and Fick cardiac output measurements, when performed. While the morphologic right atrium and morphologic right ventricle are typically the right heart structures supplying blood flow to the pulmonary artery, in congenital heart disease the subpulmonic ventricle may be a morphologic left ventricle and the subpulmonic atrium may be a morphologic left atrium. For reporting purposes, when the morphologic left ventricle or left atrium is in a subpulmonic position due to congenital heart disease, catheter placement in either of these structures is considered part of right heart catheterization and does not constitute left heart catheterization. Right heart catheterization for congenital cardiac anomalies does not typically involve thermodilution cardiac output assessments. When thermodilution cardiac output is performed in this setting, it may be separately reported using add-on code 93598. Right heart catheterization does not include right ventricular or right atrial angiography. When right ventricular or right atrial angiography is performed, use 93566. For reporting purposes, angiography of the morphologic right ventricle or morphologic right atrium is reported with 93566, whether these structures are in the standard pre-pulmonic position or in a systemic (subaortic) position. For placement of a flow directed catheter (eg, Swan-Ganz) performed for hemodynamic monitoring purposes not in conjunction with other catheterization services, use 93503. Do not report 93503 in conjunction with 93453, 93456, 93457, 93460, 93461, 93593, 93594, 93595, 93596, 93597.

Right heart catheterization for congenital heart defects may be performed in patients with normal or abnormal connections. The terms *normal* and *abnormal* native connections are used to define the variations in the anatomic connections from the great veins to the atria, atria to the ventricles, and ventricles to the great arteries. This designation as normal or abnormal is used to determine the appropriate code to report right heart catheterization services in congenital heart disease.

▶Normal native connections exist when the pathway of blood flow follows the expected course through the right and left heart chambers and great vessels (ie, superior vena cava [SVC]/inferior vena cava [IVC] to right atrium, then right ventricle, then pulmonary arteries for the right heart; left atrium to left ventricle, then aorta for the left heart). Examples of congenital heart defects with normal connections would include acyanotic defects such as isolated atrial septal defect, ventricular septal defect, or patent ductus arteriosus. Services including right heart catheterization for congenital cardiac anomalies with normal connections are reported with 93593, 93596.◄

Abnormal native connections exist when there are alternative connections for the pathway of blood flow through the heart and great vessels. Abnormal connections are typically present in patients with cyanotic congenital heart defects, any variation of single ventricle anatomy (eg, hypoplastic right or left heart, double outlet right ventricle), unbalanced atrioventricular canal (endocardial cushion) defect, transposition of the great arteries, valvular atresia, tetralogy of Fallot with or without major aortopulmonary collateral arteries (MAPCAs), total anomalous pulmonary veins, truncus arteriosus, and any lesions with heterotaxia and/or dextrocardia. Examples of right heart catheterization through abnormal connections include accessing the pulmonary arteries via surgical shunts, accessing the pulmonary circulation from the aorta via MAPCAs, or accessing isolated pulmonary arteries through a patent ductus arteriosus. Other examples would include right heart catheterization through cavopulmonary anastomoses, Fontan conduits, atrial switch conduits (Mustard/Senning), or any variations of single ventricle anatomy/physiology. Services including right heart catheterization for congenital heart defects with abnormal connections are reported with 93594, 93597.

Left heart catheterization for congenital heart defects (93595, 93596, 93597): involves catheter placement in a left-sided (systemic) cardiac chamber(s) (ventricle or atrium). The systemic chambers channel oxygenated blood to the aorta. In normal physiology, the systemic chambers include the morphologic left atrium and left ventricle. In congenital heart disease, the systemic chambers may include a morphologic right atrium or morphologic right ventricle which is connected to the aorta due to transposition or other congenital anomaly. These may be termed *subaortic* chambers. For the purposes of reporting, the term left ventricle or left atrium is meant to describe the systemic (subaortic) ventricle or atrium. When left heart catheterization is performed using either transapical puncture of the left ventricle or transseptal puncture of an intact septum, report 93462 in conjunction with 93595, 93596, 93597. Left heart catheterization for congenital heart defects does not include left ventricular/left atrial angiography when performed. Left ventriculography or left atrial angiography performed during cardiac catheterization for congenital heart defects is separately reported with 93565. For reporting purposes, angiography of the morphologic left ventricle or morphologic left atrium is reported with 93565, whether these structures are in the standard systemic (subaortic) position or in a pre-pulmonic position. For left heart catheterization only, in patients with congenital heart defects, with either normal or abnormal connections, use 93595. When combined left and right heart catheterization is performed to evaluate congenital heart defects, use 93596 for normal native connections, or 93597 for abnormal native connections.

Catheter placement and injection procedures: The work of imaging guidance, including fluoroscopy and ultrasound guidance for vascular access and to guide catheter placement for hemodynamic evaluation, is included in the cardiac catheterization for congenital heart defects codes, when performed by the same operator.

For cardiac catheterization for congenital heart defects, injection procedures are separately reportable due to the marked variability in the cardiovascular anatomy encountered.

▶When contrast injection(s) is performed in conjunction with cardiac catheterization for congenital heart defects, see injection procedure codes 93563, 93564, 93565, 93566, 93567, 93568, 93569, 93573, 93574, 93575, 93584, 93585, 93586, 93587, 93588, or use appropriate codes from the Radiology section and the Vascular Injection Procedures subsection in the Surgery/Cardiovascular System section. For venography of the IVC, report 75825. For venography of the SVC, report 75827. Venography of an anomalous or persistent SVC (93584), the azygous/hemiazygous venous system (93585), the coronary sinus (93586), or venovenous collaterals (93587, 93588) requires catheter placement(s) distinct from that required for congenital right and left heart catheterization. Therefore, 93584, 93585, 93586, 93587, 93588 include catheter placement in addition to venography. Codes 93563, 93564, 93565, 93566, 93567, 93568, 93569, 93573, 93574, 93575, 93584, 93585, 93586, 93587, 93588 include imaging supervision, interpretation, and report.

Injection procedures 93563, 93564, 93565, 93566, 93567, 93568, 93569, 93573, 93574, 93575, 93584, 93585, 93586, 93587, 93588 represent separate, identifiable services and may be reported in conjunction with one another, when appropriate. For angiography of other noncoronary and nonpulmonary arteries and veins, performed as a distinct service, use appropriate codes from the Radiology section and the Vascular Injection Procedures subsection in the Surgery/Cardiovascular System section.

Venography: Catheter placement in a normal SVC and a normal IVC is considered as part of a standard congenital cardiac catheterization. When venography of the normal IVC is performed, report 75825. When venography of the normal SVC is performed, report 75827. For coding purposes, the term "anomalous/persistent left or right SVC" refers to a second SVC on the opposite side of the chest from the first SVC. For example, in a typical cardiac anatomy, the SVC is on the right side and a persistent left SVC would be on the left side. In situs inversus, the SVC would typically be located on the left side of the chest and a persistent right SVC would be on the right side. In heterotaxy, bilateral SVCs are common. In these scenarios, venography of the first SVC would be reported with 75827, and catheter placement and venography of the persistent/anomalous SVC would be reported with 93584.

Selective catheter placement in anomalous congenital venous structures is not included in a standard congenital cardiac catheterization. Therefore, add-on codes 93584, 93585, 93586, 93587, 93588 include selective catheter placement in the specific venous structure(s) being imaged as well as venography and radiologic supervision, interpretation, and report.◄

Angiography of the native coronary arteries or bypass grafts during cardiac catheterization for congenital heart defects is reported with 93563, 93564. Catheter placement(s) in coronary artery(ies) or bypass grafts involves selective engagement of the origins of the native coronary artery(ies) or bypass grafts for the purpose of coronary angiography.

(Selective pulmonary angiography codes for cardiac catheterization [93569, 93573, 93574, 93575] include selective catheter positioning of the angiographic catheter, injection, and radiologic supervision and interpretation)

93596   Right and left heart catheterization for congenital heart defect(s) including imaging guidance by the proceduralist to advance the catheter to the target zone(s); normal native connections

93597   abnormal native connections

#✚● **93584**   Venography for congenital heart defect(s), including catheter placement, and radiological supervision and interpretation; anomalous or persistent superior vena cava when it exists as a second contralateral superior vena cava, with native drainage to heart (List separately in addition to code for primary procedure)

▶(Use 93584 in conjunction with 93593, 93594, 93596, 93597)◄

▶(Report 93584 once per session)◄

#✚● **93585**   azygos/hemiazygos venous system (List separately in addition to code for primary procedure)

▶(Use 93585 in conjunction with 93593, 93594, 93596, 93597)◄

▶(Report 93585 once per session)◄

#✚● **93586**   coronary sinus (List separately in addition to code for primary procedure)

▶(Use 93586 in conjunction with 93593, 93594, 93596, 93597)◄

▶(Report 93586 once per session)◄

#✚● **93587**   venovenous collaterals originating at or above the heart (eg, from innominate vein) (List separately in addition to code for primary procedure)

▶(Use 93587 in conjunction with 93593, 93594, 93596, 93597)◄

▶(Report 93587 once per session)◄

#✚● **93588**   venovenous collaterals originating below the heart (eg, from the inferior vena cava) (List separately in addition to code for primary procedure)

▶(Use 93588 in conjunction with 93593, 93594, 93596, 93597)◄

▶(Report 93588 once per session)◄

Rationale

Add-on codes 93584 and 93585-93588 have been established for reporting venography services to treat congenital heart defects. The Cardiac Catheterization for Congenital Heart Defects guidelines have been revised with instructions on the appropriate reporting of these procedures, including the addition of a definition of *venography*.

Abnormalities in the cardiac anatomy (eg, heterotaxy syndrome, complex single ventricle physiology, anatomy following previous Fontan surgery) may affect the performance of procedures such as diagnostic procedures, interventional procedures, and open heart surgery. Therefore, identification of cardiac abnormalities via venography is important. In addition, venography of abnormal cardiac anatomy involves different work and complexity than venography of normal cardiac anatomy. Codes 93584-93588 describe venography procedures to identify and assess cardiac anatomy when cardiac abnormalities are present. These venography procedures are add-on procedures performed during heart catheterization for congenital heart defect(s) (ie, 93593, 93594, 93596, 93597). Radiological supervision and interpretation are included, and codes 93584-93588 are reported once per session. Each of the new codes describes venography in a specific abnormal vessel or abnormal venous system as indicated in the following table:

CPT Code	Vessel or Venous System
93584	Superior vena cava
93585	Azygos/hemiazygos venous system
93586	Coronary sinus
93587	Venovenous collaterals originating *at or above* the heart (eg, from innominate vein)
93588	Venovenous collaterals originating *below* the heart (eg, from the inferior vena cava)

Inclusionary and instructional parenthetical notes have been added following each of the new codes to indicate the codes with which codes 93584-93588 are reported, and that each code is reported only once per session.

The cross-reference parenthetical note following cardiac output measurement code 93598 that direct users to the codes for contrast injections during cardiac catheterization for congenital heart defect(s) has been revised with the addition of codes 75825, 75827, and 93584-93588.

Clinical Example (93584)

A 5-month-old female with hypoplastic left heart syndrome, whose status is post-Norwood operation, is identified with an anomalous superior vena cava (SVC) during a diagnostic right and left cardiac catheterization in preparation for next-stage cavopulmonary anastomosis, has venography to aid surgical planning. [**Note:** This is an add-on code. Only consider the additional work related to achieving catheter placement and performance of anomalous superior vena cava venography.]

Description of Procedure (93584)

Insert an end-hole guide catheter through a venous sheath and, with guidewire assistance, into an SVC. Perform venography with contrast injection. If present, a second SVC that requires incorporation into a surgical cavopulmonary anastomosis is entered. (Catheter placement is reported separately with the diagnostic cardiac catheterization codes for congenital heart disease.) Repeat venography with contrast injection to delineate the vessel course.

Clinical Example (93585)

A 2-month-old male with heterotaxy syndrome has venography of the azygos or hemi-azygos vein during diagnostic right and left cardiac catheterization. [**Note:** This is an add-on code. Only consider the additional work related to achieving catheter placement and performance of azygos or hemi-azygos venography.]

Description of Procedure (93585)

Insert an end-hole guide catheter through a venous sheath and, with guidewire assistance, into the inferior vena cava (IVC). If present, a second IVC is entered. (Catheter placement is reported separately with the diagnostic cardiac catheterization codes for congenital heart disease.) Perform venography of the IVC with contrast injection to delineate its drainage.

Clinical Example (93586)

An 18-year-old female with complex single-ventricle physiology, who has undergone classic Fontan surgery, has venography of the coronary sinus during diagnostic cardiac catheterization. [**Note:** This is an add-on code. Only consider the additional work related to achieving catheter placement and performance of coronary sinus venography.]

Description of Procedure (93586)

Insert an end-hole guide catheter through a venous sheath and, with guidewire assistance, to the heart and direct into the coronary sinus. (Catheter placement is reported separately with the diagnostic cardiac catheterization codes for congenital heart disease.) Perform venography of the coronary sinus with contrast injection in the vessel coronary sinus to delineate the course.

Clinical Example (93587)

A 15-year-old female, who previously had Fontan surgery has cyanosis, is discovered with venovenous collaterals has venography performed during diagnostic cardiac catheterization. [**Note:** This is an add-on code. Only consider the additional work related to achieving catheter placement and performance of venography of venovenous collaterals originating at or above the heart.]

Description of Procedure (93587)

Insert an end-hole guide catheter through a venous sheath and, with guidewire assistance, direct into all portions of the systemic venous pathway(s) draining to the heart from the level of the heart or above. (Catheter placement is reported separately with the diagnostic cardiac catheterization codes for congenital heart disease.) Perform venography with contrast injection to delineate the course and drainage of the venovenous collaterals arising at the level of the heart or above. Repeat the process for any additional venovenous collaterals arising at the level of the heart or above and draining to the heart.

Clinical Example (93588)

A 17-year-old male, who previously had Fontan surgery has cyanosis, is discovered with venovenous collaterals has venography performed during diagnostic cardiac catheterization. [**Note:** This is an add-on code. Only consider the additional work related to achieving catheter placement and performance of venography of venovenous collaterals originating below the heart.]

Description of Procedure (93588)

Insert an end-hole guide catheter through a venous sheath and, with guidewire assistance, direct into all portions of the systemic venous pathway(s) arising from below the heart. (Catheter placement is reported separately with the diagnostic cardiac catheterization codes for congenital heart disease.) Perform venography with contrast injection to delineate the course and drainage of the venovenous collaterals. Repeat the process for any additional venovenous collaterals arising from below the heart and draining to the heart.

+ 93598 Cardiac output measurement(s), thermodilution or other indicator dilution method, performed during cardiac catheterization for the evaluation of congenital heart defects (List separately in addition to code for primary procedure)

(Use 93598 in conjunction with 93593, 93594, 93595, 93596, 93597)

(Do not report 93598 in conjunction with 93451-93461)

(For pharmacologic agent administration during cardiac catheterization for congenital heart defect[s], use 93463)

(For physiological exercise study with cardiac catheterization for congenital heart defect[s], use 93464)

(For indicator dilution studies such as thermodilution for cardiac output measurement during cardiac catheterization for congenital heart defect[s], use 93598)

▶(For contrast injections during cardiac catheterization for congenital heart defect[s], see 75825, 75827, 93563, 93564, 93565, 93566, 93567, 93568, 93569, 93573, 93574, 93575, 93584, 93585, 93586, 93587, 93588)◀

(For angiography or venography not described in the 90000 series code section, see appropriate codes from the Radiology section and the Vascular Injection Procedures subsection in the Surgery/Cardiovascular System section)

(For transseptal or transapical access of the left atrium during cardiac catheterization for congenital heart defect[s], use 93462 in conjunction with 93595, 93596, 93597, as appropriate)

Rationale

In accordance with the establishment of codes 93584-93588, the cross-reference parenthetical note for contrast injections during cardiac catheterization for congenital heart defect(s) following code 93598 has been revised to reflect these changes.

Refer to the codebook and the Rationale for codes 93584-93588 for a full discussion of these changes.

Intracardiac Electrophysiological Procedures/Studies

+ 93662 Intracardiac echocardiography during therapeutic/diagnostic intervention, including imaging supervision and interpretation (List separately in addition to code for primary procedure)

▶(Use 93662 in conjunction with 33274, 33275, 33340, 33361, 33362, 33363, 33364, 33365, 33366, 33418, 33477, 33741, 33745, 92986, 92987, 92990, 92997, 93451, 93452, 93453, 93454, 93455, 93456, 93457, 93458, 93459, 93460, 93461, 93505, 93580, 93581, 93582, 93583, 93590, 93591, 93593, 93594, 93595, 93596, 93597, 93620, 93653, 93654, 0345T, 0483T, 0484T, 0543T, 0544T, 0545T, 0795T, 0796T, 0797T, 0798T, 0799T, 0800T, 0801T, 0802T, 0803T, 0823T, 0824T, 0825T, as appropriate)◀

(Do not report 93662 in conjunction with 92961, 0569T, 0570T, 0613T)

Rationale

In accordance with the establishment of codes 0795T-0803T and 0823T-0825T, the inclusionary parenthetical note following code 93662 has been revised.

Refer to the codebook and the Rationale for codes 0795T-0803T and 0823T-0825T for a full discussion of these changes.

Neurology and Neuromuscular Procedures

Sleep Medicine Testing

95808 Polysomnography; any age, sleep staging with 1-3 additional parameters of sleep, attended by a technologist

 # 95783 younger than 6 years, sleep staging with 4 or more additional parameters of sleep, with initiation of continuous positive airway pressure therapy or bi-level ventilation, attended by a technologist

▶(For interrogation and programming of a phrenic nerve stimulator system during a polysomnogram, use 93152)◀

★ = Telemedicine   ◀ = Audio-only   + = Add-on code   ✚ = FDA approval pending   # = Resequenced code   ⊘ = Modifier 51 exempt

Rationale

In accordance with the establishment of code 93152, a cross-reference parenthetical note has been added following code 95783 to direct users to report code 93152 for interrogation and programming of a phrenic nerve stimulator system during a polysomnogram.

Refer to the codebook and the Rationale for codes 93150-93153 for a full discussion of these changes.

Electromyography

#✚ 95885 Needle electromyography, each extremity, with related paraspinal areas, when performed, done with nerve conduction, amplitude and latency/velocity study; limited (List separately in addition to code for primary procedure)

#✚ 95886 complete, five or more muscles studied, innervated by three or more nerves or four or more spinal levels (List separately in addition to code for primary procedure)

(Use 95885, 95886 in conjunction with 95907-95913)

(Do not report 95885, 95886 in conjunction with 95860-95864, 95870, 95905)

▶(Do not report 95885, 95886 for noninvasive nerve conduction guidance used in conjunction with 0766T)◀

#✚ 95887 Needle electromyography, non-extremity (cranial nerve supplied or axial) muscle(s) done with nerve conduction, amplitude and latency/velocity study (List separately in addition to code for primary procedure)

(Use 95887 in conjunction with 95907-95913)

(Do not report 95887 in conjunction with 95867-95870, 95905)

▶(Do not report 95887 for noninvasive nerve conduction guidance used in conjunction with 0766T)◀

Rationale

In accordance with the deletion of code 0768T, parenthetical notes following codes 95886 and 95887 have been revised to reflect the deleted code and to direct users to the appropriate codes for reporting transcutaneous magnetic stimulation.

Refer to the codebook and the Rationale for codes 0766T-0769T for a full discussion of these changes.

Nerve Conduction Tests

95907 Nerve conduction studies; 1-2 studies

95913 13 or more studies

▶(Do not report 95905, 95907, 95908, 95909, 95910, 95911, 95912, 95913 for noninvasive nerve conduction guidance used in conjunction with 0766T)◀

Rationale

In accordance with the deletion of code 0768T, a parenthetical note following code 95913 has been revised to reflect the deleted code and to direct users to the appropriate codes for reporting transcutaneous magnetic stimulation.

Refer to the codebook and the Rationale for codes 0766T-0769T for a full discussion of these changes.

Hydration, Therapeutic, Prophylactic, Diagnostic Injections and Infusions, and Chemotherapy and Other Highly Complex Drug or Highly Complex Biologic Agent Administration

Therapeutic, Prophylactic, and Diagnostic Injections and Infusions (Excludes Chemotherapy and Other Highly Complex Drug or Highly Complex Biologic Agent Administration)

96372 Therapeutic, prophylactic, or diagnostic injection (specify substance or drug); subcutaneous or intramuscular

▶(For administration of vaccines/toxoids, see 90460, 90461, 90471, 90472, 0001A, 0002A, 0003A, 0004A, 0011A, 0012A, 0013A, 0021A, 0022A, 0031A, 0034A, 0041A, 0042A, 0044A, 0051A, 0052A, 0053A, 0054A, 0064A, 0071A, 0072A, 0073A, 0074A, 0081A, 0082A, 0083A, 0091A, 0092A, 0093A, 0094A, 0104A, 0111A, 0112A, 0113A, 0121A, 0124A, 0134A, 0141A, 0142A, 0144A, 0151A, 0154A, 0164A, 0171A, 0172A, 0173A, 0174A)◀

Medicine 90281-99607

(Report 96372 for non-antineoplastic hormonal therapy injections)

(Report 96401 for anti-neoplastic nonhormonal injection therapy)

(Report 96402 for anti-neoplastic hormonal injection therapy)

(For intradermal cancer immunotherapy injection, see 0708T, 0709T)

(Do not report 96372 for injections given without direct physician or other qualified health care professional supervision. To report, use 99211. Hospitals may report 96372 when the physician or other qualified health care professional is not present)

(96372 does not include injections for allergen immunotherapy. For allergen immunotherapy injections, see 95115-95117)

Rationale

To accommodate the addition of new codes for reporting for COVID-19 vaccinations, the parenthetical note following code 96372 has been updated to reflect the addition of the new codes.

Refer to the codebook and the Rationale for COVID-19 vaccination administrations for a full discussion of the changes.

Chemotherapy and Other Highly Complex Drug or Highly Complex Biologic Agent Administration

Other Injection and Infusion Services

▲ **96446**   Chemotherapy administration into the peritoneal cavity via implanted port or catheter

▶(For intraoperative hyperthermic intraperitoneal chemotherapy [HIPEC], see 96547, 96548)◀

96542   Chemotherapy injection, subarachnoid or intraventricular via subcutaneous reservoir, single or multiple agents

(For radioactive isotope therapy, use 79005)

▶Codes 96547, 96548 describe the hyperthermic intraperitoneal chemotherapy (HIPEC) procedure that includes intraoperative perfusion of a heated chemotherapy agent into the abdominal cavity through catheters. The HIPEC procedure is distinct from the primary procedure and may include chemotherapy agent selection, confirmation of perfusion equipment settings for chemotherapy agent delivery, additional incision(s) for catheter and temperature probe placement, perfusion

supervision and manual agitation of the heated chemotherapy agent in the abdominal cavity during chemotherapy agent dwell time, irrigation of the chemotherapy agent, closure of wounds related to HIPEC, and documentation of the chemotherapy agent and HIPEC procedure in the medical record. Codes 96547, 96548 are add-on codes and do not include the typical preoperative, intraoperative, and postoperative work related to the primary procedure. Code 96547 is reported for the first 60 minutes of the HIPEC procedure and 96548 is reported for each additional 30 minutes.◀

+● **96547**   Intraoperative hyperthermic intraperitoneal chemotherapy (HIPEC) procedure, including separate incision(s) and closure, when performed; first 60 minutes (List separately in addition to code for primary procedure)

+● **96548**   each additional 30 minutes (List separately in addition to code for primary procedure)

▶(Use 96547, 96548 in conjunction with 38100, 38101, 38102, 38120, 43611, 43620, 43621, 43622, 43631, 43632, 43633, 43634, 44010, 44015, 44110, 44111, 44120, 44121, 44125, 44130, 44139, 44140, 44141, 44143, 44144, 44145, 44146, 44147, 44150, 44151, 44155, 44156, 44157, 44158, 44160, 44202, 44203, 44204, 44207, 44213, 44227, 47001, 47100, 48140, 48145, 48152, 48155, 49000, 49010, 49203, 49204, 49205, 49320, 58200, 58210, 58575, 58940, 58943, 58950, 58951, 58952, 58953, 58954, 58956, 58957, 58958, 58960)◀

Rationale

Intra-abdominal tumor excision followed by hyperthermic intraperitoneal chemotherapy (HIPEC) is an accepted treatment for disorders of the abdomen, such as peritoneal, mesenteric, and retroperitoneal disease. HIPEC is performed intraoperatively in which a catheter is placed in the abdomen for chemotherapy administration. Variable time is required depending on the tumor-specific drug selection. It is for this reason, add-on codes 96547 and 96548 have been established for the CPT 2024 code set.

Code 96446 was originally created to report chemotherapy administration into the peritoneal cavity through an indwelling port or catheter. For the CPT 2024 code set, code 96446 has been revised to define the work involved in code 96466 and to distinguish the chemotherapy administration performed in HIPEC by replacing "indwelling" with "implanted" in the code descriptor. In addition, add-on codes 96547 and 96548 have been established to report time duration of the HIPEC procedure. Specifically, code 96547 describes HIPEC for the first 60 minutes, and add-on code 96548 describes HIPEC for each additional 30 minutes. Codes 96547 and 96548 are add-on codes and do not include the typical preoperative, intraoperative, and postoperative work related to the primary procedure.

A cross-reference parenthetical note has been added in the Radiology and Medicine sections following codes 77605 and 96446 to direct users to codes 96547 and 96548 for HIPEC. In addition, guidelines have been added to describe work that is and is not included in the HIPEC procedure when performed.

Clinical Example (96446)

A 62-year-old female with advanced ovarian cancer, who has undergone optimal surgical debulking of her cancer and placement of an intraperitoneal catheter with or without a subcutaneous port at operation for chemotherapy on subsequent dates, presents to the office for intraperitoneal chemotherapy (other than hyperthermic intraperitoneal chemotherapy [HIPEC]) using the previously implanted peritoneal catheter.

Description of Procedure (96446)

N/A

Clinical Example (96547)

A HIPEC procedure that required 60 minutes is performed during the same operative session after the completion of a peritoneal tumor resection and cytoreduction. [**Note:** This is an add-on code. Only consider the additional work related to the first 60 minutes of the HIPEC procedure.]

Description of Procedure (96547)

After completion of the resectional component of the primary procedure, place inflow and outflow catheters. Secure catheters to the skin with sutures. Close the skin of the abdominal incision from the primary procedure over the viscera and catheters with monofilament sutures. Place patient on a cooling pad, connect the catheters to the infusion pump, and deliver heated chemotherapy into the peritoneal space. Constant external manual agitation is carried out by the surgeon throughout the chemotherapy dwell time. Additional chemotherapy is administered during this process as dictated by protocol. Following completion of HIPEC and dwell time, reopen the abdomen by removing the abdominal closure sutures. Remove the abdominal infusion catheters. Thoroughly inspect the abdomen and viscera. Inspect each of the catheter insertion sites, and close the catheter skin incisions as appropriate. Patient then undergoes completion of the separately reported primary procedure.

Clinical Example (96548)

An additional 30 minutes of HIPEC is performed after a peritoneal tumor resection and cytoreduction and a 60-minute HIPEC procedure during the same operative session. [**Note:** This is an add-on code. Only consider the additional work related to the additional 30 minutes of HIPEC.]

Description of Procedure (96548)

Code 96548 is reported for each additional 30 minutes of procedure time for HIPEC after the first 60 minutes, which is separately reported with code 96547.

96549   Unlisted chemotherapy procedure

Special Dermatological Procedures

▲ **96920**   Excimer laser treatment for psoriasis; total area less than 250 sq cm

▲ **96921**   250 sq cm to 500 sq cm

▲ **96922**   over 500 sq cm

Rationale

Codes 96920-96922 have been revised to better align with the intended use of these services exclusively for psoriasis. Specifically, parent code 96920 has been revised to include the term "Excimer" to identify the type of ultraviolet laser used to perform the service. The revision has also been made to indicate how the skin surface area is treated and to offer guidance to better understand the physician's work involved in performing the service and to prevent improper coding.

▲ = Revised code   ● = New code   ▶ ◀ = Contains new or revised text   ✂ = Duplicate PLA test   ↕ = Category I PLA   American Medical Association   **143**

Medicine 90281-99607

Physical Medicine and Rehabilitation

Modalities

Supervised

97010   Application of a modality to 1 or more areas; hot or cold packs

97014   electrical stimulation (unattended)

(For acupuncture with electrical stimulation, see 97813, 97814)

▶(For peripheral nerve transcutaneous magnetic stimulation, see 0766T, 0767T)◀

Rationale

In accordance with the deletion of codes 0768T and 0769T, a parenthetical note following code 97014 has been revised to reflect the deleted codes and to direct users to the appropriate codes for reporting transcutaneous magnetic stimulation.

Refer to the codebook and the Rationale for codes 0766T-0769T for a full discussion of these changes.

Constant Attendance

97032   Application of a modality to 1 or more areas; electrical stimulation (manual), each 15 minutes

(For transcutaneous electrical modulation pain reprocessing [TEMPR/scrambler therapy], use 0278T)

▶(For peripheral nerve transcutaneous magnetic stimulation, see 0766T, 0767T)◀

Rationale

In accordance with the deletion of codes 0768T and 0769T, a parenthetical note following code 97032 has been revised to reflect the deleted codes and to direct users to the appropriate codes for reporting transcutaneous magnetic stimulation.

Refer to the codebook and the Rationale for codes 0766T-0769T for a full discussion of these changes.

#● **97037**   low-level laser therapy (ie, nonthermal and non-ablative) for post-operative pain reduction

▶(Do not report 97037 in conjunction with 0552T)◀

▶(For dynamic thermokinetic energies therapy, infrared, use 97026)◀

Rationale

Code 97037 has been established to report low-level laser therapy for postoperative pain reduction. In addition, parenthetical notes have been added in both the Medicine and Category III sections to direct users regarding appropriate reporting.

To support the addition of this new code, two parenthetical notes have been added. The exclusionary parenthetical note precludes the reporting of code 97037 with code 0552T because this is also for reporting low-level laser therapy. In addition, an instructional parenthetical note refers to code 97026 to report infrared dynamic thermokinetic energies therapy.

Code 97037 has been placed in the Constant Attendance subsection as a child code to code 97032. The language within the descriptor specifies "low-level laser therapy" to clarify that the treatment is completely non-thermal.

Clinical Example (97037)

A 30-year-old female, who underwent breast augmentation surgery, is treated with low-level laser therapy.

Description of Procedure (97037)

N/A

97033   iontophoresis, each 15 minutes

97034   contrast baths, each 15 minutes

97035   ultrasound, each 15 minutes

97036   Hubbard tank, each 15 minutes

97037   Code is out of numerical sequence. See 97028-97034

97039   Unlisted modality (specify type and time if constant attendance)

Therapeutic Procedures

★ **97110**   Therapeutic procedure, 1 or more areas, each 15 minutes; therapeutic exercises to develop strength and endurance, range of motion and flexibility

★ **97112**   neuromuscular reeducation of movement, balance, coordination, kinesthetic sense, posture, and/or proprioception for sitting and/or standing activities

97113   aquatic therapy with therapeutic exercises

★ **97116**   gait training (includes stair climbing)

★ = Telemedicine   ◀ = Audio-only   ✚ = Add-on code   ✗ = FDA approval pending   # = Resequenced code   ⊘ = Modifier 51 exempt

(Use 96000-96003 to report comprehensive gait and motion analysis procedures)

▶(For motor-cognitive, semi-immersive virtual reality–facilitated gait training, use 97116 in conjunction with 0791T)◀

Rationale

In accordance with the establishment of Category III code 0791T, an instructional parenthetical note has been added following code 97116. This note directs users to report code 0791T in conjunction with code 97116 when motor-cognitive, semi-immersive virtual reality–facilitated gait training is performed.

Refer to the codebook and the Rationale for code 0791T for a full discussion of these changes.

97545 Work hardening/conditioning; initial 2 hours

✚ 97546 each additional hour (List separately in addition to code for primary procedure)

(Use 97546 in conjunction with 97545)

▶Caregiver Training Without the Patient Present◀

▶Caregiver training is direct, skilled intervention for the caregiver(s) to provide strategies and techniques to equip caregiver(s) with knowledge and skills to assist patients living with functional deficits. Codes 97550, 97551 are used to report the total duration of face-to-face time spent by the qualified health care professional providing training to the caregiver(s) of an individual patient without the patient present. Code 97552 is used to report group caregiver training provided to multiple sets of caregivers for multiple patients with similar conditions or therapeutic needs without the patient present.

During a skilled intervention, the caregiver(s) is trained using verbal instructions, video and live demonstrations, and feedback from the qualified health care professional on the use of strategies and techniques to facilitate functional performance and safety in the home or community without the patient present. Skilled training supports a caregiver's understanding of the patient's treatment plan, ability to engage in activities with the patient in between treatment sessions, and knowledge of external resources to assist in areas such as activities of daily living (ADLs), transfers, mobility, safety practices, problem solving, and communication.

These services do not represent therapeutic interventions requiring direct one-to-one patient contact.◀

● 97550 Caregiver training in strategies and techniques to facilitate the patient's functional performance in the home or community (eg, activities of daily living [ADLs], instrumental ADLs [iADLs], transfers, mobility, communication, swallowing, feeding, problem solving, safety practices) (without the patient present), face to face; initial 30 minutes

✚● 97551 each additional 15 minutes (List separately in addition to code for primary service)

▶(Use 97551 in conjunction with 97550)◀

● 97552 Group caregiver training in strategies and techniques to facilitate the patient's functional performance in the home or community (eg, activities of daily living [ADLs], instrumental ADLs [iADLs], transfers, mobility, communication, swallowing, feeding, problem solving, safety practices) (without the patient present), face to face with multiple sets of caregivers

Rationale

A new Category I subsection within the Physical Medicine and Rehabilitation/Therapeutic Procedures subsection, guidelines, three new Category I codes (97550- 97552) and an associated instructional parenthetical note have been added to report skilled training of caregiver strategies and techniques.

Codes 97550-97552 have been added for reporting skilled training provided by qualified health care professionals (QHPs) to caregivers without the presence of their patients regarding strategies and techniques that may be used to enable a patient to function in their home or community. For each of these services, the QHP provides skilled intervention to introduce strategies and techniques to caregivers. These strategies and techniques provide caregivers the skills, knowledge, and awareness they need to assist patients with certain conditions that may manifest in functional deficits for living in their environment. This learned knowledge and skill provide the caregiver the ability to understand, communicate, and have the competency to address day-to-day living needs of the patient, including social interaction, home safety, and how to care for themselves as they assist patients with complex needs.

The training services allow the caregiver to understand the treatment plan, to have the ability to engage in activities with the patient in-between treatment sessions, and to gain knowledge of external resources to assist with patient care.

Medicine 90281-99607

The three codes developed to identify these services include:

- A time-based code (97550) to identify 30 minutes of service and to describe caregiver training in strategies to facilitate the patient's functional performance in the home or community for the caregiver(s) of an individual patient without the patient present.

- An add-on code (97551) to identify each additional 15 minutes of these services.

- A non-time-based code (97552) for group caregiver training of multiple caregivers of multiple patients that have similar conditions/therapeutic needs.

Guidelines and an add-on parenthetical note following code 97551 have been included to define the services and provide instructions regarding the use of these codes. This includes a guideline that reiterates that these codes are not intended to be reported when "direct one-to-one patient contact" is needed.

Clinical Example (97550)

The caregiver(s) of a 75-year-old male, who has right hemiparesis and visual/perceptual and cognitive deficits because of a stroke, requires caregiver training. Patient's symptoms result in communication deficits and cognitive functioning limited to following one-step directions, making functional management difficult. Direct (one-on-one) training is provided to the caregiver(s) to facilitate management of activities of daily living (ADLs), transfers, mobility, communication, and problem solving to enable the caregiver(s) to effectively facilitate a home-management program.

Description of Procedure (97550)

The QHP provides skilled intervention as part of a therapy plan of care to introduce strategies and techniques to the caregiver(s) to assist the patient living with functional deficits and to competently guide completion of ADLs that may include patient safety instruction; identification and implementation of compensatory strategies for proper sequencing, following directions, and safe activity completion; graded interventions focusing on motor, process, communication, and other skills that affect functional activity performance; problem-solving approaches to adapt to unusual tasks; environmental adaptation training; use of individualized visual or verbal cueing, memory devices (eg, picture lists), sequenced directions, or other approaches to enable completion of activities; or training in use of equipment or assistive devices for self-care/home management. The QHP guides and assesses return demonstration by the caregiver(s) of

activity or task performance required to ensure safety and efficient completion. The QHP addresses the caregiver's questions and concerns and provides resources as needed. The QHP documents caregiver(s) training in the medical record.

Clinical Example (97551)

The caregiver(s) of a 75-year-old male, who has right hemiparesis and visual/perceptual and cognitive deficits because of a stroke, requires additional caregiver training. Patient's symptoms result in communication deficits and cognitive functioning limited to following one-step directions, making functional management difficult. Direct (one-on-one) training is provided to the caregiver(s) to facilitate management of ADLs, transfers, mobility, communication, and problem solving to enable the caregiver to effectively facilitate a home-management program. The caregiver(s) requires an additional 15 minutes of training beyond the initial 30 minutes. [**Note:** This is an add-on code. Only consider the additional work related to caregiver training in strategies and techniques to facilitate patient's functional performance.]

Description of Procedure (97551)

The QHP continues to provide skilled intervention as part of the therapy plan of care to introduce strategies and techniques to the caregiver(s) to assist patient living with functional deficits and to competently guide completion of ADLs that may include patient safety instruction; identification and implementation of compensatory strategies for proper sequencing, following directions, and safe activity completion; graded interventions focusing on motor, process, communication, and other skills that affect functional activity performance; problem-solving approaches to adapt to unusual tasks; environmental adaptation training; use of individualized visual or verbal cueing, memory devices (eg, picture lists), sequenced directions, or other approaches to enable completion of activities; or training in use of equipment or assistive devices for self-care/home management. The QHP guides and assesses return demonstration by the caregiver(s) of activity or task performance required to ensure safety and efficient completion. The QHP addresses the caregiver's questions and concerns and provides resources as needed. [**Note:** This is an add-on code. Only consider the additional work spent by the QHP performing caregiver functional skills training beyond the initial 30 minutes reported with code 97550.]

★ = Telemedicine   ◀ = Audio-only   ✦ = Add-on code   ⊮ = FDA approval pending   # = Resequenced code   ⊘ = Modifier 51 exempt

Clinical Example (97552)

The caregiver(s) of a 75-year-old male, who has right hemiparesis and visual/perceptual, communication, and cognitive deficits because of a stroke, participates in group-based training to facilitate and support patient's functional performance in management of ADLs, transfers, mobility, communication, and problem solving in the home or community. The training provides the caregivers the opportunity to ask questions and engage in group problem solving around caregiver challenges.

Description of Procedure (97552)

The QHP initiates group-based skilled intervention as part of a therapy plan of care to introduce strategies and techniques to the caregivers to assist patient living with functional deficits and to competently guide completion of ADLs that may include patient safety instruction; identification and implementation of compensatory strategies for proper sequencing, following directions, and safe activity completion; graded interventions focusing on motor, process, communication, and other skills that affect functional activity performance; problem-solving approaches to adapt to unusual tasks; environmental adaptation training; use of individualized visual or verbal cueing, memory devices (eg, picture lists), sequenced directions, or other approaches to enable completion of activities; or training in use of equipment or assistive devices for self-care/home management. As appropriate, the QHP facilitates group problem solving to enhance generalizability of concepts across participants. The QHP guides and assesses return demonstration by the caregivers of activity or task performance required to ensure safety and efficient completion. The QHP addresses the caregivers' questions and concerns and provides resources as needed. The QHP documents caregivers' training in the medical record.

▲ = Revised code   ● = New code   ▶ ◀ = Contains new or revised text   ✄ = Duplicate PLA test   ↑↓ = Category I PLA   American Medical Association   **147**

Medicine 90281-99607

Notes

Category II Codes

See the Introduction section of the CPT code set for a complete list of the dates of release and implementation.

The superscripted numbers included at the end of each code descriptor direct users to the measure developers that are associated with these footnotes, whose names and Web addresses are listed below.

▶1. For more information on measures developed by the Physician Consortium for Performance Improvement (PCPI), see the appropriate payer website.

2. National Committee on Quality Assurance (NCQA), Health Employer Data Information Set (HEDIS˚), www.ncqa.org.

3. The Joint Commission (TJC), https://www. jointcommission.org.

4. For more information on measures developed by the National Diabetes Quality Improvement Alliance (NDQIA), see the appropriate payer website.

5. For more information on measures developed as joint measures from Physician Consortium for Performance Improvement (PCPI) and the National Committee on Quality Assurance (NCQA), visit the NCQA website at www.ncqa.org.

6. The Society of Thoracic Surgeons at www.sts.org and National Quality Forum, www.qualityforum.org.

7. Optum, www.optum.com.

8. American Academy of Neurology, https://www.aan. com/practice/quality-measurements or quality@aan. com.

9. College of American Pathologists (CAP), https:// www.cap.org/advocacy/quality-payment-program-for-pathologists/mips-for-pathologists/2023-pathology-quality-measures.

10. American Gastroenterological Association (AGA), www.gastro.org/quality.

11. American Society of Anesthesiologists (ASA), www. asahq.org.

12. American College of Gastroenterology (ACG), www. gi.org; American Gastroenterological Association (AGA), www.gastro.org; and American Society for Gastrointestinal Endoscopy (ASGE), www.asge.org.◀

Rationale

To address several incorrect or outdated web addresses listed for the organizations whose measures are used with Category II codes for compliance, the outdated web addresses have been replaced with current web addresses. These revised web addresses may either provide the measure information directly or redirect users to other sources for the needed information for reporting specific measures.

Category II 0042T-0713T

Notes

Category III Codes

Summary of Additions, Deletions, and Revisions

The summary of changes shows the actual changes that have been made to the code descriptors.

New codes appear with a bullet (●) and are indicated as "Code added." Revised codes are preceded with a triangle (▲). Within revised codes, or if a code symbol has been deleted, the deleted language and code symbol appear with a ~~strikethrough~~, while new text appears underlined.

The ✚ symbol is used to identify codes for vaccines that are pending FDA approval. The # symbol is used to identify codes that have been resequenced. CPT add-on codes are annotated by the ✚ symbol. The ⃠ symbol is used to identify codes that are exempt from the use of modifier 51. The ★ symbol is used to identify codes that may be used for reporting telemedicine services. The ✕ symbol is used to identify a proprietary laboratory analyses (PLA) test that has an identical descriptor as another PLA test. A PLA code that satisfies Category I code criteria and has been accepted by the CPT Editorial Panel is annotated with the ↕ symbol. The ◀ symbol is used to identify codes that may be used to report audio-only telemedicine services when appended by modifier 93 (see Appendix T).

Code	Description
0404T	~~Transcervical uterine fibroid(s) ablation with ultrasound guidance, radiofrequency~~
0424T	~~Insertion or replacement of neurostimulator system for treatment of central sleep apnea; complete system (transvenous placement of right or left stimulation lead, sensing lead, implantable pulse generator)~~
0425T	~~sensing lead only~~
0426T	~~stimulation lead only~~
0427T	~~pulse generator only~~
0428T	~~Removal of neurostimulator system for treatment of central sleep apnea; pulse generator only~~
0429T	~~sensing lead only~~
0430T	~~stimulation lead only~~
0431T	~~Removal and replacement of neurostimulator system for treatment of central sleep apnea, pulse generator only~~
0432T	~~Repositioning of neurostimulator system for treatment of central sleep apnea; stimulation lead only~~
0433T	~~sensing lead only~~
0434T	~~Interrogation device evaluation implanted neurostimulator pulse generator system for central sleep apnea~~
0435T	~~Programming device evaluation of implanted neurostimulator pulse generator system for central sleep apnea; single session~~
0436T	~~during sleep study~~
0465T	~~Suprachoroidal injection of a pharmacologic agent (does not include supply of medication)~~
# ▲0640T	Noncontact near-infrared spectroscopy ~~studies of flap or wound~~ (eg, for measurement of deoxyhemoglobin, oxyhemoglobin, and ratio of tissue oxygenation), other than for screening for peripheral arterial disease, ~~[StO$_2$]);~~ image acquisition, interpretation, and report; ~~image acquisition, interpretation and report, each flap or wound~~first anatomic site

Category III 0042T-0713T

Code	Description
0641T	~~Noncontact near-infrared spectroscopy studies of flap or wound (eg, for measurement of deoxyhemoglobin, oxyhemoglobin, and ratio of tissue oxygenation [StO$_2$]); image acquisition only, each flap or wound~~
0642T	~~Noncontact near-infrared spectroscopy studies of flap or wound (eg, for measurement of deoxyhemoglobin, oxyhemoglobin, and ratio of tissue oxygenation [StO$_2$]); interpretation and report only, each flap or wound~~
#+●0859T	Code added
#●0860T	Code added
0499T	~~Cystourethroscopy, with mechanical dilation and urethral therapeutic drug delivery for urethral stricture or stenosis, including fluoroscopy, when performed~~
0501T	~~Noninvasive estimated coronary fractional flow reserve (FFR) derived from coronary computed tomography angiography data using computation fluid dynamics physiologic simulation software analysis of functional data to assess the severity of coronary artery disease; data preparation and transmission, analysis of fluid dynamics and simulated maximal coronary hyperemia, generation of estimated FFR model, with anatomical data review in comparison with estimated FFR model to reconcile discordant data, interpretation and report~~
0502T	~~data preparation and transmission~~
0503T	~~analysis of fluid dynamics and simulated maximal coronary hyperemia, and generation of estimated FFR model~~
0504T	~~anatomical data review in comparison with estimated FFR model to reconcile discordant data, interpretation and report~~
0508T	~~Pulse-echo ultrasound bone density measurement resulting in indicator of axial bone mineral density, tibia~~
▲0517T	~~pulse generator~~both component~~(s)~~ of pulse generator (battery and~~/or~~ transmitter) only
#●0861T	Code added
▲0518T	~~Removal of only pulse generator component(s) (battery and/or transmitter) or wireless cardiac stimulator for left ventricular pacing~~battery component only
#●0862T	Code added
#●0863T	Code added
▲0519T	Removal and replacement of pulse generator for wireless cardiac stimulator for left ventricular pacing, including device interrogation and programming; ~~pulse generator~~both component~~(s)~~ (battery and~~/or~~ transmitter)
▲0520T	~~pulse generator~~battery component~~(s)~~ only~~(battery and/or transmitter), including placement of a new electrode~~
0533T	~~Continuous recording of movement disorder symptoms, including bradykinesia, dyskinesia, and tremor for 6 days up to 10 days; includes set-up, patient training, configuration of monitor, data upload, analysis and initial report configuration, download review, interpretation and report~~
0534T	~~set-up, patient training, configuration of monitor~~
0535T	~~data upload, analysis and initial report configuration~~
0536T	~~download review, interpretation and report~~
▲0587T	Percutaneous implantation or replacement of integrated single device neurostimulation system for bladder dysfunction including electrode array and receiver or pulse generator, including analysis, programming, and imaging guidance when performed, posterior tibial nerve
▲0588T	Revision or removal of percutaneously placed integrated single device neurostimulation system for bladder dysfunction including electrode array and receiver or pulse generator, including analysis, programming, and imaging guidance when performed, posterior tibial nerve

★ = Telemedicine   ◀ = Add-on code   ✚ = Add-on code   ⊿ = FDA approval pending   # = Resequenced code   ⊘ = Modifier 51 exempt

Code	Description
▲0589T	Electronic analysis with simple programming of implanted integrated neurostimulation system <u>for bladder dysfunction</u> (eg, electrode array and receiver), including contact group(s), amplitude, pulse width, frequency (Hz), on/off cycling, burst, dose lockout, patient-selectable parameters, responsive neurostimulation, detection algorithms, closed-loop parameters, and passive parameters, when performed by physician or other qualified health care professional, posterior tibial nerve, 1-3 parameters
▲0590T	Electronic analysis with complex programming of implanted integrated neurostimulation system <u>for bladder dysfunction</u> (eg, electrode array and receiver), including contact group(s), amplitude, pulse width, frequency (Hz), on/off cycling, burst, dose lockout, patient-selectable parameters, responsive neurostimulation, detection algorithms, closed-loop parameters, and passive parameters, when performed by physician or other qualified health care professional, posterior tibial nerve, 4 or more parameters
▲0656T	<u>Anterior lumbar or thoracolumbar</u> <del>V</del>vertebral body tethering<del>, anterior</del>; up to 7 vertebral segments
▲0657T	8 or more vertebral segments
#●0790T	Code added
~~0715T~~	~~Percutaneous transluminal coronary lithotripsy (List separately in addition to code for primary procedure)~~
#✚●0827T	Code added
#✚●0828T	Code added
#✚●0829T	Code added
#✚●0830T	Code added
#✚●0831T	Code added
#✚●0832T	Code added
#✚●0833T	Code added
#✚●0834T	Code added
#✚●0835T	Code added
#✚●0836T	Code added
#✚●0837T	Code added
#✚●0838T	Code added
#✚●0839T	Code added
#✚●0840T	Code added
#✚●0841T	Code added
#✚●0842T	Code added
#✚●0843T	Code added
#✚●0844T	Code added
#✚●0845T	Code added
#✚●0846T	Code added
#✚●0847T	Code added

Category III 0042T-0713T

Code	Description
#+●0848T	Code added
#+●0849T	Code added
#+●0850T	Code added
#+●0851T	Code added
#+●0852T	Code added
#+●0853T	Code added
#+●0854T	Code added
#+●0855T	Code added
#+●0856T	Code added
▲0766T	Transcutaneous magnetic stimulation by focused low-frequency electromagnetic pulse, peripheral nerve, ~~initial treatment,~~ with identification and marking of the treatment location, including noninvasive electroneurographic localization (nerve conduction localization), when performed; first nerve
+▲0767T	each additional nerve (List separately in addition to code for primary procedure)
~~0768T~~	~~Transcutaneous magnetic stimulation by focused low-frequency electromagnetic pulse, peripheral nerve, subsequent treatment, including noninvasive electroneurographic localization (nerve conduction localization), when performed; first nerve~~
~~0769T~~	~~each additional nerve (List separately in addition to code for primary procedure)~~
~~0775T~~	~~Arthrodesis, sacroiliac joint, percutaneous, with image guidance, includes placement of intra-articular implant(s) (eg, bone allograft[s], synthetic device[s])~~
●0784T	Code added
●0785T	Code added
●0786T	Code added
●0787T	Code added
●0788T	Code added
●0789T	Code added
+●0791T	Code added
●0792T	Code added
●0793T	Code added
●0794T	Code added
●0795T	Code added
●0796T	Code added
●0797T	Code added
●0798T	Code added
●0799T	Code added
●0800T	Code added

★ = Telemedicine ◀ = Add-on code + = Add-on code ⚡ = FDA approval pending # = Resequenced code ⊘ = Modifier 51 exempt

Code	Description
●0801T	Code added
●0802T	Code added
●0803T	Code added
●0804T	Code added
●0805T	Code added
●0806T	Code added
●0807T	Code added
●0808T	Code added
0809T	~~Arthrodesis, sacroiliac joint, percutaneous or minimally invasive (indirect visualization), with image guidance, placement of transfixing device(s) and intra-articular implant(s) including allograft or synthetic device(s)~~
●0810T	Code added
●0811T	Code added
●0812T	Code added
●0813T	Code added
●0814T	Code added
●0815T	Code added
●0816T	Code added
●0817T	Code added
●0818T	Code added
●0819T	Code added
●0820T	Code added
✚●0821T	Code added
✚●0822T	Code added
●0823T	Code added
●0824T	Code added
●0825T	Code added
●0826T	Code added
✚●0857T	Code added
●0858T	Code added
●0864T	Code added
●0865T	Code added
✚●0866T	Code added

Category III 0042T-0713T

Category III Codes

0278T   Transcutaneous electrical modulation pain reprocessing (eg, scrambler therapy), each treatment session (includes placement of electrodes)

▶(For peripheral nerve transcutaneous magnetic stimulation, see 0766T, 0767T)◀

Rationale

In accordance with the deletion of codes 0768T and 0769T, a parenthetical note following code 0278T has been revised to reflect the deleted codes and to direct users to the appropriate codes for reporting transcutaneous magnetic stimulation.

Refer to the codebook and the Rationale for codes 0766T and 0767T for a full discussion of these changes.

▶(0404T has been deleted)◀

▶(For transcervical radiofrequency ablation of uterine fibroid[s], including intraoperative ultrasound guidance and monitoring, use 58580)◀

Rationale

Code 0404T has been deleted from the Category III section and parenthetical notes have been added to denote this deletion and to direct users to code 58580 for transcervical radiofrequency ablation of uterine fibroid(s), including intraoperative ultrasound guidance and monitoring.

Refer to the codebook and the Rationale for code 58580 for a full discussion of these changes.

Phrenic Nerve Stimulation System

▶(0424T, 0425T, 0426T, 0427T have been deleted)◀

▶(For insertion of a phrenic nerve stimulator transvenous sensing lead, use 33277)◀

▶(For removal and replacement of phrenic nerve stimulator pulse generator, use 33287)◀

▶(For removal and replacement of phrenic nerve stimulator transvenous stimulation or sensing lead[s], use 33288)◀

▶(0428T, 0429T, 0430T have been deleted)◀

▶(For removal of phrenic nerve stimulator sensing or stimulation lead[s], use 33279)◀

▶(For removal of phrenic nerve stimulator pulse generator, use 33280)◀

▶(0431T has been deleted)◀

▶(For removal and replacement of phrenic nerve stimulator pulse generator, use 33287)◀

▶(0432T, 0433T have been deleted)◀

▶(For repositioning of phrenic nerve stimulator transvenous lead[s], use 33281)◀

▶(0434T has been deleted)◀

▶(For interrogation device evaluation of implanted phrenic nerve stimulator system, use 93153)◀

▶(0435T, 0436T have been deleted)◀

▶(For interrogation and programming of implanted phrenic nerve stimulator system, use 93151)◀

▶(For interrogation and programming of implanted phrenic nerve stimulator system during a polysomnography, use 93152)◀

Rationale

In accordance with the deletion of Category III codes 0424T-0436T for insertion, removal and replacement, repositioning, and interrogation and programming, and the addition of Category I codes 33276-33288 and 93150-93153, several parenthetical notes have been added in the Category III section to direct reporting for phrenic nerve stimulator services.

Refer to the codebook and the Rationale for codes 33276-33288 and 93150-93153 for a full discussion of these changes.

▶(0465T has been deleted)◀

▶(For suprachoroidal injection of a pharmacologic agent, use 67516)◀

Rationale

In accordance with the conversion of Category III code 0465T to Category I code 67516, a deletion parenthetical note and a cross-reference parenthetical note have been added to reflect these changes.

Refer to the codebook and the Rationale for code 67516 for a full discussion of these changes.

▶Noncontact near-infrared spectroscopy is used to measure cutaneous vascular perfusion. Codes 0640T, 0859T describe noncontact near-infrared spectroscopy for measurement of cutaneous vascular perfusion (other than for screening for peripheral arterial disease) that does not require direct contact of the spectrometer sensors with the patient's skin. Codes 0640T, 0859T may only be reported once, when performing noncontact near-infrared spectroscopy of multiple wounds in one anatomic site (eg, multiple diabetic ulcers involving the plantar surface of the foot). For noncontact near-infrared spectroscopy studies for screening for peripheral arterial disease, use 0860T.◄

#▲ 0640T   Noncontact near-infrared spectroscopy (eg, for measurement of deoxyhemoglobin, oxyhemoglobin, and ratio of tissue oxygenation), other than for screening for peripheral arterial disease, image acquisition, interpretation, and report; first anatomic site

►(Do not report 0640T in conjunction with 0860T)◄

#+● 0859T   each additional anatomic site (List separately in addition to code for primary procedure)

►(Use 0859T in conjunction with 0640T)◄

►(Report 0640T, 0859T only once, when performing noncontact near-infrared spectroscopy of multiple wounds in one anatomic site)◄

►(For noncontact near-infrared spectroscopy studies for screening for peripheral arterial disease, use 0860T)◄

►(0641T, 0642T have been deleted)◄

►(For noncontact near-infrared spectroscopy studies other than for screening for peripheral arterial disease, see 0640T, 0859T)◄

#● 0860T   Noncontact near-infrared spectroscopy (eg, for measurement of deoxyhemoglobin, oxyhemoglobin, and ratio of tissue oxygenation), for screening for peripheral arterial disease, including provocative maneuvers, image acquisition, interpretation, and report, one or both lower extremities

►(Do not report 0860T in conjunction with 0640T)◄

►(For noncontact near-infrared spectroscopy studies other than for screening for peripheral arterial disease, see 0640T, 0859T)◄

Rationale

Code 0640T has been revised; codes 0641T and 0642T and associated references have been deleted; and two new Category III codes (0859T, 0860T) have been established to report services for noncontact near-infrared spectroscopy. In addition, guidelines have been revised and parenthetical notes have been added to accommodate the addition of the new codes and the instructions for reporting these new services.

Codes 0640T and 0859T identify noncontact near-infrared spectroscopy services when they are performed for reasons other than screening for peripheral arterial disease. These services include image acquisition, interpretation, and report. Code 0860T identifies noncontact near-infrared spectroscopy services screening

for peripheral arterial disease. This service also differs from the services represented by codes 0640T and 0859T because it includes provocative maneuvers for one or both lower extremities. To accommodate these additions, codes 0641T and 0642T have been deleted.

The language in code 0640T has been revised to reflect its intended use: (1) for the first anatomic site where the procedure is performed (instead of by "flap" or "wound"); and (2) for when it's used for other than screening for peripheral arterial disease. Additional deletions within the code descriptor (eg, "[StO$_2$]" and relocation of the semicolon ";") have been included to accommodate the instruction for intended use and to capture common elements within the parent portion of the code family. Add-on code 0859T has been added to allow reporting for each additional anatomic site.

The introductory guidelines have been updated to explain what is noncontact near-infrared spectroscopy and how it may be reported, and new parenthetical notes have been added to reflect appropriate use according to: (1) anatomic site; (2) the number of times this service may be reported; and (3) direction regarding what code to use for noncontact near-infrared spectroscopy studies for screening for peripheral arterial disease (0860T).

New parenthetical notes provide instruction regarding mutual exclusion of these services and conventional instruction regarding the use of the add-on code.

Clinical Example (0640T)

A 65-year-old male presents with a 10-cm^2 left heel ulcer. Noncontact near-infrared spectroscopy images are obtained of the patient's left heel.

Description of Procedure (0640T)

Power on and calibrate the noncontact near-infrared spectrometer. Log in and enter the patient's information. Prepare the area of interest, ensuring it is fully exposed, clean, and dry. Position the spectrometer over the area of interest and acquire images. Review and manipulate the images and note the biomarker values. Incorporate the interpretation of the spectroscopy images in a report and add the report to the patient's record.

Clinical Example (0859T)

A 65-year-old male with diabetes who has underçgone noncontact near-infrared spectroscopy of the left foot is noted to have a right plantar ulcer and undergoes noncontact near-infrared spectroscopy of the involved right foot. [**Note:** This is an add-on code. Only consider the additional work related to the noncontact near-infrared spectroscopy of the right foot.]

Category III 0042T-0713T

Description of Procedure (0859T)

Prepare the area of interest, ensuring it is fully exposed, clean, and dry. Position the spectrometer over the area of interest and acquire images. Review and manipulate the images and note the biomarker values. Incorporate the interpretation of the spectroscopy images and biomarker values in a report and add the report to the patient's record.

Clinical Example (0860T)

A 69-year-old male with type 2 diabetes mellitus and a recent ankle-brachial index showing 1.05 ratio undergoes screening for bilateral lower extremity peripheral arterial disease using noncontact near-infrared spectroscopy imaging.

Description of Procedure (0860T)

Place the patient on the examination table in the supine position. Power on and calibrate the noncontact near-infrared spectrometer. Log in and enter the patient's information. Expose the first leg to be examined and capture baseline noncontact near-infrared spectrometer images of that leg. Elevate the leg to a minimum of 30° for 3 minutes, assuring that the limb is above the level of the patient's heart. After 3 minutes, return the leg to the original position and obtain post-elevation noncontact near-infrared spectrometer images. Repeat the same steps for the opposite leg. Review and manipulate the images and note the biomarker values. Incorporate the interpretation of the spectroscopy images and biomarker values in a report and add the report to the patient's record.

▶(0499T has been deleted)◀

▶(For cystourethroscopy with mechanical urethral dilation and urethral therapeutic drug delivery by drug-coated balloon catheter for urethral stricture or stenosis, including fluoroscopy, use 52284)◀

Rationale

In accordance with the conversion of Category III code 0499T to Category I code 52284, a deletion parenthetical note and a cross-reference parenthetical note have been added to the Category III section.

Refer to the codebook and the Rationale for code 52284 for a full discussion of these changes.

▶(0501T, 0502T, 0503T, 0504T have been deleted)◀

▶(For noninvasive estimate of coronary fractional flow reserve [FFR] derived from augmentative software analysis of the data set from a coronary computed tomography angiography, with interpretation and report by a physician or other qualified health care professional, use 75580)◀

Rationale

Codes 0501T-0504T have been deleted from the Category III section and three parenthetical notes have been deleted and replaced with two new parenthetical notes to accommodate the establishment of code 75580.

Refer to the codebook and the Rationale for code 75580 for a full discussion of these changes.

Automated quantification and characterization of coronary atherosclerotic plaque is a service in which coronary computed tomographic angiography (CTA) data are analyzed using computerized algorithms to assess the extent and severity of coronary artery disease. The computer-generated findings are provided in an interactive format to the physician or other qualified health care professional who performs the final review and report. The coronary CTA is performed and interpreted as a separate service and is not included in the service of automated analysis of coronary CTA.

\# 0623T   Automated quantification and characterization of coronary atherosclerotic plaque to assess severity of coronary disease, using data from coronary computed tomographic angiography; data preparation and transmission, computerized analysis of data, with review of computerized analysis output to reconcile discordant data, interpretation and report

\# 0624T   data preparation and transmission

\# 0625T   computerized analysis of data from coronary computed tomographic angiography

\# 0626T   review of computerized analysis output to reconcile discordant data, interpretation and report

(Use 0623T, 0624T, 0625T, 0626T one time per coronary computed tomographic angiogram)

(Do not report 0623T in conjunction with 0624T, 0625T, 0626T)

(Do not report 0623T, 0624T, 0625T, 0626T in conjunction with 76376, 76377)

▶(For noninvasive estimate of coronary fractional flow reserve [FFR] derived from augmentative software analysis of the data set from a coronary computed tomography angiography, with interpretation and report by a physician or other qualified health care professional, use 75580)◀

Category III 0042T-0713T

Rationale

In accordance with the deletion of codes 0501T-0504T and the establishment of code 75580, the cross-reference parenthetical note following code 0626T has been revised.

Refer to the codebook and the Rationale for code 75580 for a full discussion of these changes.

#✚ 0523T   Intraprocedural coronary fractional flow reserve (FFR) with 3D functional mapping of color-coded FFR values for the coronary tree, derived from coronary angiogram data, for real-time review and interpretation of possible atherosclerotic stenosis(es) intervention (List separately in addition to code for primary procedure)

(Use 0523T in conjunction with 93454, 93455, 93456, 93457, 93458, 93459, 93460, 93461)

(Do not report 0523T more than once per session)

▶(Do not report 0523T in conjunction with 75580, 76376, 76377, 93571, 93572)◀

Rationale

In accordance with the deletion of codes 0501T-0504T and the establishment of code 75580, the exclusionary parenthetical note following code 0523T has been revised.

Refer to the codebook and the Rationale for code 75580 for a full discussion of these changes.

▶(0508T has been deleted)◀

▶(For pulse-echo ultrasound bone density measurement resulting in indicator of axial bone mineral density, tibia, use 76999)◀

Rationale

In accordance with the CPT guidelines for archiving Category III codes, code 0508T has been deleted and instructions added to report code 76999, *Unlisted ultrasound procedure (eg, diagnostic, interventional),* for pulse-echo ultrasound bone-density measurement resulting in indicator of axial bone mineral density, tibia. A cross-reference parenthetical note has been added to reflect these changes.

Wireless Cardiac Stimulation System for Left Ventricular Pacing

▶A wireless cardiac stimulator system for left ventricular pacing functions by sensing right ventricular pacing output from a previously implanted conventional device (pacemaker or defibrillator, with univentricular or biventricular leads), and then transmitting an ultrasound pulse to a wireless electrode implanted on the endocardium of the left ventricle, which then emits a left ventricular pacing pulse. In combination, the left ventricular and right ventricular pacemakers provide biventricular cardiac pacing.

The complete wireless left ventricular pacing system consists of a wireless endocardial left ventricle electrode and a pulse generator. The pulse generator has two components: a transmitter and a battery. The electrode is typically implanted transarterially into the left ventricular wall and powered wirelessly using ultrasound delivered by a subcutaneously implanted transmitter. Two subcutaneous pockets are created on the chest wall, one for the battery and one for the transmitter, and these two components are connected by a subcutaneously tunneled cable.

Patients with a wireless cardiac stimulator who also have a conventional pacing device require programming/interrogation of their existing conventional device, as well as the wireless device. The wireless cardiac stimulator is programmed and interrogated with its own separate programmer and settings.

Code 0515T describes insertion of a complete wireless cardiac stimulator system (electrode and pulse generator, which includes transmitter and battery) for left ventricular pacing, including interrogation, programming, pocket creation, relocation, and all echocardiography, left ventriculography, and fluoroscopic imaging to guide the procedure, when performed. For insertion of only the electrode of a wireless cardiac stimulator for left ventricular pacing, use 0516T. For insertion of both components of a new pulse generator (battery and transmitter), use 0517T.

A wireless cardiac stimulator for left ventricular pacing may need to be removed, relocated, or replaced. The electrode component of the stimulator typically is not removed once implanted. For removal of both components of the pulse generator (battery and transmitter) without replacement, use 0861T. For removal of only the battery component of the pulse generator without replacement, use 0518T. For relocation of the pulse generator, use 0862T for relocation of the battery component or 0863T for relocation of the transmitter component. For removal and replacement of both components of the pulse generator, use 0519T. For removal and replacement of only the battery component, use 0520T.

Category III 0042T-0713T

All catheterization, angiography, and imaging guidance (including transthoracic or transesophageal echocardiography) required to complete a wireless cardiac stimulator procedure is included in 0515T, 0516T, 0517T, 0518T, 0519T, 0520T, 0861T, 0862T, 0863T. Do not report 76000, 76998, 93303-93355, 93452, 93453, 93458, 93459, 93460, 93461, 93565, 93586, 93595, 93596, 93597 in conjunction with 0515T, 0516T, 0517T, 0518T, 0519T, 0520T, 0795T, 0796T, 0797T, 0798T, 0799T, 0800T, 0801T, 0802T, 0803T, 0823T, 0824T, 0825T, 0861T, 0862T, 0863T.◄

Do not report left heart catheterization codes (93452, 93453, 93458, 93459, 93460, 93461, 93595, 93596, 93597) for delivery of a wireless cardiac stimulator electrode into the left ventricle.

0515T Insertion of wireless cardiac stimulator for left ventricular pacing, including device interrogation and programming, and imaging supervision and interpretation, when performed; complete system (includes electrode and generator [transmitter and battery])

0516T electrode only

▲ **0517T** both components of pulse generator (battery and transmitter) only

▶(Do not report 0515T, 0516T, 0517T in conjunction with 0518T, 0519T, 0520T, 0521T, 0522T, 0861T, 0862T, 0863T)◄

#● **0861T** Removal of pulse generator for wireless cardiac stimulator for left ventricular pacing; both components (battery and transmitter)

▶(Do not report 0861T in conjunction with 0515T, 0516T, 0517T, 0518T, 0519T, 0520T, 0521T, 0522T, 0862T, 0863T)◄

▲ **0518T** battery component only

▶(Do not report 0518T in conjunction with 0515T, 0516T, 0517T, 0519T, 0520T, 0521T, 0861T, 0862T, 0863T)◄

#● **0862T** Relocation of pulse generator for wireless cardiac stimulator for left ventricular pacing, including device interrogation and programming; battery component only

▶(Do not report 0862T in conjunction with 0515T, 0517T, 0518T, 0519T, 0520T, 0521T, 0522T, 0861T)◄

#● **0863T** transmitter component only

▶(Do not report 0863T in conjunction with 0515T, 0517T, 0518T, 0519T, 0520T, 0521T, 0522T, 0861T)◄

▲ **0519T** Removal and replacement of pulse generator for wireless cardiac stimulator for left ventricular pacing, including device interrogation and programming; both components (battery and transmitter)

▲ **0520T** battery component only

▶(Do not report 0519T, 0520T in conjunction with 0515T, 0516T, 0517T, 0518T, 0521T, 0522T, 0861T, 0862T, 0863T)◄

0521T Interrogation device evaluation (in person) with analysis, review and report, includes connection, recording, and disconnection per patient encounter, wireless cardiac stimulator for left ventricular pacing

▶(Do not report 0521T in conjunction with 0515T, 0516T, 0517T, 0518T, 0519T, 0520T, 0522T, 0861T, 0862T, 0863T)◄

0522T Programming device evaluation (in person) with iterative adjustment of the implantable device to test the function of the device and select optimal permanent programmed values with analysis, including review and report, wireless cardiac stimulator for left ventricular pacing

▶(Do not report 0522T in conjunction with 0515T, 0516T, 0517T, 0518T, 0519T, 0520T, 0521T, 0861T, 0862T, 0863T)◄

0523T Code is out of numerical sequence. See 0496T-0507T

Rationale

Codes 0861T-0863T have been established to identify reporting for removal and relocation services of components of a wireless cardiac stimulator of the left ventricle. In addition, codes 0517T-0520T have been revised to accommodate the addition of the new codes and to better specify all component services that may be provided for these devices. The guidelines and parenthetical notes listed for these services have also been revised to clarify the different services of insertion, removal, revision, replacement, and programming for left ventricular pacing services.

Codes 0861T-0863T have been established to better differentiate services of removal and relocation services that may be provided for left ventricular pacing devices. These codes identify removal services for both components of the pulse generator (0861T), as well as relocation services for the battery component only (0862T) and transmitter component only (0863T). In addition, codes 0517T-0520T have been revised to include language that better specifies the type of service and component(s) that are being addressed by usage of each code.

Guideline language for wireless cardiac stimulation for left ventricular pacing has been revised to accommodate additional instructions regarding left ventricular pacing functions and differentiate it from conventional pacing devices. The language identifies how left ventricular pacing is used in combination with conventional right ventricular pacemakers to provide biventricular cardiac pacing. The existing guidelines have also been revised to be more specific in defining components of the left ventricular pacing services. This includes the addition of terms that better describe the services, language that identifies efforts that are inherently included for the procedure (eg, left ventriculography and fluoroscopic imaging), and coding instruction for reporting insertion of elements of these devices, such as the use of code 0516T for insertion of only the electrode of a wireless cardiac stimulator for left ventricular pacing and how to code for insertion of both components (ie, battery and transmitter [0517T]). In addition, new guideline language explains how removals, relocations, and replacements of these devices are performed, components that may not be removed as part of a replacement, and how to code for removals/relocations/replacements of components for left ventricular pacing.

The parenthetical notes that have been added or revised regarding these services are exclusionary and commonly restrict reporting for services that overlap. In some locations, existing parenthetical notes have been amended by adding codes that should be excluded from reporting with other services because of the overlap in services performed. In other instances, new parenthetical notes have been added to mirror existing parentheticals for consistency in restriction of services that are mutually excluded or services that may otherwise not be reported together.

Clinical Example (0517T)

A 65-year-old female has ischemic cardiomyopathy, ejection fraction 28%, QRS 165 ms, left bundle branch block, and New York Heart Association class III congestive heart failure. The patient meets class I indications for biventricular pacing for cardiac resynchronization therapy (CRT). A conventional CRT defibrillator (CRT-D) device has previously been implanted with no improvement. As the patient is a nonresponder to conventional CRT, insertion of a wireless cardiac stimulator transmitter and battery for left ventricular pacing is now planned.

Description of Procedure (0517T)

Obtain informed consent from the patient. Bring the patient to the electrophysiology laboratory and anesthetize to achieve deep sedation. Perform transthoracic echocardiography (TTE) imaging to verify the appropriate intercostal location to implant the transmitter. Prepare and drape the skin. Make skin incisions for the transmitter and battery, and create two pockets. Utilize a tunneling tool to place a routing tube from the battery pocket to the medial incision. Insert the transmitter's cable into the routing tube and pull through the tunnel to the battery pocket. Position the transmitter medially in the channel and secure. Connect the battery to the cable and then secure in the battery pocket. Close wounds with appropriate sutures. Evaluate the system for biventricular capture functionality with the programmer. Perform the programming device evaluation only when the electrode is implanted before the time of transmitter and battery insertion.

Clinical Example (0518T)

A 65-year-old female with a previously implanted wireless cardiac stimulator system for left ventricle (LV) pacing develops a mild infection of the battery subcutaneous pocket. The pulse generator battery is removed followed by antibiotic treatment. A new pulse generator battery insertion will be performed after the infection has been resolved.

Description of Procedure (0518T)

Make an incision along the previous implant incision scar. Access the existing pocket, and take care to remove the battery from the pocket. Using a torque wrench, disconnect the transmitter cable. A cap is placed over the connector pin of the transmitter cable. Close wound with appropriate sutures.

Clinical Example (0519T)

A 65-year-old female with a previously implanted wireless cardiac stimulator system for LV pacing presents at follow-up, at which time it suggests insufficient biventricular pacing secondary to transmitter malfunction. After discussion with the patient, it is agreed to proceed with removal and replacement of the transmitter and battery.

Description of Procedure (0519T)

Obtain informed consent from the patient. Bring the patient to the electrophysiology laboratory and anesthetize to achieve deep sedation. Perform TTE imaging to verify the appropriate intercostal location to implant the new transmitter. Prepare and drape the skin. For the battery replacement, make an incision along the previous implant incision scar. Access the existing battery pocket, and take care to remove the battery from the pocket. Using a torque wrench, disconnect the transmitter cable from the battery. Make an incision along the previous transmitter implant incision scar. Access the existing transmitter pocket and carefully remove the sutures securing the transmitter. Remove the transmitter from the existing pocket. Make a new skin incision at the site of the new transmitter implant, and create pocket. Use a tunneling tool to place a routing tube from the battery pocket to the medial incision. Insert the transmitter's cable into the routing tube and pull through the tunnel to the battery pocket. Position the transmitter medially in the channel and secure.

Category III 0042T-0713T

Clinical Example (0520T)

A 65-year-old female with a previously implanted wireless cardiac stimulator system for LV pacing presents at follow-up, at which time the battery is found to be at end of life. After discussion with the patient, it is agreed to proceed with battery replacement.

Description of Procedure (0520T)

Obtain informed consent from the patient. Bring the patient to the electrophysiology laboratory and anesthetize. Prepare and drape the skin. Make an incision along the previous battery implant incision scar. Access the existing pocket, and take care to remove the battery from the pocket. Using a torque wrench, disconnect the transmitter cable from the battery. Inspect the transmitter cable connector and battery header connection for any fluid or material inside; no issues noted. Insert the transmitter cable into the new battery and tighten set screws. Place the battery into the existing pocket and secure with two sutures. Evaluate the system for biventricular capture functionality with the programmer. Confirm biventricular pacing with previous settings. Close wounds with appropriate sutures.

Clinical Example (0861T)

A 72-year-old male with a previously implanted wireless cardiac stimulator system for LV pacing develops a mild infection of the subcutaneous transmitter pocket. The transmitter and battery are removed followed by antibiotic treatment.

Description of Procedure (0861T)

Make an incision along both the previous transmitter and battery implant incision scars. Access the existing transmitter pocket, and take care to remove transmitter from the pocket. Access the existing battery pocket, and take care to remove the battery from the pocket. Using a torque wrench, disconnect the transmitter cable from the battery. Close wounds with appropriate sutures.

Clinical Example (0862T)

A 68-year-old male with a previously implanted wireless cardiac stimulator system for LV pacing has erosion of the subcutaneous pocket of the battery. A new subcutaneous pocket is created, the existing pocket is opened, and the battery is removed and placed in the new pocket.

Description of Procedure (0862T)

Make an incision along the previous implant incision scar. Access the existing pocket, and take care to remove the battery from the pocket. Using a torque wrench, disconnect the transmitter cable from the battery. Using

sharp and blunt technique, create a new pocket in a different location. Connect the device battery to the cable and then secure in the battery pocket. Close wound in appropriate sutures.

Evaluate the system for biventricular capture functionality with the programmer. Perform the evaluation only when the electrode is implanted before the time of transmitter and battery insertion.

Clinical Example (0863T)

A 68-year-old male with a previously implanted wireless cardiac stimulator system for LV pacing experiences reverse remodeling and now has lung encroachment, requiring repositioning of the transmitter within the same intercostal space to optimize communication with the electrode.

Description of Procedure (0863T)

Make an incision along the previous implant incision scar. Access the existing pocket, and take care to remove the sutures securing the transmitter, adjust the transmitter position appropriately and resecure using new sutures. Close wound with appropriate sutures.

Evaluate the system for biventricular capture functionality with the programmer. Perform the evaluation only when the electrode is implanted before the time of transmitter and battery insertion.

▶(0533T, 0534T, 0535T, 0536T have been deleted)◀

▶(For continuous recording of movement disorder symptoms including bradykinesia, dyskinesia, and tremor for 6 days up to 10 days, use 95999)◀

Rationale

In accordance with the CPT guidelines for archiving Category III codes, codes 0533T-0536T have been deleted and instructions have been added to report code 95999, *Unlisted neurological or neuromuscular diagnostic procedure,* for continuous recording of movement disorder symptoms, including bradykinesia, dyskinesia, and tremor for 6 to 10 days. A cross-reference parenthetical note has been added to reflect these changes.

0552T   Low-level laser therapy, dynamic photonic and dynamic thermokinetic energies, provided by a physician or other qualified health care professional

▶(Do not report 0552T in conjunction with 97037)◀

▶(For low-level laser therapy [ie, nonthermal and non-ablative] for post-operative pain, use 97037)◀

★=Telemedicine ◀=Add-on code ✚=Add-on code ⁄✓=FDA approval pending #=Resequenced code ⊘=Modifier 51 exempt

Rationale

In accordance with the establishment of code 97037, two parenthetical notes have been added following code 0552T. An exclusionary parenthetical note precludes the reporting of code 0552T with code 97037 because it is also reported for low-level laser therapy, and the instructional parenthetical note refers users to code 97037 when low-level laser therapy for postoperative pain reduction is performed.

Refer to the codebook and the Rationale for code 97037 for a full discussion of these changes.

▲ **0587T** Percutaneous implantation or replacement of integrated single device neurostimulation system for bladder dysfunction including electrode array and receiver or pulse generator, including analysis, programming, and imaging guidance when performed, posterior tibial nerve

►(Do not report 0587T in conjunction with 64555, 64566, 64575, 64590, 64596, 95970, 95971, 95972, 0588T, 0589T, 0590T, 0816T, 0817T)◄

▲ **0588T** Revision or removal of percutaneously placed integrated single device neurostimulation system for bladder dysfunction including electrode array and receiver or pulse generator, including analysis, programming, and imaging guidance when performed, posterior tibial nerve

►(Do not report 0588T in conjunction with 64555, 64566, 64575, 64590, 64598, 95970, 95971, 95972, 0587T, 0589T, 0590T, 0818T, 0819T)◄

▲ **0589T** Electronic analysis with simple programming of implanted integrated neurostimulation system for bladder dysfunction (eg, electrode array and receiver), including contact group(s), amplitude, pulse width, frequency (Hz), on/off cycling, burst, dose lockout, patient-selectable parameters, responsive neurostimulation, detection algorithms, closed-loop parameters, and passive parameters, when performed by physician or other qualified health care professional, posterior tibial nerve, 1-3 parameters

►(Do not report 0589T in conjunction with 43647, 43648, 43881, 43882, 61850-61888, 63650, 63655, 63661, 63662, 63663, 63664, 63685, 63688, 64553-64595, 95970, 95971, 95972, 95976, 95977, 95983, 95984, 0587T, 0588T, 0590T, 0788T)◄

▲ **0590T** Electronic analysis with complex programming of implanted integrated neurostimulation system for bladder dysfunction (eg, electrode array and receiver), including contact group(s), amplitude, pulse width, frequency (Hz), on/off cycling, burst, dose lockout, patient-selectable parameters, responsive neurostimulation, detection algorithms, closed-loop parameters, and passive parameters, when performed by physician or other qualified health care professional, posterior tibial nerve, 4 or more parameters

►(Do not report 0590T in conjunction with 43647, 43648, 43881, 43882, 61850-61888, 63650, 63655, 63661, 63662, 63663, 63664, 63685, 63688, 64553-64595, 95970, 95971, 95972, 95976, 95977, 95983, 95984, 0587T, 0588T, 0589T, 0788T)◄

Rationale

The codes for insertion or replacement (0587T), revision or removal (0588T), and programming (0589T, 0590T) of a percutaneously placed integrated single device neurostimulation system have been revised by the addition of terminology that reflects their use for treatment of bladder dysfunction. Parenthetical notes have been revised to provide instruction regarding restrictions for reporting these codes. The term "percutaneously placed" has been added to code 0588T to differentiate it from open procedures for the posterior tibial nerve. Codes 0818T and 0819T have been added to the exclusionary parenthetical note following code 0588T to restrict reporting of these procedures together.

Refer to the codebook and the Rationale for codes 64590-64598 for a full discussion of these changes.

0619T Cystourethroscopy with transurethral anterior prostate commissurotomy and drug delivery, including transrectal ultrasound and fluoroscopy, when performed

►(Do not report 0619T in conjunction with 52000, 52441, 52442, 52450, 52500, 52601, 52630, 52640, 52647, 52648, 52649, 53850, 53852, 53854, 76872)◄

Rationale

In accordance with the deletion of Category III code 0499T and the establishment of code 52284, the cross-reference parenthetical note following code 0619T has been revised to reflect these changes.

Refer to the codebook and the Rationale for code 52284 for a full discussion of these changes.

0632T Percutaneous transcatheter ultrasound ablation of nerves innervating the pulmonary arteries, including right heart catheterization, pulmonary artery angiography, and all imaging guidance

(Do not report 0632T in conjunction with 36013, 36014, 36015, 75741, 75743, 75746, 93451, 93453, 93456, 93460, 93503, 93505, 93568, 93593, 93594, 93596, 93597)

▲ = Revised code   ● = New code   ► ◄ = Contains new or revised text   ✕ = Duplicate PLA test   ↕ = Category I PLA   American Medical Association   **163**

Category III 0042T-0713T

▶(For percutaneous transcatheter thermal ablation of nerves innervating the pulmonary arteries, including right heart catheterization, pulmonary artery angiography, and all imaging guidance, use 0793T)◀

Rationale

In accordance with the establishment of code 0793T, a cross-reference parenthetical note has been added following code 0632T.

Refer to the codebook and the Rationale for code 0793T for a full discussion of these changes.

▲ **0656T**   Anterior lumbar or thoracolumbar vertebral body tethering; up to 7 vertebral segments

▲ **0657T**   8 or more vertebral segments

(Do not report 0656T, 0657T in conjunction with 22800, 22802, 22804, 22808, 22810, 22812, 22818, 22819, 22845, 22846, 22847)

▶(For vertebral body tethering of the thoracic spine, see 22836, 22837)◀

#● **0790T**   Revision (eg, augmentation, division of tether), replacement, or removal of thoracolumbar or lumbar vertebral body tethering, including thoracoscopy, when performed

▶(For revision, replacement, or removal of thoracic vertebral body tethering, use 22838)◀

Rationale

In accordance with the establishment of codes 22836-22838, codes 0656T and 0657T have been revised to capture the work of "anterior lumbar or thoracolumbar" for vertebral body tethering (VBT) procedures. In addition, to mirror the code structure to include a code to report the revision of a VBT (22838), which was created for codes 22836-22838, code 0790T has been added. Parenthetical notes have been added to instruct how to report thoracic VBT procedures.

Refer to the codebook and Rationale for codes 22836-22838 for a full discussion of these changes.

Clinical Example (0656T)

A 12-year-old skeletally immature female is diagnosed with thoracolumbar idiopathic scoliosis and has been either unsuccessful or intolerant to bracing. The curve magnitude and remaining growth suggest continued progression without intervention is likely. A vertebral body tethering (VBT) construct is applied from T11 to L3 to provide initial coronal correction through tensioning.

Description of Procedure (0656T)

Identify the scoliotic curve, the levels to be instrumented, implant sizing/selection, and the target initial correction. Gain surgical access through the preferred approach as restricted by the levels being instrumented (ie, retroperitoneal, minimally invasive or open, including possible rib resection). Dissect or retract the diaphragm, allowing access to the pleural cavity. The procedure should follow a standard anesthesia protocol but may require a single-lung ventilation technique and lung deflation to allow access depending on the curve location. Using an ultrasonic scalpel or a thermal device, dissect the iliopsoas muscle from the lateral aspect of the vertebral bodies and identify the segmental vessels along the vertebrae to be instrumented. At seven vertebral segments or less, coagulate the segmental vessels and expose the lateral aspect of the vertebral bodies intended for instrumentation. Dissection to release the diaphragm may be required if the construct will extend proximally to the lower thoracic vertebrae. Confirm the trajectory and placement on the vertebral body at all levels prior to anchor insertion, screw preparation, and screw insertion using direct visualization, intraoperative fluoroscopy, or computed tomography (CT) image guidance. Owing to difficulty avoiding the iliac crest and variable vascular anatomy, caution should be taken if extending instrumentation distal to L3. Secure a cord to the most cranial screw and segmentally tensioned, maintaining compression by tightening set screws at the adjacent levels. Following final tensioning, perform closure and place a chest tube.

Clinical Example (0657T)

A 12-year-old skeletally immature female is diagnosed with thoracolumbar idiopathic scoliosis and has been either unsuccessful or intolerant to bracing. The curve magnitude and remaining growth suggest continued progression without intervention is likely. A VBT construct is applied from T9 to L4 to provide initial coronal correction through tensioning.

Description of Procedure (0657T)

Identify the scoliotic curve, the levels to be instrumented, implant sizing/selection, and the target initial correction. Gain surgical access through the preferred approach as restricted by the levels being instrumented (ie, retroperitoneal, minimally invasive or open, including possible rib resection). Dissect or retract the diaphragm , allowing access to the pleural cavity. The procedure should follow a standard anesthesia protocol but may require a single-lung ventilation technique and lung deflation to allow access depending on the curve location. Using an ultrasonic scalpel or a thermal device, dissect the iliopsoas muscle from the lateral aspect of the vertebral bodies and identify the segmental vessels along the vertebrae to be instrumented. At eight vertebral segments or more, coagulate the segmental vessels and expose the lateral aspect of the vertebral bodies intended for instrumentation. Dissection to release the diaphragm may be required if the construct will extend proximally to the lower thoracic vertebrae. Confirm the trajectory and placement on the vertebral body at all levels prior to anchor insertion, screw preparation, and screw insertion using direct visualization, intraoperative fluoroscopy, or CT image guidance. Owing to difficulty avoiding the iliac crest and variable vascular anatomy, caution should be taken if extending instrumentation distal to L3. Secure a cord to the most cranial screw and segmentally tensioned, maintaining compression by tightening set screws at the adjacent levels. Following final tensioning, perform closure and place a chest tube.

Clinical Example (0790T)

A 12-year-old skeletally immature female, who is 2 years post-primary-tethering procedure, presents with radiographic evidence of a broken tether device and an increase in the size of the scoliosis. The patient has remaining skeletal growth. The patient is referred for removal of the broken tether and placement of a new VBT construct to provide coronal correction.

Description of Procedure (0790T)

The procedure should follow a standard anesthesia protocol but may require a single-lung ventilation technique and lung deflation to allow access depending on the curve location. Gain surgical access through the preferred approach as restricted by the levels being instrumented (ie, retroperitoneal, minimally invasive or open, including possible rib resection). Dissect or retract the diaphragm, allowing access to the pleural cavity. Using an ultrasonic scalpel or a thermal device, dissect the iliopsoas muscle from the lateral aspect of the vertebral bodies. Inspect the cord and assess for any areas of breakage. Remove set screws and remove the broken cord. Assess the vertebral body screws. Remove or replace any loose vertebral body screws. May add new vertebral body screws at adjacent levels. Confirm the trajectory and placement on the vertebral body at all levels prior to anchor insertion, screw preparation, and screw insertion using fluoroscopy or CT image guidance. Owing to difficulty avoiding the iliac crest and variable vascular anatomy, caution should be taken if extending instrumentation distal to L3. Secure a cord to the most cranial screw and segmentally tensioned, maintaining compression by tightening set screws at the adjacent levels. Following final tensioning, perform closure and place a chest tube.

0710T Noninvasive arterial plaque analysis using software processing of data from non-coronary computerized tomography angiography; including data preparation and transmission, quantification of the structure and composition of the vessel wall and assessment for lipid-rich necrotic core plaque to assess atherosclerotic plaque stability, data review, interpretation and report

(Do not report 0710T in conjunction with 0711T, 0712T, 0713T)

0711T data preparation and transmission

0712T quantification of the structure and composition of the vessel wall and assessment for lipid-rich necrotic core plaque to assess atherosclerotic plaque stability

0713T data review, interpretation and report

▶(Do not report 0710T, 0711T, 0712T, 0713T in conjunction with 75580, 0623T, 0624T, 0625T, 0626T)◀

Rationale

In accordance with the deletion of codes 0501T-0504T and the establishment of code 75580, the exclusionary parenthetical note following code 0713T has been revised to reflect these changes.

Refer to the codebook and the Rationale for code 75580 for a full discussion of these changes.

▶(0715T has been deleted)◀

▶(For percutaneous transluminal coronary lithotripsy, use 92972)◀

Rationale

To accommodate the addition of code 92972, code 0715T has been deleted. In addition, a parenthetical note directing use of code 92972 has been added.

Refer to the codebook and the Rationale for code 92972 for a full description of these changes.

Digital Pathology Digitization Procedures

Digital pathology is a dynamic, image-based environment that enables the acquisition, management, and interpretation of pathology information generated from digitized glass microscope slides.

▶Glass microscope slides are scanned by clinical staff, and captured whole-slide images (either in real-time or stored in a computer server or cloud-based digital image archival and communication system) are used for digital examination for pathologic diagnosis distinct from direct visualization through a microscope. Static digital photographic and photomicrographic imaging or digital video streaming of any portion of a glass microscope slide on mobile smartphone and tablet devices does not constitute a digital pathology digitization procedure.

Digitization of glass microscope slides enables remote examination by the pathologist and/or in conjunction with the use of artificial intelligence (AI) algorithms. Category III add-on codes 0751T-0763T, 0827T-0856T may be reported in addition to the appropriate Category I service code when the digitization procedure of glass microscope slides is performed and reported in conjunction with the Category I code for the primary service. Each Category III add-on code is reported as a one-to-one unit of service for each primary pathology service code.◄

Do not report the Category III codes in this subsection solely for archival purposes (eg, after the Category I service has already been performed and reported), solely for educational purposes (eg, when services are not used for individual patient reporting), solely for developing a database for training or validation of AI algorithms, or solely for clinical conference presentations (eg, tumor board interdisciplinary conferences).

+ 0751T Digitization of glass microscope slides for level II, surgical pathology, gross and microscopic examination (List separately in addition to code for primary procedure)

(Use 0751T in conjunction with 88302)

+ 0763T Digitization of glass microscope slides for morphometric analysis, tumor immunohistochemistry (eg, Her-2/neu, estrogen receptor/progesterone receptor), quantitative or semiquantitative, per specimen, each single antibody stain procedure, manual (List separately in addition to code for primary procedure)

(Use 0763T in conjunction with 88360)

#+● 0827T Digitization of glass microscope slides for cytopathology, fluids, washings, or brushings, except cervical or vaginal; smears with interpretation (List separately in addition to code for primary procedure)

►(Use 0827T in conjunction with 88104)◄

#+● 0828T simple filter method with interpretation (List separately in addition to code for primary procedure)

►(Use 0828T in conjunction with 88106)◄

#+● 0829T Digitization of glass microscope slides for cytopathology, concentration technique, smears, and interpretation (eg, Saccomanno technique) (List separately in addition to code for primary procedure)

►(Use 0829T in conjunction with 88108)◄

#+● 0830T Digitization of glass microscope slides for cytopathology, selective-cellular enhancement technique with interpretation (eg, liquid-based slide preparation method), except cervical or vaginal (List separately in addition to code for primary procedure)

►(Use 0830T in conjunction with 88112)◄

#+● 0831T Digitization of glass microscope slides for cytopathology, cervical or vaginal (any reporting system), requiring interpretation by physician (List separately in addition to code for primary procedure)

►(Use 0831T in conjunction with 88141)◄

►(Do not report 0831T in conjunction with 88141, when digitization of glass microscope slides is performed using an automated, computer-assisted screening-imaging system)◄

#+● 0832T Digitization of glass microscope slides for cytopathology, smears, any other source; screening and interpretation (List separately in addition to code for primary procedure)

►(Use 0832T in conjunction with 88160)◄

#+● 0833T preparation, screening and interpretation (List separately in addition to code for primary procedure)

►(Use 0833T in conjunction with 88161)◄

#+● 0834T extended study involving over 5 slides and/or multiple stains (List separately in addition to code for primary procedure)

►(Use 0834T in conjunction with 88162)◄

#+● 0835T Digitization of glass microscope slides for cytopathology, evaluation of fine needle aspirate; immediate cytohistologic study to determine adequacy for diagnosis, first evaluation episode, each site (List separately in addition to code for primary procedure)

►(Use 0835T in conjunction with 88172)◄

►(Do not report 0835T in conjunction with 88172, when 0837T is reported in conjunction with 88173)◄

#+● 0836T immediate cytohistologic study to determine adequacy for diagnosis, each separate additional evaluation episode, same site (List separately in addition to code for primary procedure)

►(Use 0836T in conjunction with 88177)◄

►(Do not report 0836T in conjunction with 88177, when 0837T is reported in conjunction with 88173)◄

#+● 0837T interpretation and report (List separately in addition to code for primary procedure)

►(Use 0837T in conjunction with 88173)◄

#+● 0838T Digitization of glass microscope slides for consultation and report on referred slides prepared elsewhere (List separately in addition to code for primary procedure)

►(Use 0838T in conjunction with 88321)◄

Category III 0042T–0713T

▶(Do not report 0838T in conjunction with 88321 for referred digitized glass microscope slides prepared elsewhere)◀

#+● 0839T Digitization of glass microscope slides for consultation and report on referred material requiring preparation of slides (List separately in addition to code for primary procedure)

▶(Use 0839T in conjunction with 88323)◀

▶(Do not report 0839T in conjunction with 88323 for referred digitized glass microscope slides prepared elsewhere)◀

#+● 0840T Digitization of glass microscope slides for consultation, comprehensive, with review of records and specimens, with report on referred material (List separately in addition to code for primary procedure)

▶(Use 0840T in conjunction with 88325)◀

▶(Do not report 0840T in conjunction with 88325 for referred digitized glass microscope slides prepared elsewhere)◀

#+● 0841T Digitization of glass microscope slides for pathology consultation during surgery; first tissue block, with frozen section(s), single specimen (List separately in addition to code for primary procedure)

▶(Use 0841T in conjunction with 88331)◀

#+● 0842T each additional tissue block with frozen section(s) (List separately in addition to code for primary procedure)

▶(Use 0842T in conjunction with 88332)◀

#+● 0843T cytologic examination (eg, touch preparation, squash preparation), initial site (List separately in addition to code for primary procedure)

▶(Use 0843T in conjunction with 88333)◀

#+● 0844T cytologic examination (eg, touch preparation, squash preparation), each additional site (List separately in addition to code for primary procedure)

▶(Use 0844T in conjunction with 88334)◀

#+● 0845T Digitization of glass microscope slides for immunofluorescence, per specimen; initial single antibody stain procedure (List separately in addition to code for primary procedure)

▶(Use 0845T in conjunction with 88346)◀

#+● 0846T each additional single antibody stain procedure (List separately in addition to code for primary procedure)

▶(Use 0846T in conjunction with 88350)◀

#+● 0847T Digitization of glass microscope slides for examination and selection of retrieved archival (ie, previously diagnosed) tissue(s) for molecular analysis (eg, *KRAS* mutational analysis) (List separately in addition to code for primary procedure)

▶(Use 0847T in conjunction with 88363)◀

▶(Do not report 0847T in conjunction 88363, when digitization of glass microscope slides has been previously reported)◀

#+● 0848T Digitization of glass microscope slides for in situ hybridization (eg, FISH), per specimen; initial single probe stain procedure (List separately in addition to code for primary procedure)

▶(Use 0848T in conjunction with 88365)◀

#+● 0849T each additional single probe stain procedure (List separately in addition to code for primary procedure)

▶(Use 0849T in conjunction with 88364)◀

#+● 0850T each multiplex probe stain procedure (List separately in addition to code for primary procedure)

▶(Use 0850T in conjunction with 88366)◀

#+● 0851T Digitization of glass microscope slides for morphometric analysis, in situ hybridization (quantitative or semiquantitative), manual, per specimen; initial single probe stain procedure (List separately in addition to code for primary procedure)

▶(Use 0851T in conjunction with 88368)◀

#+● 0852T each additional single probe stain procedure (List separately in addition to code for primary procedure)

▶(Use 0852T in conjunction with 88369)◀

#+● 0853T each multiplex probe stain procedure (List separately in addition to code for primary procedure)

▶(Use 0853T in conjunction with 88377)◀

#+● 0854T Digitization of glass microscope slides for blood smear, peripheral, interpretation by physician with written report (List separately in addition to code for primary procedure)

▶(Use 0854T in conjunction with 85060)◀

▶(Do not report 0854T in conjunction with 85060, when digitization of glass microscope slides is performed using an automated, computer-assisted cell-morphology imaging analyzer)◀

#+● 0855T Digitization of glass microscope slides for bone marrow, smear interpretation (List separately in addition to code for primary procedure)

▶(Use 0855T in conjunction with 85097)◀

#+● 0856T Digitization of glass microscope slides for electron microscopy, diagnostic (List separately in addition to code for primary procedure)

▶(Use 0856T in conjunction with 88348)◀

Category III 0042T-0713T

Rationale

Thirty Category III add-on codes (0827T-0856T) have been established to report additional clinical staff work and service requirements associated with digitizing glass microscope slides for primary diagnosis. These codes have been added to the current Digital Pathology Digitization Procedures subsection. The Digital Pathology Digitization Procedures guidelines have also been revised to further define digital pathology and to outline the appropriate reporting of these codes.

Digital pathology refers to systems in which slides are scanned into a computer so they can be examined digitally rather than directly visualized through a microscope. Digitization of glass microscope slides facilitates/enables remote examination by the pathologist. Add-on codes (0827T-0856T) may be reported in addition to the appropriate Category I service when the digitization of glass microscope slides is performed. An instructional parenthetical note has been added following each Category III code referencing the appropriate Category I code with which it may be reported.

The Category III Digital Pathology Digitization Procedures guidelines have been revised to indicate that the images captured are "whole-slide" images to clarify that static digital photographic and photomicrographic imaging or digital video streaming of any portion of a glass microscope slide on mobile smartphone and tablet devices does not constitute a digital pathology digitization procedure and that each code (0827T-0856T) is reported as a one-to-one unit of service for each primary pathology service code.

Instructional parenthetical notes have been added following codes 85060, 85097, 88104, 88106, 88108, 88112, 88141, 88160-88162, 88172, 88173, 88177, 88321, 88323, 88325, 88331-88334, 88346, 88348, 88350, 88363-88366, 88368, 88369, and 88377, directing users to the appropriate Category III code when the digitization of glass microscope slides is performed.

The digitization add-on codes for codes 88346 to 88377 are similar to other glass digitization add-on codes in terms of being whole-slide imaging. A glass slide would need to be digitized in order for a pathologist to remotely review it using digital pathology.

Clinical Example (0827T)

A 60-year-old male with hemoptysis has a cytologic examination performed using bronchoscopic brushings obtained from a left main stem bronchus mass. Glass microscope slide digitization is performed. [**Note:** This is an add-on code. Only consider the additional work related to 0827T glass microscope slide digitization.]

Description of Procedure (0827T)

Scan glass microscope slides using a digital slide imaging system and store the images.

Clinical Example (0828T)

A 70-year-old male with hematuria has a cytologic examination performed using bladder washings obtained during cystoscopic examination. Glass microscope slide digitization is performed. [**Note:** This is an add-on code. Only consider the additional work related to 0828T glass microscope slide digitization.]

Description of Procedure (0828T)

Scan glass microscope slides using a digital slide imaging system and store the images.

Clinical Example (0829T)

A 72-year-old male smoker with a history of urothelial carcinoma of the bladder has a cytologic examination performed using his voided urine specimen. Glass microscope slide digitization is performed. [**Note:** This is an add-on code. Only consider the additional work related to 0829T glass microscope slide digitization].

Description of Procedure (0829T)

Scan glass microscope slides using a digital slide imaging system and store the images.

Clinical Example (0830T)

An elderly male with a history of high-grade papillary urothelial carcinoma, who is post Bacillus Calmette–Guérin therapy, submitted a surveillance urine specimen and a cellular enhancement preparation is processed from the urine sediment. Glass microscope slide digitization is performed. [**Note:** This is an add-on code. Only consider the additional work related to 0830T glass microscope slide digitization.]

Description of Procedure (0830T)

Scan glass microscope slides using a digital slide imaging system and store the images.

Clinical Example (0831T)

A 27-year-old female's specimen was sent for a Pap test and the cytotechnologist at the laboratory identifies abnormal cells requiring physician evaluation and interpretation. Glass microscope slide digitization is performed. [**Note:** This is an add-on code. Only consider the additional work related to 0831T glass microscope slide digitization].

Description of Procedure (0831T)

Scan glass microscope slides using a digital slide imaging system and store the images.

Clinical Example (0832T)

A 66-year-old male with cough and hemoptysis has a cytopathologic examination of his sputum sample without centrifugation. Glass microscope slide digitization is performed. [**Note:** This is an add-on code. Only consider the additional work related to 0832T glass microscope slide digitization.]

Description of Procedure (0832T)

Scan glass microscope slides using a digital slide imaging system and store the images.

Clinical Example (0833T)

A 66-year-old male with cough and hemoptysis has a cytopathologic examination of his sputum sample without centrifugation. Glass microscope slide digitization is performed. [**Note:** This is an add-on code. Only consider the additional work related to 0833T glass microscope slide digitization.]

Description of Procedure (0833T)

Scan glass microscope slides using a digital slide imaging system and store the images.

Clinical Example (0834T)

A 66-year-old male with cough and hemoptysis has a cytopathologic examination of his sputum sample without centrifugation. Glass microscope slide digitization is performed. [**Note:** This is an add-on code. Only consider the additional work related to 0834T glass microscope slide digitization.]

Description of Procedure (0834T)

Scan glass microscope slides using a digital slide imaging system and store the images.

Clinical Example (0835T)

A 56-year-old male with chronic obstructive pulmonary disease (COPD) has a fine-needle aspiration performed for evaluation of a 1.0-cm lung nodule. The physician is asked to immediately evaluate the smears to determine if the specimen is adequate to make a definitive diagnosis. Glass microscope slide digitization is performed. [**Note:** This is an add-on code. Only consider the additional work related to 0835T glass microscope slide digitization.]

Description of Procedure (0835T)

Scan glass microscope slides using a digital slide imaging system and store the images.

Clinical Example (0836T)

A 56-year-old male with COPD, closely following a previous aspirate specimen that was found inadequate for diagnosis, has a fine-needle aspiration performed for evaluation of a 1.0-cm lung nodule. The physician is asked to immediately evaluate additional smears to determine if the specimen is adequate to make a definitive diagnosis. Glass microscope slide digitization is performed. [**Note:** This is an add-on code. Only consider the additional work related to 0836T glass microscope slide digitization.]

Description of Procedure (0836T)

Scan glass microscope slides using a digital slide imaging system and store the images.

Clinical Example (0837T)

A 56-year-old male with COPD has a definitive diagnosis of a 1.0-cm lung nodule with interpretation and written report. Glass microscope slide digitization is performed. [**Note:** This is an add-on code. Only consider the additional work related to 0837T glass microscope slide digitization.]

Description of Procedure (0837T)

Scan glass microscope slides using a digital slide imaging system and store the images.

Clinical Example (0838T)

A 70-year-old female presents with a skin lesion on the posterior neck. On routine microscopic examination, biopsy reveals a tumor composed of poorly differentiated neoplastic cells. A panel of immunohistochemical stains is not conclusive as to the lineage of the tumor when reviewed by the submitting pathologist. The routine microscopic slides and immunohistochemical stains are sent to a consulting pathologist for evaluation. Glass microscope slide digitization is performed. [**Note:** This is an add-on code. Only consider the additional work related to 0838T glass microscope slide digitization.]

Description of Procedure (0838T)

Scan glass microscope slides using a digital slide imaging system and store the images.

Clinical Example (0839T)

A 66-year-old male presents with a pigmented skin lesion and undergoes biopsy. Microscopic examination reveals a melanocytic neoplasm with the differential diagnosis of dysplastic nevus vs melanoma. The routine microscopic slides and blocks are referred to a consultant pathologist. After examining the submitted microscopic slides, the consultant pathologist orders multiple deeper hematoxylin and eosin (H&E)–stained sections cut from the blocks, examines the sections with the microscope, and renders a diagnosis. Glass microscope slide digitization is performed. [**Note:** This is an add-on code. Only consider the additional work related to 0839T glass microscope slide digitization.]

Description of Procedure (0839T)

Scan glass microscope slides using a digital slide imaging system and store the images.

Clinical Example (0840T)

A 65-year-old female presents with a liver mass and undergoes needle-core biopsy. Microscopic examination reveals a tumor composed of poorly differentiated malignant cells. Immunohistochemical stains are performed to determine the cell of origin; however, the results are inconclusive. Slides including H&E–stained slides and paraffin blocks, as well as multiple immunohistochemical-stained slides, and medical records, including laboratory and imaging studies and history and physical examination findings, are referred to a consulting pathologist who renders a diagnosis. Glass microscope slide digitization is performed. [**Note:** This is an add-on code. Only consider the additional work related to 0840T glass microscope slide digitization.]

Description of Procedure (0840T)

Scan glass microscope slides using a digital slide imaging system and store the images.

Clinical Example (0841T)

A 68-year-old female has a resection margin of 1.2-cm malignant skin neoplasm (initial tissue block) removed from her face for frozen-section assessment. Glass microscope slide digitization is performed. [**Note:** This is an add-on code. Only consider the additional work related to 0841T glass microscope slide digitization.]

Description of Procedure (0841T)

Scan glass microscope slides using a digital slide imaging system and store the images.

Clinical Example (0842T)

A 57-year-old male has a resection margin of 2.5-cm malignant skin neoplasm (each additional tissue block) removed from his back for frozen-section assessment. Glass microscope slide digitization is performed. [**Note:** This is an add-on code. Only consider the additional work related to 0842T glass microscope slide digitization.]

Description of Procedure (0842T)

Scan glass microscope slides using a digital slide imaging system and store the images.

Clinical Example (0843T)

A 65-year-old male with a peribronchial mass undergoes a needle biopsy, and an immediate evaluation is requested. Touch preparations of the specimen are made. Glass microscope slide digitization is performed. [**Note:** This is an add-on code. Only consider the additional work related to 0843T glass microscope slide digitization.]

Description of Procedure (0843T)

Scan glass microscope slides using a digital slide imaging system and store the images.

Clinical Example (0844T)

A 67-year-old female with a 1-cm lung mass undergoes biopsy of a right lung lesion; needle cores are procured from two areas of the tumor. These are received in a single-specimen container on saline-moistened gauze. Immediate evaluation is requested, and touch preparations of one-needle core are made and are not diagnostic. Touch preparations are made from the second-needle core and separately interpreted. Glass microscope slide digitization is performed. [**Note:** This is an add-on code. Only consider the additional work related to 0844T glass microscope slide digitization.]

Description of Procedure (0844T)

Scan glass microscope slides using a digital slide imaging system and store the images.

Clinical Example (0845T)

A 65-year-old female presents with bullous dermatitis. An immunoglobulin G (IgG) immunofluorescent antibody stain procedure is performed on the skin biopsy specimen. Glass microscope slide digitization is performed. [**Note:** This is an add-on code. Only consider the additional work related to 0845T glass microscope slide digitization.]

★ = Telemedicine   ◀ = Add-on code   ✚ = Add-on code   ✘ = FDA approval pending   # = Resequenced code   ⊘ = Modifier 51 exempt

Description of Procedure (0845T)

Scan glass microscope slides using a digital slide imaging system and store the images.

Clinical Example (0846T)

A 65-year-old female presents with bullous dermatitis. An IgA immunofluorescent antibody stain procedure is performed on the skin biopsy specimen. Glass microscope slide digitization is performed. [**Note:** This is an add-on code. Only consider the additional work related to 0846T glass microscope slide digitization.]

Description of Procedure (0846T)

Scan glass microscope slides using a digital slide imaging system and store the images.

Clinical Example (0847T)

A 56-year-old male had a colectomy for a colonic adenocarcinoma 2 years ago. The laboratory processed the surgical specimen and issued a surgical pathology report. The patient now presents with probable liver metastases, which was diagnosed clinically. The patient's oncologist requests that the pathologist send tissue to a reference laboratory for KRAS gene mutation analysis. Glass microscope slide digitization is performed. [**Note:** This is an add-on code. Only consider the additional work related to 0847T glass microscope slide digitization.]

Description of Procedure (0847T)

Scan glass microscope slides using a digital slide imaging system and store the images.

Clinical Example (0848T)

A 68-year-old male with a history of kidney transplant presents with lymphadenopathy and undergoes biopsy. A lymphoproliferative process is identified histologically. A stained slide of the lymph node biopsy is analyzed by fluorescence in situ hybridization (FISH) for the presence of Epstein-Barr virus-encoded RNAs (EBERs). Glass microscope slide digitization is performed. [**Note:** This is an add-on code. Only consider the additional work related to 0848T glass microscope slide digitization.]

Description of Procedure (0848T)

Scan glass microscope slides using a digital slide imaging system and store the images.

Clinical Example (0849T)

A 60-year-old male with a history of lung transplant develops pneumonitis and undergoes transbronchial biopsy. A lung tissue section has been examined for the presence of EBERs using in situ hybridization (ISH). Another tissue section is examined for cytomegalovirus by ISH. Glass microscope slide digitization is performed. [**Note:** This is an add-on code. Only consider the additional work related to 0849T glass microscope slide digitization.]

Description of Procedure (0849T)

Scan glass microscope slides using a digital slide imaging system and store the images.

Clinical Example (0850T)

A 67-year-old male with lymphadenopathy presents for biopsy. The lymph node biopsy histologically shows features suggestive of malignant lymphoma. A stained slide is analyzed by FISH for IGH@/BCL2 translocation using DNA probes for both IGH@ and BCL2. Glass microscope slide digitization is performed. [**Note:** This is an add-on code. Only consider the additional work related to 0850T glass microscope slide digitization.]

Description of Procedure (0850T)

Scan glass microscope slides using a digital slide imaging system and store the images.

Clinical Example (0851T)

A 60-year-old male presents with a suspected plasma cell dyscrasia. ISH is performed on a bone marrow specimen to assess for the relative kappa light chain mRNA expression using manual technology. Glass microscope slide digitization is performed. [**Note:** This is an add-on code. Only consider the additional work related to 0851T glass microscope slide digitization.]

Description of Procedure (0851T)

Scan glass microscope slides using a digital slide imaging system and store the images.

Clinical Example (0852T)

A 60-year-old male presents with a suspected plasma cell dyscrasia. ISH is performed on a bone marrow specimen to assess for relative lambda light chain mRNA expression using manual technology. Glass microscope slide digitization is performed. [**Note:** This is an add-on code. Only consider the additional work related to 0852T glass microscope slide digitization.]

Description of Procedure (0852T)

Scan glass microscope slides using a digital slide imaging system and store the images.

Clinical Example (0853T)

A 54-year-old female has been diagnosed with invasive ductal carcinoma of the breast. A stained slide of the breast tumor is analyzed by FISH, quantifying the copy number of the HER2 and centromere 17 (CEP 17) signals using manual technology. Glass microscope slide digitization is performed. [**Note:** This is an add-on code. Only consider the additional work related to 0853T glass microscope slide digitization.]

Description of Procedure (0853T)

Scan glass microscope slides using a digital slide imaging system and store the images.

Clinical Example (0854T)

A 72-year-old male presents with abnormal peripheral blood leukocytes and hemoglobin of 11 g/dl. Peripheral smear slide is submitted for digitization. Glass microscope slide digitization is performed. [**Note:** This is an add-on code. Only consider the additional work related to 0854T glass microscope slide digitization.]

Description of Procedure (0854T)

Scan glass microscope slides using a digital slide imaging system and store the images.

Clinical Example (0855T)

A 67-year-old male with a history of treated acute myeloid leukemia with rare circulating blasts, requiring bone marrow aspirate assessment. Bone marrow aspirate slide is submitted for digitization. Glass microscope slide digitization is performed. [**Note:** This is an add-on code. Only consider the additional work related to 0855T glass microscope slide digitization.]

Description of Procedure (0855T)

Scan glass microscope slides using a digital slide imaging system and store the images.

Clinical Example (0856T)

A 50-year-old male kidney transplant recipient with persistent allograph dysfunction undergoes a renal allograph biopsy. Biopsy tissue specimen is submitted for electron microscopy evaluation. Glass microscope slide digitization is performed. [**Note:** This is an add-on code. Only consider the additional work related to 0856T glass microscope slide digitization.]

Description of Procedure (0856T)

Scan glass microscope slides using a digital slide imaging system and store the images.

▶Codes 0766T, 0767T describe transcutaneous magnetic stimulation that is performed to treat chronic nerve pain and provided by a physician or other qualified health care professional. The selected nerve is mapped and localized using magnetic stimulation at the time of each treatment and the appropriate amplitude of magnetic stimulation is defined. Noninvasive electroneurography (nerve conduction) may be used as guidance to confirm the precise localization of the selected nerve and, when performed, should not be separately reported as a diagnostic study. A separate diagnostic nerve conduction study performed prior to the decision to treat with transcutaneous magnetic stimulation may be separately reported.◀

▲ **0766T** Transcutaneous magnetic stimulation by focused low-frequency electromagnetic pulse, peripheral nerve, with identification and marking of the treatment location, including noninvasive electroneurographic localization (nerve conduction localization), when performed; first nerve

+▲ **0767T** each additional nerve (List separately in addition to code for primary procedure)

(Use 0767T in conjunction with 0766T)

(Do not report 0766T, 0767T in conjunction with 95885, 95886, 95887, 95905, 95907, 95908, 95909, 95910, 95911, 95912, 95913, for nerve conduction used as guidance for transcutaneous magnetic stimulation therapy)

(Do not report 0766T, 0767T in conjunction with 64566, 90867, 90868, 90869, 97014, 97032, 0278T, for the same nerve)

(For posterior tibial neurostimulation, percutaneous needle electrode, use 64566)

(For therapeutic repetitive transcranial magnetic stimulation [TMS] treatment, see 90867, 90868, 90869)

(For application of a modality to one or more areas, electrical stimulation [unattended], use 97014)

(For application of a modality to one or more areas, electrical stimulation [manual], each 15 minutes, use 97032)

(For transcutaneous electrical modulation pain reprocessing [eg, scrambler therapy], each treatment session [includes placement of electrodes], use 0278T)

▶(0768T, 0769T have been deleted)◀

▶(For transcutaneous magnetic stimulation by focused low-frequency electromagnetic pulse, peripheral nerve, see 0766T, 0767T)◀

★ = Telemedicine ◀ = Add-on code ✛ = Add-on code ⟋ = FDA approval pending # = Resequenced code ⊘ = Modifier 51 exempt

Rationale

In the Category III section, codes reporting transcutaneous magnetic stimulation by focused low-frequency electromagnetic pulse (0768T, 0769T) have been deleted and codes 0766T and 0767T revised.

In accordance with the deletion of codes 0768T and 0769T, several parenthetical notes have been moved to follow code 0767T to direct users to the appropriate codes for reporting transcutaneous magnetic stimulation. In addition, the parenthetical note following code 0278T has been revised to reflect the deleted codes. Finally, guidelines have been revised to provide guidance on the appropriate reporting of these codes.

Category III codes 0766T and 0767T were used to report transcutaneous magnetic stimulation of a peripheral nerve by focused low-frequency electromagnetic pulse with noninvasive electroneurographic localization since its creation for the CPT 2023 code set. However, the service has since continued to evolve so much so that there is no longer a difference between the initial and subsequent treatment. Therefore, codes 0768T and 0769T have been deleted.

The parenthetical note and guideline revisions reflect the updates in clinical practice for these services. The cross reference to other services/procedures and deletion of the term "initial" in codes 0766T and 0767T have been made to reflect the lack of markation of the skin and obtaining photographs, which were procedures that differentiated initial services from subsequent services.

Clinical Example (0766T)

A 62-year-old male 5 years post-inguinal hernia repair surgery presents with left groin pain (continuous, throbbing, worse with activity and 7/10 on a pain scale). The patient is diagnosed with left groin neuroma, with palpable neuroma (1.5 × 1 cm), and paresthesia in the distribution of the genital branch of the left genitofemoral nerve. CT scan showed no hernia recurrence. Previous pain management therapies were unsuccessful.

Description of Procedure (0766T)

Position the patient to allow access to the nerve being treated. Place the transcutaneous magnetic stimulation coil over the position of the targeted nerve as determined initially by local bony/anatomic guidance. Use the coil to map the exact position of the nerve to be treated, applying magnetic stimulation to elicit a response that identifies the nerve to be treated. Determine sensory and/or motor thresholds by careful micromovements of the coil and mapping of the response. Assess the response using fractional increases in the magnetic field intensity

with pulses initiated by using the coil-trigger button. This threshold and mapping process allows identification of the exact treatment point and the optimum magnetic field intensity (reduced from where the field intensity produces paresthesia and/or motor activation in the patient's region of pain). Noninvasive electroneurography (nerve conduction) may also be used to localize the nerve (not separately reportable). Once correct positioning and mapping are achieved, initiate treatment and maintain for 13 to 15 minutes. Monitor the patient during this therapy to make sure the stimulation remains over the correct position. If needed, the coil may be repositioned to maintain optimum application to the target nerve.

Clinical Example (0767T)

A 51-year-old female with a history of Crohn's disease and multiple abdominal surgeries presents with right lower quadrant pain along a surgical incision site, rated as 5/10 on narcotic therapy. Two neuromas (1.5 × 1.25 cm and 1.5 × 1.0 cm) are palpable. Tactile allodynia to light stroking is present. [**Note:** This is an add-on code. Only consider the additional service specific to localizing and defining the treatment parameters and treatment of the second neuroma.]

Description of Procedure (0767T)

A separate nerve is targeted for therapy after the initial nerve is identified and treated (separately reported).

Reposition the patient as necessary to allow access to the separate nerve being treated. Place the transcutaneous magnetic stimulation coil over the expected position of the targeted nerve as determined initially by local bony/anatomic guidance. The coil is used to map the exact position of the nerve to be treated, applying magnetic stimulation to elicit a response that identifies the nerve to be treated. Determine sensory and/or motor thresholds by careful micromovements of the coil and mapping of the response. Assess the response using fractional increases in the magnetic field intensity, with pulses initiated by using the coil-trigger button. This threshold and mapping process allows identification of the exact treatment point and the optimum magnetic field intensity (reduced from where the field intensity produces paresthesia and/or motor activation in the patient's region of pain). Noninvasive electroneurography (nerve conduction) may also be used to localize the nerve (not separately reportable). Once correct positioning and mapping are achieved, initiate the treatment and maintain for 13 to 15 minutes. Monitor the patient during this therapy to make sure the stimulation remains over the correct position. The coil may be repositioned if needed to maintain optimum application to the target nerve.

Category III 0042T-0713T

▶(0775T has been deleted)◀

▶(For percutaneous arthrodesis of the sacroiliac joint, see 27278, 27279)◀

Rationale

Code 0775T and its associated guidelines and parenthetical notes have been deleted to accommodate the addition of code 27278 for reporting percutaneous sacroiliac (SI) joint fusion using placement of an intra-articular implant(s).

The changes made for reporting this procedure are associated with the changes made to update reporting for hybrid percutaneous SI joint fixations, ie, percutaneous SI joint fixations that use both a transfixation device and intra-articular implant(s).

Refer to the codebook and the Rationale for code 27278 for a full discussion of these changes.

0783T Transcutaneous auricular neurostimulation, set-up, calibration, and patient education on use of equipment

● **0784T** Insertion or replacement of percutaneous electrode array, spinal, with integrated neurostimulator, including imaging guidance, when performed

● **0785T** Revision or removal of neurostimulator electrode array, spinal, with integrated neurostimulator

● **0786T** Insertion or replacement of percutaneous electrode array, sacral, with integrated neurostimulator, including imaging guidance, when performed

● **0787T** Revision or removal of neurostimulator electrode array, sacral, with integrated neurostimulator

● **0788T** Electronic analysis with simple programming of implanted integrated neurostimulation system (eg, electrode array and receiver), including contact group(s), amplitude, pulse width, frequency (Hz), on/off cycling, burst, dose lockout, patient-selectable parameters, responsive neurostimulation, detection algorithms, closed-loop parameters, and passive parameters, when performed by physician or other qualified health care professional, spinal cord or sacral nerve, 1-3 parameters

▶(Do not report 0788T in conjunction with 43647, 43648, 43881, 43882, 61850-61888, 63650, 63655, 63661, 63662, 63663, 63664, 63685, 63688, 64553-64595, 64596, 64598, 95970, 95971, 95972, 95976, 95977, 95983, 95984, 0587T, 0588T, 0589T, 0590T, 0784T, 0785T, 0786T, 0787T, 0789T)◀

● **0789T** Electronic analysis with complex programming of implanted integrated neurostimulation system (eg, electrode array and receiver), including contact group(s), amplitude, pulse width, frequency (Hz), on/off cycling, burst, dose lockout, patient-selectable parameters, responsive neurostimulation, detection algorithms, closed-loop parameters, and passive parameters, when performed by physician or other qualified health care professional, spinal cord or sacral nerve, 4 or more parameters

▶(Do not report 0789T in conjunction with 43647, 43648, 43881, 43882, 61850-61888, 63650, 63655, 63661, 63662, 63663, 63664, 63685, 63688, 64553-64595, 64596, 64598, 95970, 95971, 95972, 95976, 95977, 95983, 95984, 0587T, 0588T, 0589T, 0590T, 0784T, 0785T, 0786T, 0787T, 0788T)◀

Rationale

Codes 0784T-0789T have been added to enable reporting of percutaneous insertion/replacement of integrated neurostimulator electrode arrays of the spine (0784T) and sacrum (0786T), as well as revisions and removals of the same (0785T, 0787T).

Refer to the codebook and the Rationale for codes 64590-64598 and 0816T-0819T for a full discussion of these changes.

Clinical Example (0784T)

A 60-year-old male with intractable back and leg pain after lumbar fusion had unsuccessful conservative treatment for pain management. He underwent a successful trial of a percutaneously placed spinal cord stimulator electrode array. He is referred for placement of a neurostimulator that includes an electrode array, which is placed through the same access site.

Description of Procedure (0784T)

Make a skin incision and use electrocautery to obtain hemostasis. Make a subcutaneous pocket to facilitate the implantation of the neurostimulator. Through the same access site, place the electrode array percutaneously in the epidural space utilizing fluoroscopy. Test the electrode array for impedance and paresthesia. When the position is confirmed, place the remainder of the total neurostimulator into the subcutaneous pocket and anchor in place. Check the wound for hemostasis and then irrigate copiously. Close the wound in layers and apply a sterile dressing. Transport the patient to the recovery room.

Clinical Example (0785T)

A 57-year-old male who has benefited from a spinal neurostimulator needs to have the stimulator revised due to migration.

Description of Procedure (0785T)

Make an incision to reopen the old pocket for the neurostimulator and achieve hemostasis. Re-suture the neurostimulator in the pocket to prevent migration. Check the wound again for hemostasis and then irrigate copiously. Close the wound in layers and apply a sterile dressing. Transport the patient to the recovery room.

Clinical Example (0786T)

A 57-year-old male with debilitating urge incontinence voids hourly. Conservative remedies have been unsuccessful. A percutaneous test stimulation of the sacral nerve is successful, and placement of a permanent neurostimulator with an integrated electrode array is planned.

Description of Procedure (0786T)

Approximate levels of the sacral foramina using fluoroscopy. Anesthetize skin and periosteum and pass an electrically insulated 3- or 5-inch needle percutaneously into the foramen. Connect an external screener (power source) to the foramen needle by a separate cable and grounding source. Discern and document specific biologic responses to stimulation of the sacral spinal nerve 2 (S2) and no activity for S4 (desired responses are S2 and S3). Exchange a 3-0 temporary electrode through the lumen of the foramen needle, leaving only the integrated neurostimulator and electrode in place. Perform retesting to confirm response. Place dressing to secure the electrode in place. Perform a hard X ray to confirm the lead position.

Clinical Example (0787T)

A 47-year-old male, who has benefited from a sacral nerve neurostimulator, needs to have the electrode array with integrated neurostimulator revised due to migration of the lead.

Description of Procedure (0787T)

Make incisions near the sacral foramen to access the electrode array with integrated neurostimulator. Proceed with dissection to the sensor lead placed through the sacral foramen. Once identified, remove the lead and integrated neurostimulator from its subcutaneous tunnel. Carefully dissect the stimulator array free of the sacral nerve. Irrigate the wounds. Close the surgical incisions in a layered fashion and apply dressings.

Clinical Example (0788T)

A 61-year-old male with a condition that requires nerve stimulation returns for simple programming of the implanted integrated neurostimulation system in which three or fewer of the parameters are adjusted.

Description of Procedure (0788T)

Link the programmer with the patient's programmer (handheld device) and interrogate the patient's neurostimulator device. Review preset program settings by switching the handheld programmer between programs and recording patient sensation. Change the lead configuration, and adjust and maintain the amplitude when stimulation is felt, as appropriate. If inappropriate, repeat the process until the appropriate response is obtained. Three parameters are assessed and changed as necessary. The new program is resynchronized with the patient's handheld programmer.

Clinical Example (0789T)

A 58-year-old male with a condition that requires nerve stimulation returns for complex programming of the implanted integrated neurostimulation system in which four or more parameters are adjusted.

Description of Procedure (0789T)

Link the programmer with the patient's programmer (ie, handheld device) and interrogate the patient's neurostimulator device. Review the preset program settings by switching the patient's handheld programmer between programs and recording the patient's sensation. Change the lead configuration and, as appropriate, change the amplitude until stimulation is felt. The resulting configuration is maintained. If inappropriate, repeat the process until the appropriate response is obtained. Four or more parameters are assessed and changed as necessary. The new program is resynchronized with the patient's handheld programmer.

0790T	Code is out of numerical sequence. See 0656T-0659T
✚● 0791T	Motor-cognitive, semi-immersive virtual reality–facilitated gait training, each 15 minutes (List separately in addition to code for primary procedure)

▶(Use 0791T in conjunction with 97116)◀

▲=Revised code ●=New code ▶◀=Contains new or revised text ✖=Duplicate PLA test ↕=Category I PLA   American Medical Association   **175**

Category III 0042T-0713T

Rationale

A new Category III add-on code (0791T) has been established to report motor-cognitive, semi-immersive virtual reality–facilitated gait training.

Code 0791T may be reported in addition to code 97116. Code 97116 describes therapeutic procedure (gait training of one or more areas for each 15 minutes, including stair climbing), and code 0791T describes combined motor and cognitive training for gait rehabilitation. During this procedure, the patient is exercising decision making, memory, attention, and response time while negotiating virtual obstacles.

The patient sees a representation of their feet movement in a simulated environment displayed on a television screen placed in front of the treadmill. The patient engages with different cognitive tasks during ambulation, such as navigating to different locations in the simulated environment, remembering objects that appear along the virtual path, ignoring attention distractors, spotting different objects, etc.

Clinical Example (0791T)

A 66-year-old female with gait impairment, history of falls, and declining motor and cognitive function is referred for motor-cognitive, semi-immersive virtual reality (VR)-facilitated gait training. [**Note:** This is an add-on code related to gait training.]

Description of Procedure (0791T)

During treadmill-based gait training, the physician, qualified health care professional (QHP), or their clinical staff configures the semi-immersive VR-simulation system, which consists of a television, depth camera, operator touchscreen, and a dedicated computer to meet the patient's specific functional level and the therapeutic goals. Position the camera to track the movement of the patient's feet while the patient is walking on the treadmill. Start the treadmill, and the patient starts to walk while simultaneously participating in the semi-immersive VR experience. The patient's feet movements are represented in the VR simulation and projected to the patient on the screen, providing the patient with real-time feedback on performance. The patient experiences different virtual obstacles that require the patient to modulate gait to successfully negotiate the obstacles projected on the screen while attending to cognitively demanding tasks. (Code 0791T represents each 15 minutes of practice expense in conjunction with code 97116.)

● **0792T**   Application of silver diamine fluoride 38%, by a physician or other qualified health care professional

Rationale

Category III code 0792T has been established to report application of silver diamine fluoride (SDF). Application of SDF is intended for treatment of dental cavities in children and adults. It may also result in reduction of new dental caries.

Code 99188 differs from code 0792T because code 99188 is reported for the application of topical fluoride varnish to all tooth surfaces for dental caries prevention. Code 0792T is specific to the SDF application to the carious lesions, a service commonly performed for much smaller and specific areas to arrest active tooth decay.

Clinical Example (0792T)

A 2-year-old female presents with severe early childhood caries. The physician or other QHP applies silver diamine fluoride topically to the caries lesions (cavities).

Description of Procedure (0792T)

Identify the presence of a dental caries lesion visually upon physical examination. Isolate the tooth with gauze, and gently clean and dry the cavity with cotton. Apply a drop of silver diamine fluoride to the decayed tooth surface with a disposable microbrush. Isolate the area for 1 minute and blot the excess agent with cotton. Treat other carious lesions, if present.

● **0793T**   Percutaneous transcatheter thermal ablation of nerves innervating the pulmonary arteries, including right heart catheterization, pulmonary artery angiography, and all imaging guidance

▶(Do not report 0793T in conjunction with 75746, 93503, 93568)◀

▶(For percutaneous transcatheter ultrasound ablation of nerves innervating the pulmonary arteries, including right heart catheterization, pulmonary artery angiography, and all imaging guidance, use 0632T)◀

Rationale

Code 0793T has been established to report percutaneous transcatheter thermal ablation of nerves innervating the pulmonary arteries.

Thermal ablation of nerves innervating the pulmonary arteries is performed to treat diagnoses, such as pulmonary arterial hypertension. Prior to the establishment of code 0793T, no CPT code exists to describe thermal ablation of the nerves innervating the pulmonary arteries. Existing code 0632T describes ablation of these nerves using ultrasound; however, code 0632T does not include thermal ablation. Code 0793T includes right heart catheterization, pulmonary artery angiography, and all imaging guidance. An exclusionary parenthetical note has been added restricting use of code 0793T with codes 75746, 93503, and 93568. A cross-reference parenthetical note has been added directing users to code 0632T for percutaneous transcatheter ultrasound ablation of nerves innervating the pulmonary arteries, including right heart catheterization, pulmonary artery angiography, and all imaging guidance.

Clinical Example (0793T)

A 40-year-old female presents with World Health Organization functional class III pulmonary hypertension, pericardial effusion, and an enlarged right atrium and ventricle. Mean pulmonary arterial pressure was 55 mm Hg (by right heart catheterization) with a pulmonary vascular resistance of 10 Wood units. The patent is refractory to pulmonary vasodilators.

Description of Procedure (0793T)

The interventional cardiologist performs a right heart catheterization using the femoral venous access with an 8-French long sheath placed into the pulmonary artery. Perform hemodynamic measurements and blood oxygen pressure/saturation determinations from the right atrium, right ventricle, and pulmonary artery. Use pulmonary angiography to define the main right and left pulmonary arteries for ablation catheter placement.

Select an appropriate pulmonary artery denervation (PADN) diameter ablation catheter, insert and push along the transseptal guiding introducer sheath into the main pulmonary artery. Slightly rotate and push the handle of the PADN catheter in a clockwise direction to position it at the ostium of the left pulmonary artery (level 1 of ablation, <2 mm distal to the orifice). Select and confirm the appropriate ablation targets with each of the ablation target's temperature at least 45° centigrade (maximum temperature is 60° centigrade). After ablation at this level, counterclockwise rotation and withdrawing the handle will allow the circular tip to slide down to the distal bifurcation area of the main pulmonary artery (level 2 of ablation, <2 mm proximal to the bifurcation level). Next rotate and push the handles until the circular tip jumps into level 3 of ablation (<2 mm distal to the ostial right pulmonary artery). Perform hemodynamic measurements and blood oxygen pressure/saturation determinations from the right atrium, right ventricle, and pulmonary artery after the ablations. Procedural success is defined as a reduction in the mean pulmonary artery pressure of ≥10 mm Hg (as measured by a Swan-Ganz catheter) and there are no complications.

▶Pharmaco-oncologic Algorithmic Treatment Ranking◀

▶Code 0794T (pharmaco-oncologic treatment ranking) represents rules based algorithm–generated match scores that rank available monotherapies and drug combinations according to their ability to target the patient's specific cancer biomarkers. These pharmaco-oncologic treatment ranking options are based only on current Food and Drug Administration (FDA)-approved drugs but may include both on-label and off-label uses for targeted therapies, and additional information may also be provided on potential active clinical trials that include specifically matched, currently available, therapy options. Code 0794T includes time spent by the physician, other qualified health care professional, or clinical staff in submitting the patient's clinical and existing molecular, laboratory, or pathology result data for algorithmic assessment. Only existing result data should be submitted without alteration of original results and interpretations (eg, variant calls or expression markers) from those separately reported by the original performing clinical laboratories and should not include genomic sequencing raw data files for re-evaluation. The algorithmic program generates a report that is used by the physician or other qualified health care professional to inform treatment choices.◀

● **0794T**   Patient-specific, assistive, rules-based algorithm for ranking pharmaco-oncologic treatment options based on the patient's tumor-specific cancer marker information obtained from prior molecular pathology, immunohistochemical, or other pathology results which have been previously interpreted and reported separately

Rationale

A new Category III code (0794T) has been established to report a patient-specific, assistive, rules-based algorithm for ranking pharmaco-oncologic treatment options. A new subsection, "Pharmaco-oncologic Algorithmic Treatment Ranking," and its associated guidelines have also been established to define pharmaco-oncologic treatment ranking and outline the appropriate reporting of this code.

This analytic process provides physicians or other QHPs with personalized, specific, and verifiable information to assist them in ranking and determining the appropriate treatment for hematology and oncology patients.

Pharmaco-oncologic treatment ranking represents a rules-based algorithm-generated match scores that rank available monotherapies and drug combinations according to their ability to target the patient's specific cancer biomarkers. The time spent by the physician, other QHP, or clinical staff in submitting the patient's clinical and existing molecular, laboratory, or pathology result data for algorithmic assessment is included in code 0794T.

Clinical Example (0794T)

A 50-year-old female with hormone-positive advanced breast cancer, who has not responded to two prior therapeutic regimens, is referred for algorithmic ranking of pharmaco-oncologic treatment options.

Description of Procedure (0794T)

The physician submits tumor-specific and next-generation sequencing data (if available) into the technology platform, excluding the two failed therapies from the scoring system. The algorithm generates a report with match scores that rank available monotherapies and drug combinations according to their ability to target the patient's specific cancer biomarkers, which are used to inform subsequent treatment choices. Data are submitted without alteration of original results and interpretations and do not include genomic sequencing raw data files.

►Dual-Chamber Leadless Pacemaker◄

►A complete dual-chamber leadless pacemaker system includes two pulse generators, each with a built-in battery and electrode. Implantation of this system is performed using a catheter under fluoroscopic guidance via transvenous access. One pacemaker is implanted in the right atrium, and one is implanted in the right ventricle. Rarely, for clinical reasons, a complete dual-chamber leadless pacemaker system may be completed in stages, with one pacemaker implanted into the right ventricle at the initial procedure and the other implanted into the right atrium at a subsequent session. An existing single-chamber right ventricular leadless pacemaker may be upgraded to a complete dual-chamber leadless pacemaker system by implantation of a right atrial leadless pacemaker.

For insertion of a complete dual-chamber leadless pacemaker system, report 0795T. For insertion of a leadless pacemaker into the right atrium when a single-chamber right ventricular leadless pacemaker already exists, in order to complete the dual-chamber leadless

pacemaker system, report 0796T. For insertion of only the right ventricular pacemaker component of a dual-chamber leadless pacemaker system, report 0797T. For removal of a complete dual-chamber leadless pacemaker system, report 0798T. For removal of only the right atrial leadless pacemaker component of a complete dual-chamber leadless pacemaker, report 0799T. For removal of only the right ventricular leadless pacemaker component of a complete dual-chamber leadless pacemaker, report 0800T. For removal and replacement of a complete dual-chamber leadless pacemaker system, report 0801T. For removal and replacement of only one pacemaker component of a complete dual-chamber leadless pacemaker system, report 0802T for the right atrial pacemaker component or 0803T for the right ventricular pacemaker component.

Right heart catheterization (93451, 93453, 93456, 93457, 93460, 93461, 93593, 93594, 93596, 93597) may not be reported in conjunction with dual-chamber leadless pacemaker codes 0795T, 0796T, 0797T, 0798T, 0799T, 0800T, 0801T, 0802T, 0803T, unless complete right heart catheterization is performed for an indication distinct from the dual-chamber leadless pacemaker procedure.

For programming device evaluation of a dual-chamber leadless pacemaker system, report 0804T. Device evaluation code 93279 may not be reported in conjunction with dual-chamber leadless pacemaker system codes 0795T, 0796T, 0797T, 0798T, 0799T, 0800T, 0801T, 0802T, 0803T.

Radiological supervision and interpretation, fluoroscopy (76000, 77002), ultrasound guidance for vascular access (76937), right ventriculography (93566), and femoral venography (75820) are included in the leadless pacemaker procedures, when performed.◄

● **0795T**   Transcatheter insertion of permanent dual-chamber leadless pacemaker, including imaging guidance (eg, fluoroscopy, venous ultrasound, right atrial angiography, right ventriculography, femoral venography) and device evaluation (eg, interrogation or programming), when performed; complete system (ie, right atrial and right ventricular pacemaker components)

►(Do not report 0795T in conjunction with 75820, 76000, 76937, 77002, 93566, 0796T, 0797T)◄

● **0796T**   right atrial pacemaker component (when an existing right ventricular single leadless pacemaker exists to create a dual-chamber leadless pacemaker system)

● **0797T**   right ventricular pacemaker component (when part of a dual-chamber leadless pacemaker system)

►(Do not report 0795T, 0796T, 0797T in conjunction with 33274, 75820, 76000, 76937, 77002, 93566)◄

▶(Do not report 0795T, 0796T, 0797T in conjunction with 93451, 93453, 93456, 93457, 93460, 93461, 93593, 93594, 93596, 93597, 93598, unless complete right heart catheterization is performed for indications distinct from the leadless pacemaker procedure)◀

● **0798T** Transcatheter removal of permanent dual-chamber leadless pacemaker, including imaging guidance (eg, fluoroscopy, venous ultrasound, right atrial angiography, right ventriculography, femoral venography), when performed; complete system (ie, right atrial and right ventricular pacemaker components)

● **0799T** right atrial pacemaker component

● **0800T** right ventricular pacemaker component (when part of a dual-chamber leadless pacemaker system)

▶(Do not report 0798T, 0799T, 0800T in conjunction with 75820, 76000, 76937, 77002, 93451, 93453, 93456, 93457, 93460, 93461, 93566, 93593, 93594, 93596, 93597)◀

▶(Do not report 0799T, 0800T in conjunction with 33275, 0798T)◀

● **0801T** Transcatheter removal and replacement of permanent dual-chamber leadless pacemaker, including imaging guidance (eg, fluoroscopy, venous ultrasound, right atrial angiography, right ventriculography, femoral venography) and device evaluation (eg, interrogation or programming), when performed; dual-chamber system (ie, right atrial and right ventricular pacemaker components)

● **0802T** right atrial pacemaker component

● **0803T** right ventricular pacemaker component (when part of a dual-chamber leadless pacemaker system)

▶(Do not report 0801T, 0802T, 0803T in conjunction with 33274, 33275, 75820, 76000, 76937, 77002, 93451, 93453, 93456, 93457, 93460, 93461, 93566, 0795T, 0796T, 0797T, 0798T, 0799T, 0800T)◀

▶(Do not report 33274, 33275 when right ventricular single-chamber leadless pacemaker is part of a dual-chamber leadless pacemaker system)◀

● **0804T** Programming device evaluation (in person) with iterative adjustment of implantable device to test the function of device and to select optimal permanent programmed values, with analysis, review, and report, by a physician or other qualified health care professional, leadless pacemaker system in dual cardiac chambers

▶(Do not report 0804T in conjunction with 0795T, 0796T, 0797T, 0798T, 0799T, 0800T, 0801T, 0802T, 0803T)◀

Rationale

A new Category III subsection, new guidelines, and 10 Category III codes have been established to report transcatheter permanent dual-chamber leadless pacemaker procedures.

A dual-chamber leadless pacemaker system consists of two pulse generators that have built-in batteries and electrodes. The dual-chamber system is used to treat diagnoses, such as sinus node disease and atrioventricular node disease. In addition, patients who have a single, right ventricular chamber leadless pacemaker and who experience sinus-node dysfunction and pacemaker syndrome may require an upgrade from a single-chamber system to a dual-chamber leadless pacemaker. In these scenarios, the single-chamber leadless system (the existing right ventricular leadless pacemaker) is kept or retained and a right atrial leadless pacemaker is inserted to create the dual-chamber system.

Typically, insertion of the complete (right atrial and right ventricular) dual-chamber system is performed at the same session and reported with code 0795T. However, in instances in which the pacemakers are inserted in separate sessions, the right ventricular pacemaker is inserted at an initial session and reported with code 0797T. The right atrial pacemaker is inserted at a subsequent session and reported with code 0796T.

Codes 0798T-0800T describe removal of the pacemaker. Codes 0801T-0803T describe removal and replacement of the pacemaker. Codes 0795T-0803T include imaging guidance (eg, fluoroscopy, venous ultrasound, right atrial angiography, right ventriculography, femoral venography) and device evaluation (eg, interrogation or programming) when performed.

Code 0804T describes in-person programming device evaluation of the dual-chamber leadless pacemaker system, with iterative adjustment to test device function and to select optimal permanent programmed values. Code 0804T includes analysis, review, and report by a physician or other QHP. Code 0804T may not be reported with codes 0795T-0803T, because device evaluation is included in these codes when performed at the time of the procedure.

It is important to note that procedures for single-chamber pacemakers that are *not* part of a dual-chamber leadless pacemaker system are reported using different CPT codes. Specifically, insertion or replacement of a right ventricular leadless pacemaker that is not part of a dual-chamber is reported with code 33274, and removal is reported with code 33275. Codes 0823T-0826T have been established to report right atrial leadless pacemaker procedures when the pacemaker is *not* part of a dual-chamber system. (See the following table for a summary of which of these new codes should be reported.)

Refer to the codebook and the Rationale for codes 0823T-0826T for a full discussion of these changes.

Insertion Procedure		
	Dual-Chamber System	**Single-Chamber System (when not part of dual-chamber system)**
Right atrial and right ventricular	0795T	–
Right atrial	0796T	0823T
Right ventricular	0797T	33724 (**Note:** 33274 describes insertion or replacement)

Removal Procedure Only		
	Dual-Chamber System	**Single-Chamber System (when not part of dual-chamber system)**
Right atrial and right ventricular	0798T	–
Right atrial	0799T	0824T
Right ventricular	0800T	33275

Removal and Replacement Procedure		
	Dual-Chamber System	**Single-Chamber System (when not part of dual-chamber system)**
Right atrial and right ventricular	0801T	–
Right atrial	0802T	0825T
Right ventricular	0803T	33274

Clinical Example (0795T)

A 72-year-old male presents with persistent dizziness and shortness of breath. He is diagnosed with sinus node disease and atrioventricular (AV) node disease, and a dual-chamber leadless pacemaker is recommended.

Description of Procedure (0795T)

In the electrophysiology laboratory, sedate or anesthetize the patient, as clinically appropriate. Prepare the femoral region and administer local anesthesia. Depending on the leadless pacemaker system, place surface electrocardiogram (ECG) electrodes or programming heads on the patient's chest and connect to the external pacemaker programmer. Prior to insertion into the target chambers, load the pacemaker onto a catheter—one for each target chamber, the right atrium, and right ventricle. Obtain access via a guidewire in the femoral vein. Ultrasound guidance may be used, and femoral venography may be performed to identify the anatomy. After sequential dilation and upsizing the femoral sheath, including a small incision if needed, insert the leadless pacemaker introducer into the femoral vein and remove the guidewire. Under fluoroscopic guidance, insert the first leadless pacemaker delivery catheter into the femoral vein through the introducer. Using steering and deflection, advance the delivery catheter through the inferior vena cava (IVC) to the right ventricle. Contrast agent may be injected through the catheter to identify the anatomy. With the catheter still attached and prior to fixation of the device, a test may be performed to ensure mechanical stability of leadless pacemaker. Electrical measurements, including intrinsic cardiac signal, can be measured and captured threshold can be performed via communication to the device from the programmer to assess device function. Perform mapping using the delivery catheter for accurate device placement. Then fix the leadless pacemaker to the endocardium. After fixation, the pacemaker is undocked from the delivery system but still connected via tethers. Use the external programmer to measure pacing-capture threshold, sensing amplitude, and impedance. As needed, reposition and re-engage the pacemaker within the target chamber under fluoroscopic guidance. Once appropriate parameters and adequate fixation are confirmed, the tether is released, and the pacemaker is released from the delivery catheter. This process is repeated for the leadless pacemaker placement in the atrium. Remove the tether, delivery catheter, and sheath. Close the access site with a nonabsorbable single figure-of-eight stitch or by other means.

Clinical Example (0796T)

A 72-year-old male with a history of AV node disease and previously implanted right ventricular leadless pacemaker develops palpitations and shortness of breath due to sinus node dysfunction and pacemaker syndrome. Upgrade to a dual-chamber leadless pacemaker using the existing right ventricular leadless pacemaker is recommended.

Description of Procedure (0796T)

In the electrophysiology laboratory, sedate or anesthetize the patient, as clinically appropriate. Prepare the femoral region and administer local anesthesia. Depending on the leadless pacemaker system, surface ECG electrodes or programming heads may be placed on the patient's chest and connected to the external pacemaker programmer. Prior to insertion into the right atrium, load the pacemaker onto a catheter. Obtain access via a guidewire in the femoral vein. Ultrasound guidance may be used, and femoral venography may be performed to identify the anatomy. After sequential dilation and upsizing the femoral sheath, including a small incision if needed, insert the leadless pacemaker introducer into the femoral vein and remove the guidewire. Under fluoroscopic guidance, insert the leadless pacemaker delivery catheter into the femoral vein through the introducer. Using steering and deflection, advance the delivery catheter through the IVC to the right atrium. Contrast agent may be injected through the catheter to identify right atrial anatomy. Perform mapping using the delivery catheter for accurate device placement in the right atrium. Then fix the leadless pacemaker to the endocardium. With the catheter still attached and prior to fixation of the device, a test may be performed to ensure mechanical stability of leadless pacemaker. After fixation, the pacemaker is undocked from the delivery system but still connected via tethers. Use the external programmer to measure pacing-capture threshold, sensing amplitude, and impedance. As needed, reposition and re-engage the pacemaker within the target chamber under fluoroscopic guidance. Once appropriate parameters and adequate fixation are confirmed, the tether is released, and the pacemaker is released from the delivery catheter. If the patient has an existing ventricular leadless pacemaker in place that is compatible, pair the atrial leadless pacemaker to communicate with the existing ventricular leadless pacemaker prior to closure of venous access. Remove the delivery catheter and sheath, and close the access site with a nonabsorbable single figure-of-eight stitch or by other means.

Clinical Example (0797T)

A 90-year-old male with previously implanted dual-chamber leadless pacemaker for AV node disease was found to have right ventricular leadless pacemaker failure. Given the risks of right ventricular leadless pacemaker extraction in this elderly patient, implantation of a right ventricular leadless pacemaker to complete the dual-chamber leadless system is recommended.

Description of Procedure (0797T)

In the electrophysiology laboratory, sedate or anesthetize the patient, as clinically appropriate. Interrogation of the existing leadless atrial pacemaker demonstrates normal function. Prepare the femoral region and administer local anesthesia. Depending on the leadless pacemaker system, surface ECG electrodes or programming heads may be placed on the patient's chest and connected to the external pacemaker programmer. Prior to insertion into the right ventricle, load the pacemaker onto a catheter. Obtain access via a guidewire in the femoral vein. Ultrasound guidance may be used, and femoral venography may be performed to identify the anatomy. After sequential dilation and upsizing the femoral sheath, including a small incision if needed, insert the leadless pacemaker introducer into the femoral vein and remove the guidewire. Under fluoroscopic guidance, the leadless pacemaker delivery catheter is then inserted into the femoral vein through the introducer. Using steering and deflection, advance the delivery catheter through the IVC to the right ventricle. Contrast agent may be injected through the catheter to identify right ventricular anatomy. Perform mapping using the delivery catheter for accurate device placement in the right ventricle. Then fix the leadless pacemaker to the endocardium (eg, by rotation of device to secure in right ventricular endocardium). With the catheter still attached and prior to fixation of the device, a test may be performed to ensure mechanical stability of leadless pacemaker. After fixation, the pacemaker is undocked from the delivery system but still connected via tethers. Use the external programmer to measure pacing-capture threshold, sensing amplitude, and impedance. As needed, reposition and re-engage the pacemaker within the target chamber under fluoroscopic guidance. Once appropriate parameters and adequate fixation are confirmed, the tether is released, and the pacemaker is released from the delivery catheter. Pair the ventricular leadless pacemaker to communicate with the existing atrial leadless pacemaker prior to closure of venous access. Remove the delivery catheter and sheath, and close the access site with a nonabsorbable single figure-of-eight stitch or by other means.

Clinical Example (0798T)

A 72-year-old male had a dual-chamber leadless pacemaker system placed 2 years ago. He has developed significantly worsening congestive heart failure. The decision is made to remove the leadless pacemaker in favor of placing a CRT device to simultaneously treat both the sinus node disease and the heart failure.

Description of Procedure (0798T)

In the electrophysiology laboratory, prepare the femoral region and administer local anesthesia. Obtain access via a guidewire in the femoral vein. Ultrasound guidance may be used, and femoral venography may be performed to identify the anatomy. Advance a guidewire via the femoral vein into the vena cava. After sequential dilation and upsizing the femoral sheath, including a small incision if needed, insert the leadless pacemaker retrieval introducer into the femoral vein and remove the guidewire. Under fluoroscopic guidance, insert the leadless pacemaker retrieval catheter into the femoral vein through the introducer. Using steering and deflection, advance the retrieval catheter under fluoroscopic guidance through the IVC to the right atrium and through the tricuspid valve into the right ventricle. Then engage the leadless pacemaker by the retrieval catheter with a snare. After confirming under fluoroscopy that the retrieval mechanism is engaged and secure, remove the coupled retrieval catheter and leadless pacemaker.

This process is repeated to remove the leadless pacemaker capsule from the right atrium. Using steering and deflection, advance the retrieval catheter through the IVC to the right atrium. The leadless pacemaker is then engaged by the retrieval catheter. After confirming under fluoroscopy that the retrieval mechanism is engaged and secure, remove the coupled retrieval catheter and leadless pacemaker. Close the access site with a nonabsorbable single figure-of-eight stitch or by other means.

Clinical Example (0799T)

A 72-year-old male had a dual-chamber leadless pacemaker system placed 2 years ago. The patient has developed endocarditis, and there is evidence of vegetation on the right atrial leadless pacemaker. Right atrial leadless pacemaker removal is recommended.

Description of Procedure (0799T)

In the electrophysiology laboratory, prepare the femoral region and administer local anesthesia. Obtain access via a guidewire in the femoral vein. Ultrasound guidance may be used, and femoral venography may be performed to identify the anatomy. Advance a guidewire via the femoral vein into the vena cava. After sequential dilation and upsizing the femoral sheath, including a small incision if needed, insert the leadless pacemaker introducer into the femoral vein and remove the guidewire. Under fluoroscopic guidance, insert the leadless pacemaker retrieval catheter into the femoral vein through the introducer. Using steering and deflection, advance the retrieval catheter under fluoroscopic guidance to the target chamber, the right atrium. The leadless pacemaker is then engaged by the retrieval catheter with a snare.

After confirming under fluoroscopy that the retrieval catheter is appropriately secured to leadless pacemaker, disengage the leadless pacemaker from the endocardium using the retrieval catheter, and remove the coupled retrieval catheter and leadless pacemaker. Close the access site with a nonabsorbable single figure-of-eight stitch or by other means.

Clinical Example (0800T)

A 72-year-old male had a dual-chamber leadless pacemaker system placed 2 years ago. The patient has developed endocarditis, and there is evidence of vegetation on the right ventricular leadless pacemaker. Right ventricular leadless pacemaker removal is recommended.

Description of Procedure (0800T)

In the electrophysiology laboratory, prepare the femoral region and administer local anesthesia. Obtain access via a guidewire in the femoral vein. Ultrasound guidance may be used, and femoral venography may be performed to identify the anatomy. Advance a guidewire via the femoral vein into the vena cava. After sequential dilation and upsizing the femoral sheath, including a small incision if needed, insert the leadless pacemaker introducer into the femoral vein and remove the guidewire. Under fluoroscopic guidance, insert the leadless pacemaker retrieval catheter into the femoral vein through the introducer. Using steering and deflection, advance the retrieval catheter under fluoroscopic guidance to the target chamber, the right ventricle. The leadless pacemaker is then engaged by the retrieval catheter with a snare. After confirming under fluoroscopy that the retrieval catheter is appropriately secured to leadless pacemaker, disengage the leadless pacemaker from endocardium using the retrieval catheter, and remove the coupled retrieval catheter and leadless pacemaker. Close the access site with a nonabsorbable single figure-of-eight stitch or by other means.

Clinical Example (0801T)

A 90-year-old male with sinus node dysfunction and progressive AV block had a dual-chamber leadless pacemaker system implanted more than 10 years ago. Routine interrogation demonstrates battery depletion in both atrial and ventricular leadless pacemakers. Removal and replacement of both atrial and ventricular leadless pacemakers are recommended.

Description of Procedure (0801T)

In the electrophysiology laboratory, prepare the femoral region and administer local anesthesia. Obtain access via a guidewire in the femoral vein. Ultrasound guidance may be used, and femoral venography may be performed

Category III 0042T-0713T

to identify the anatomy. Advance a guidewire via the femoral vein into the vena cava. After sequential dilation and upsizing the femoral sheath, including a small incision if needed, insert the leadless pacemaker retrieval introducer into the femoral vein and remove the guidewire. Under fluoroscopic guidance, insert the leadless pacemaker retrieval catheter into the femoral vein through the introducer. Using steering and deflection, advance the retrieval catheter under fluoroscopic guidance through the IVC to the right atrium. The leadless pacemaker is then engaged by the retrieval catheter with a snare. After confirming under fluoroscopy that the retrieval mechanism is engaged and secure, remove the coupled retrieval catheter and leadless pacemaker.

Prior to insertion into the target chambers, load the pacemaker onto a catheter for placement into the right atrium. Under fluoroscopic guidance, insert the leadless pacemaker delivery catheter into the femoral vein through the introducer. Using steering and deflection, advance the delivery catheter through the IVC to the right atrium. Contrast agent may be injected through the catheter to identify the anatomy in the right atrium. The leadless pacemaker is then fixed to the endocardium. With the catheter still attached and prior to fixation of the device, a test may be performed to ensure mechanical stability of the leadless pacemaker. After fixation, the pacemaker is undocked from the delivery system but still connected via tethers. Use the external programmer to measure pacing-capture threshold, sensing amplitude, and impedance. As needed, reposition and re-engage the pacemaker within the target chamber under fluoroscopic guidance. Once appropriate parameters and adequate fixation are confirmed, the tether is released, and the pacemaker is released from the delivery catheter. Remove the tether, delivery catheter, and sheath. Repeat this process for removal and replacement of the right ventricular leadless pacemaker component. Close the access site with a nonabsorbable single figure-of-eight stitch or by other means.

Clinical Example (0802T)

A 90-year-old male with sinus node dysfunction and progressive AV block had a dual-chamber leadless pacemaker system implanted more than 10 years ago. Routine interrogation demonstrates battery depletion in the atrial leadless pacemaker. Removal and replacement of the atrial pacemakers are recommended.

Description of Procedure (0802T)

In the electrophysiology laboratory, prepare the femoral region and administer local anesthesia. Obtain access via a guidewire in the femoral vein. Ultrasound guidance may be used, and femoral venography may be performed to identify the anatomy. Advance a guidewire via the

femoral vein into the vena cava. After sequential dilation and upsizing the femoral sheath, including a small incision if needed, insert the leadless pacemaker retrieval introducer into the femoral vein and remove the guidewire. Under fluoroscopic guidance, insert the leadless pacemaker retrieval catheter into the femoral vein through the introducer. Using steering and deflection, advance the retrieval catheter under fluoroscopic guidance through the IVC to the right atrium. The leadless pacemaker is then engaged by the retrieval catheter with a snare. After confirming under fluoroscopy that the retrieval mechanism is engaged and secure, remove the coupled retrieval catheter and leadless pacemaker.

Prior to insertion into the target chambers, load the pacemaker onto a catheter for placement into the right atrium. Under fluoroscopic guidance, insert the leadless pacemaker delivery catheter into the femoral vein through the introducer. Using steering and deflection, advance the delivery catheter through the IVC to the right atrium. Contrast agent may be injected through the catheter to identify the anatomy in the right atrium. The leadless pacemaker is then fixed to the endocardium. With the catheter still attached and prior to fixation of the device, a test may be performed to ensure mechanical stability of the leadless pacemaker. After fixation, the pacemaker is undocked from the delivery system but still connected via tethers. Use the external programmer to measure pacing-capture threshold, sensing amplitude, and impedance. As needed, reposition and re-engage the pacemaker within the target chamber under fluoroscopic guidance. Once appropriate parameters and adequate fixation are confirmed, release the tether, and the pacemaker is released from the delivery catheter. Remove the tether, delivery catheter, and sheath. Close the access site with a nonabsorbable single figure-of-eight stitch or by other means.

Clinical Example (0803T)

A 90-year-old male with sinus node dysfunction and progressive AV block had a dual-chamber leadless pacemaker system implanted more than 10 years ago. Routine interrogation demonstrates battery depletion in the ventricular leadless pacemaker. Removal and replacement of the ventricular pacemaker is recommended.

Description of Procedure (0803T)

In the electrophysiology laboratory, prepare the femoral region and administer local anesthesia. Obtain access via a guidewire in the femoral vein. Ultrasound guidance may be used, and femoral venography may be performed to identify the anatomy. Advance a guidewire via the femoral vein into the vena cava. After sequential dilation and upsizing the femoral sheath, including a small

▲ = Revised code   ● = New code   ▶◀ = Contains new or revised text   ✳ = Duplicate PLA test   ↕ = Category I PLA   American Medical Association   **183**

Category III 0042T-0713T

incision if needed, insert the leadless pacemaker retrieval introducer into the femoral vein and remove the guidewire. Under fluoroscopic guidance, insert the leadless pacemaker retrieval catheter into the femoral vein through the introducer. Using steering and deflection, advance the retrieval catheter under fluoroscopic guidance through the IVC to the right ventricle. The leadless pacemaker is then engaged by the retrieval catheter with a snare. After confirming under fluoroscopy that the retrieval mechanism is engaged and secure, remove the coupled retrieval catheter and leadless pacemaker.

Prior to insertion into the target chambers, load the pacemaker onto a catheter for placement into the right ventricle. Under fluoroscopic guidance, insert the leadless pacemaker delivery catheter into the femoral vein through the introducer. Using steering and deflection, advance the delivery catheter through the IVC to the right ventricle. Contrast agent may be injected through the catheter to identify the anatomy in the right ventricle. The leadless pacemaker is then fixed to the endocardium. With the catheter still attached and prior to fixation of the device, a test may be performed to ensure mechanical stability of the leadless pacemaker. After fixation, the pacemaker is undocked from the delivery system but still connected via tethers. Use the external programmer to measure pacing-capture threshold, sensing amplitude, and impedance. As needed, reposition and re-engage the pacemaker within the target chamber under fluoroscopic guidance. Once appropriate parameters and adequate fixation are confirmed, the tether is released, and the pacemaker is released from the delivery catheter. Remove the tether, delivery catheter, and sheath. Close the access site with a nonabsorbable single figure-of-eight stitch or by other means.

Clinical Example (0804T)

A 72-year-old male with a history of sinus node dysfunction and progressive AV block had a dual-chamber leadless pacemaker system placed. Subsequent interrogation and programming device evaluation are performed in person to test the device's function and select the most favorable permanent programmed values.

Description of Procedure (0804T)

Perform an interrogation and programming device evaluation in person in a health care setting to test the device's function and select the most favorable permanent programmed values. Retrieve stored and measured data regarding the device's battery, capture and sensing function, heart rhythm, implant communication settings, and other programmed parameters using a programmer. Assess this information to discern system performance and settings for rhythm

treatment, as well as to determine the pacemaker's current programming. If necessary, adjust the sensing value, rate response, upper and lower heart rates, AV intervals, pacing voltage and pulse duration, implant communication settings, and diagnostics.

▶Codes 0805T, 0806T are used to report transcatheter superior and inferior vena cava prosthetic valve implantation (ie, caval valve implantation [CAVI]).

Codes 0805T, 0806T include the work, when performed, of vascular access, placing the access sheath, transseptal puncture, advancing the caval valve delivery systems into position, repositioning the device(s) as needed, and deploying the device(s).

Angiography and radiological supervision and interpretation performed to guide CAVI (eg, guiding device placement and documenting completion of the intervention) are included in these codes.

Diagnostic right and left heart catheterization codes (93451, 93452, 93453, 93456, 93457, 93458, 93459, 93460, 93461, 93593, 93594, 93595, 93596, 93597, 93598) should **not** be used with 0805T, 0806T to report:

1. Contrast injections, angiography, road-mapping, and/or fluoroscopic guidance for the transcatheter CAVI,

2. Left ventricular angiography to assess tricuspid regurgitation for guidance of the transcatheter CAVI, or

3. Right and left heart catheterization for hemodynamic measurements before, during, and after transcatheter superior and inferior vena cava prosthetic valve implantation for guidance.

Diagnostic right and left heart catheterization codes (93451, 93452, 93453, 93456, 93457, 93458, 93459, 93460, 93461, 93593, 93594, 93595, 93596, 93597, 93598) and diagnostic coronary angiography codes (93454, 93455, 93456, 93457, 93458, 93459, 93460, 93461, 93563, 93564) may be reported with 0805T, 0806T, representing separate and distinct services from CAVI, if:

1. No prior study is available and a full diagnostic study is performed, or

2. A prior study is available, but as documented in the medical record:

    a. There is inadequate visualization of the anatomy and/or pathology, or

    b. The patient's condition with respect to the clinical indication has changed since the prior study, or

    c. There is a clinical change during the procedure that requires new evaluation.

For same session or same day diagnostic cardiac catheterization services, the appropriate diagnostic cardiac catheterization code(s) may be reported by appending modifier 59 indicating separate and distinct procedural service from the transcatheter superior and inferior vena cava prosthetic valve implantation procedures.

Percutaneous coronary interventional therapeutic procedures may be reported separately, when performed.

When transcatheter ventricular support is required in conjunction with CAVI, the appropriate ventricular assist device (VAD) procedure codes (33990, 33991, 33992, 33993, 33995, 33997) or balloon pump insertion codes (33967, 33970, 33973) may be reported.

When cardiopulmonary bypass is performed in conjunction with CAVI, 0805T and 0806T may be reported with the appropriate add-on code for percutaneous peripheral bypass (33367), open peripheral bypass (33368), or central bypass (33369).◀

● **0805T**   Transcatheter superior and inferior vena cava prosthetic valve implantation (ie, caval valve implantation [CAVI]); percutaneous femoral vein approach

● **0806T**   open femoral vein approach

▶(Do not report 0805T, 0806T in conjunction with 33210, 33211, for temporary pacemaker insertion)◀

▶(Do not report 0805T, 0806T in conjunction with 93451, 93453, 93456, 93457, 93460, 93461, 93503, 93566, 93593, 93594, 93596, 93597, for diagnostic right heart catheterization procedures intrinsic to the superior and inferior vena cava valve implantations)◀

▶(Do not report 0805T, 0806T in conjunction with 93662, for imaging guidance with intracardiac echocardiography)◀

Rationale

Two new Category III codes (0805T, 0806T) have been established to report transcatheter superior and inferior vena cava prosthetic value implantation. In addition, new introductory guidelines and exclusionary parenthetical notes have been added to direct users regarding the appropriate use of codes 0805T and 0806T.

Guidelines included for the new codes provide information regarding: (1) the intended use of these services; (2) all the services included as part of the procedures: (a) services that should not be separately reported (eg, contrast injections, left ventricular angiography to assess tricuspid regurgitation, and right and left heart catheterization for hemodynamic measurements) and (b) when diagnostic catheterization of the right and left heart and for coronary angiography may be separately reported in conjunction with codes 0805T and 0806T; (3) how to report diagnostic cardiac catheterization and transcatheter superior and inferior vena cava prosthetic valve implantation procedures performed on the same session or same day; (4) how to separately report percutaneous

coronary interventional therapeutic procedures; (5) how to separately report transcatheter ventricular support when performed with caval valve implantation (CAVI); and (6) how to separately report cardiopulmonary bypass when performed in combination with CAVI.

Code 0805T describes transcatheter superior and inferior vena cava prosthetic valve implantation using a percutaneous formal vein approach, and code 0806T identifies the open femoral vein approach.

To provide further instruction regarding the intended use of these new codes, three parenthetical notes have been added. The first exclusionary parenthetical note excludes reporting new codes in conjunction with codes 33210 and 33211 for temporary pacemaker insertion. The second exclusionary parenthetical note restricts reporting these new codes in conjunction with diagnostic right heart catheterization codes. The third exclusionary parenthetical note restricts reporting the new codes in conjunction with code 93662 for imaging guidance with intracardiac echocardiography.

Clinical Example (0805T)

An 80-year-old male presents with New York Heart Association (NYHA) class 3 heart failure (fatigue, edema) and with severe tricuspid valve regurgitation (TVR). The patient was treated with diuretics to decrease volume overload, pulmonary vasodilators, and other guideline-directed medical therapies, which remain inadequate. To reduce the systemic effects of the patient's severe TVR, it is decided to implant both a superior and IVC valve via a percutaneous femoral vein approach with monitored anesthesia care.

Description of Procedure (0805T)

Access the left and right femoral veins percutaneously and insert a 6-French introducer sheath into each. Via the left femoral vein access, place a pulmonary catheter through the sheath into the right pulmonary artery (rPA) to mark the crossing of the rPA with the superior vena cava (SVC). Introduce a 6-French pigtail catheter in the right femoral vein and obtain an angiogram of the SVC. Exchange the pigtail catheter for a straight 0.036-inch stiff guidewire with a soft tip. Make a small right-sided skin incision at or near the introducer sheath to accommodate the larger 27-French delivery system. Hydrate the SVC valve (bioprosthesis) and advance the delivery system over the guidewire through the right femoral vein and the IVC into the right atrium and the SVC. Place the upper part of the undeployed SVC valve in the confluence of the SVC/right atrium with the belly of the SVC valve positioned above the rPA crossing. Confirm the valve position under fluoroscopic and echocardiographic visualization. Once confirmation is made, partially deploy the uppermost 20 mm of the valve. Then make a full deployment by unsheathing the bioprosthesis using the delivery system. Then close and remove the delivery system while keeping the guidewire in place. Take pressure measurements to ensure correct bioprosthesis functioning. Remove the catheter in the rPA to avoid interference with the IVC valve and position in the suprahepatic vein to help mark IVC valve positioning. Properly hydrate and load the IVC delivery system and bioprosthesis over the guidewire at the right puncture site. Position the undeployed IVC bioprosthesis at the height of the diaphragm with the skirt of the bioprosthesis visible just above the hepatic vein inflow. Alignment of the constrained segment of the IVC bioprosthetic frame with the cavo-atrial junction is accomplished by carefully pulling back the catheter. Using intraprocedural mapping and a safety margin of 5 mm, positioning of the bioprosthesis is then made to avoid a high- or low-valve position to prevent hepatic vein obstruction or paravalvular regurgitation. Then slowly deploy the IVC bioprosthesis using the delivery system. After positioning of the IVC bioprosthesis, confirm under fluoroscopy and withdraw the delivery system to the femoral vein where the delivery capsule is closed and removed.

Remove all catheters and introducer sheaths post-deployment of both the SVC and IVC bioprostheses. Close the access site per hospital protocol. Administer anticoagulation and/or antiplatelet therapy intraprocedurally.

Clinical Example (0806T)

An 80-year-old female presents with NYHA class 3 heart failure and with severe TVR. The patient was treated with diuretics to decrease volume overload, pulmonary vasodilators, and other guideline-directed medical therapy (for secondary TVR attributable to heart failure with reduced left ventricular ejection fraction), which remains inadequate. To reduce TVR, SVC and IVC valves are implanted via an open femoral vein approach.

Description of Procedure (0806T)

Access the left and right femoral veins via an open femoral approach and insert a 6-French introducer sheath into each femoral vein. Place a pulmonary catheter through the sheath and into the rPA to mark the crossing of the rPA with the SVC. Introduce a 6-French pigtail catheter in the right femoral vein and an angiogram of the SVC is obtained. The pigtail catheter is then exchanged for a straight 0.036-inch stiff guidewire with a soft tip. Make a small skin incision at or near the introducer sheath. Hydrate the SVC valve (bioprosthesis), and advance the delivery system over the guidewire through the femoral vein and the IVC into the right atrium and the SVC. Place the upper part of the SVC valve in the confluence of the SVC/right atrium

with the belly of the SVC valve positioned above the rPA crossing. Confirm the valve position under fluoroscopic and echocardiographic visualization. Once confirmation is made, partially deploy the uppermost 20 mm of the valved. Then make full deployment by unsheathing the bioprosthesis using the delivery system. The delivery system is then closed and removed while keeping the guidewire in place. Take pressure measurements to ensure correct bioprosthesis functioning. Reposition the catheter in the rPA into a suprahepatic vein for reference in placing the prosthetic IVC valve.

Then properly hydrate and load the IVC delivery system and bioprosthesis over the guidewire at the right puncture site. Position the IVC bioprosthesis at the height of the diaphragm with the skirt of the bioprosthesis visible just above the hepatic vein inflow. Alignment of the constrained segment of the IVC bioprosthetic frame with the cavo-atrial junction is accomplished by carefully pulling back the catheter. Using intraprocedural mapping and a safety margin of 5 mm, positioning of the bioprosthesis is then made to avoid a high- or low-valve position to prevent hepatic vein obstruction or paravalvular regurgitation. Then slowly deploy the IVC bioprosthesis using the delivery system. After deploying the IVC bioprosthesis, confirm the position under fluoroscopy and withdraw the delivery system to the femoral vein where the delivery capsule is closed and removed.

Remove all catheters and introducer sheaths post-deployment of both the SVC and IVC bioprostheses. Close the access site per hospital protocol. Administer anticoagulation and/or antiplatelet therapy intraprocedurally.

● **0807T**   Pulmonary tissue ventilation analysis using software-based processing of data from separately captured cinefluorograph images; in combination with previously acquired computed tomography (CT) images, including data preparation and transmission, quantification of pulmonary tissue ventilation, data review, interpretation and report

▶(Do not report 0807T in conjunction with 76000, 78579, 78582, 78598)◀

● **0808T**   in combination with computed tomography (CT) images taken for the purpose of pulmonary tissue ventilation analysis, including data preparation and transmission, quantification of pulmonary tissue ventilation, data review, interpretation and report

▶(Do not report 0808T in conjunction with 71250, 71260, 71270, 71271, 76000, 78579, 78582, 78598)◀

★ = Telemedicine   ◀ = Add-on code   ✚ = Add-on code   ✗ = FDA approval pending   # = Resequenced code   ⦸ = Modifier 51 exempt

Rationale

Two Category III codes (0807T, 0808T) have been established to report pulmonary tissue ventilation analysis using software-based processing of data from cinefluorographic images.

Codes 0807T and 0808T use image processing technology to quantify ventilation of pulmonary function. Code 0807T is intended to identify the analysis using computed tomographic (CT) images that already exist, and code 0808T identifies provision of the service on CT images that have been obtained specifically for this purpose.

An exclusionary parenthetical note following code 0807T has been added to preclude the reporting of this code with fluoroscopy, pulmonary ventilation imaging, pulmonary ventilation and perfusion imaging, and quantitative differential pulmonary perfusion. An additional exclusionary parenthetical note following code 0808T has been added to preclude the reporting of this code with diagnostic CT of the thorax, screening tomography of the thorax, fluoroscopy, pulmonary ventilation imaging, pulmonary ventilation and perfusion imaging, and quantitative differential pulmonary perfusion. The codes included within the exclusionary notes differ according to whether the services are mutually exclusive (ie, pulmonary ventilation imaging, perfusion testing [78579, 78582, 78598] vs pulmonary tissue ventilation analysis [0808T] or are inherently included [ie, CT that is included as part of 0808T]).

Clinical Example (0807T)

A 72-year-old male with COPD is no longer adequately controlled with medical therapy. His physician orders pulmonary ventilation analysis using software-based processing of data from cinefluorographic images in combination with previously obtained CT images.

Description of Procedure (0807T)

Obtain five cinefluorographic images of the lung for the purpose of pulmonary ventilation analysis, and upload images to an image routing system. (Acquisition of these images is included in the code and not separately reported.) The image routing system then identifies corresponding images from a previously obtained CT scan of the chest. The images are then transmitted to the analysis engine via standard digital imaging communications in medicine protocols for pulmonary ventilation analysis. Perform pulmonary ventilation analysis using specialized analysis software and advanced engineering computation. All results from the pulmonary ventilation analysis are included in a

structured quantitative report. Send the results report to a QHP for review and interpretation. The QHP considers all data in the results report and dictates a medical report.

Clinical Example (0808T)

A 73-year-old male with COPD is no longer adequately controlled with medical therapy. He undergoes a CT of the chest. His physician orders pulmonary ventilation analysis using assistive software-based processing of data from cinefluorographic images in combination with concurrently obtained CT images.

Description of Procedure (0808T)

Obtain five cinefluorographic images of the lung and CT of the chest for the purpose of pulmonary ventilation analysis, and upload images to an image routing system. (Acquisition of these images is included in the code and not separately reported.) The image routing system identifies corresponding images between the cinefluorographic exam and CT and transmits these images to the analysis engine via standard digital imaging communications in medicine protocols for pulmonary ventilation analysis. Perform pulmonary ventilation analysis using specialized analysis software and advanced engineering computation. All results from the pulmonary ventilation analysis are included in a structured quantitative report. Send the results report to a QHP for review and interpretation. The QHP considers all data in the results report and dictates a medical report.

►(0809T has been deleted)◄

►(For percutaneous arthrodesis of the sacroiliac joint, see 27278, 27279)◄

Rationale

Code 0809T and its associated parenthetical notes and guidelines have been deleted. Code 0809T has been deleted to accommodate the addition of new Category I code 27278 to identify the percutaneous intra-articular SI joint fusion procedures.

Refer to the codebook and the Rationale for code 27278 for a full discussion of these changes.

▲ = Revised code   ● = New code   ► ◄ = Contains new or revised text   ✖ = Duplicate PLA test   ↕ = Category I PLA   American Medical Association   **187**

Category III 0042T-0713T

● **0810T**   Subretinal injection of a pharmacologic agent, including vitrectomy and 1 or more retinotomies

►(Report medication separately)◄

►(Do not report 0810T in conjunction with 67036, 67039, 67040, 67041, 67042, 67043)◄

Rationale

Category III code 0810T has been established to report subretinal injection of a pharmacologic agent, including vitrectomy and one or more retinotomies.

This code describes the delivery of a pharmaceutical agent into the posterior portion of the eye. In order to target the drug for appropriate response, fluid is first removed via vitrectomy, one or more retinotomies are performed, and then the drug is injected into the subretinal space. Prior to the addition of code 0810T, none of the existing ophthalmic injection codes accurately describe the procedure or reference the correct area of ophthalmic anatomy.

A parenthetical note following the new code has been added to indicate that medication can be reported separately. An exclusionary parenthetical note has been added to preclude the reporting of code 0810T with vitrectomy procedures.

Clinical Example (0810T)

A 24-year-old male diagnosed with retinitis pigmentosa-associated vision loss is being treated with subretinal gene-modification therapy via injection in the right eye.

Description of Procedure (0810T)

The surgeon performs a conjunctival peritomy to expose the sclera. Next, a standard three-port vitrectomy is performed using a trocar to enter the globe through the sclera in the inferotemporal quadrant. Place an infusion cannula through the inferotemporal trocar and verify correct placement by inspection. Similarly, insert trocars both superonasally and superotemporally to allow passage of the vitrector and the fiberoptic light source through separate openings. Insert the vitrector and light pipe, and visualize within the eye under wide-angle viewing system. Infuse a balanced salt solution during the procedure to maintain intraocular pressure. Remove core vitreous with the vitrectomy instrument and induce a posterior vitreous detachment. Shave peripheral vitreous as close as is safe to the vitreous base, allowing complete removal of the vitreous. Thoroughly examine peripheral fundus with scleral depression to visualize any possible retinal tears, which are repaired with laser or cryoretinopexy.

Draw the prepared medication (reported separately) into the microdose injection syringe. Using a magnifying contact lens or under the wide-angle view, insert a 38G to 41G subretinal cannula through the trocar and advance into the subretinal space via a small retinotomy immediately above the superior temporal vascular arcade to deliver the gene therapy agent. Perform additional retinotomies inferior to the inferior vascular arcade or temporal to the macula. Direct subretinal injection to the area of viable retina. Then rinse vitreous cavity with fluid-fluid exchange. Air fluid exchange may be performed to propagate the subretinal blebs to the posterior pole. Document location and extent of subretinal blebs. Then remove trocars, and massage conjunctiva over each opening. Close any leaking sclerotomies with an interrupted 7-0 polyglactin suture. Administer subtenon corticosteroid, subconjunctival corticosteroid, and subconjunctival antibiotic. Remove the lid speculum, and apply topical corticosteroid and antibiotic solution. Place a sterile wound dressing and an eye shield over the eye.

● **0811T**   Remote multi-day complex uroflowmetry (eg, calibrated electronic equipment); set-up and patient education on use of equipment

● **0812T**   device supply with automated report generation, up to 10 days

►(Do not report 0811T, 0812T more than once per episode of care)◄

►(Do not report 0811T, 0812T in conjunction with 51736, 51741, 99453, 99454)◄

Rationale

Category III codes 0811T and 0812T have been established to report remote multiday complex uroflowmetry.

Code 0811T describes the initial set-up and patient education on the use of the equipment, and code 0812T describes supply of the device for up to 10 days with automated report generation. These codes differ from the remote physiologic monitoring codes as they are for collection of data up to 10 days (typically 7-10), whereas codes 99453 and 99454 require at least 16 days of remote monitoring.

Two parenthetical notes have been added following these codes. One specifically indicates that these codes can only be reported once per episode of care, and the other note precludes the reporting of codes 0811T and 0812T with simple uroflowmetry and complex uroflowmetry and with the physiologic monitoring codes.

★ = Telemedicine   ◄ = Add-on code   ✚ = Add-on code   ✗ = FDA approval pending   # = Resequenced code   ⊘ = Modifier 51 exempt

Category III 0042T-0713T

Clinical Example (0811T)

A 50-year-old male presents with lower urinary tract symptoms. The physician prescribes a remote uroflow test for 7 to 10 days.

Description of Procedure (0811T)

The physician orders a remote multiday uroflow test. The physician or clinical staff instructs the patient on the use of the device.

Clinical Example (0812T)

A 50-year-old male presents with lower urinary tract symptoms. The physician prescribes a remote uroflow test for 7 to 10 days.

Description of Procedure (0812T)

N/A

● **0813T** Esophagogastroduodenoscopy, flexible, transoral, with volume adjustment of intragastric bariatric balloon

▶(Do not report 0813T in conjunction with 43197, 43198, 43235, 43241, 43247, 43290, 43291)◀

Rationale

Category III code 0813T has been established to report the volume adjustment of an intragastric bariatric device. To support the addition of the new code, a parenthetical note has been added to guide users with the appropriate reporting of this code.

There are existing codes to report implantation and explantation of a gastric balloon but not for adjustment of a gastric balloon. This code is intended to identify the volume adjustment of the balloon device. In addition, the parenthetical note restricts reporting of this service in conjunction with other related services.

Clinical Example (0813T)

A 44-year-old female with obesity previously underwent adjustable gastric balloon placement. The patient requires either a balloon-volume decrease for refractory intolerance to prevent premature balloon removal or a balloon-volume increase for diminished balloon effect with weight-loss plateau or weight regain.

Description of Procedure (0813T)

Under conscious sedation, perform an endoscopy to evaluate the esophagus, stomach, and duodenum for any abnormalities. Identify the intragastric balloon and achieve access to the interior of the balloon via the device

valve. Adjust balloon volume with addition or reduction as indicated for desired clinical effect. Then withdraw the endoscope.

● **0814T** Percutaneous injection of calcium-based biodegradable osteoconductive material, proximal femur, including imaging guidance, unilateral

▶(Do not report 0814T in conjunction with 26992, 77002)◀

Rationale

Category III code 0814T has been established to report percutaneous injection of calcium-based biodegradable osteoconductive material. Additional instructions have been added to indicate that code 0814T should not be reported with codes 26992 and 77002 because incision for access and imaging guidance are inherently included. In addition, code 0814T should be reported for unilateral procedures.

Prior to 2024, there were no CPT codes that captured the work performed to implant a new osteo-enhancement material designed to strengthen the proximal femur and reduce fragility fractures of the hip. The new procedure described by Category III code 0814T involves implanting a calcium-based, osteoconductive material under imaging guidance into the lateral femoral cortex to form new bone in voids in the proximal femur of patients with disorders such as osteoporosis.

Clinical Example (0814T)

An 82-year-old female presents with a hip fracture occurring from low-energy trauma. She has the non-fractured hip treated with an injection of a calcium-based biodegradable osteoconductive material during the same operative session as the hip fracture–repair surgery.

Description of Procedure (0814T)

Place the patient in a supine position with the hip to be treated in neutral extension with the femoral neck parallel to the floor. Provide local anesthesia to the area of the incision. Make a 1- to 2-cm skin incision to allow access to the lateral femoral cortex. Insert the tissue protector, canulated centering obturator, and guide pin into the incision up to the lateral femoral cortex, and confirm position of tissue protector with fluoroscopy. Advance the guide pin under fluoroscopic guidance until it reaches the apex of the femoral neck. Remove the centering obturator and insert the provided 5.3-mm cannulated drill over the guide pin up to the lateral femoral cortex. Drill over the guide pin to the proximal intersection of the compressive and tensile trabeculae.

Remove the drill and tissue protector, and insert the blunt probe debrider. Define the margins of the enhancement site using the debrider, and perform suction and irrigation of the enhancement site to clear the area and create space for the injection. Mix the triphasic, calcium-based, osteoconductive material according to instructions and fill the syringe. Total volume added to syringes should be between 20 and 25 ml. Injection of the material should be completed within 5 minutes from when the powder components are mixed. Insert the injection cannula. Under fluoroscopic guidance, inject proximal to distal with continuous retraction of the cannula. Stop injecting when the injection material reaches the lateral cortex. Monitor for injection-material leakage under fluoroscopy during injection. Remove the injection cannula and close the incision.

● **0815T**   Ultrasound-based radiofrequency echographic multi-spectrometry (REMS), bone-density study and fracture-risk assessment, 1 or more sites, hips, pelvis, or spine

Rationale

Category III code 0815T has been established to report non-ionizing energy, ultrasound-based radiofrequency echographic multi-spectrometry (REMS) for bone-density study and fracture-risk assessment.

Prior to 2024, there were no existing codes to report the use of non-ionizing energy, ultrasound-based REMS for bone-density study and fracture-risk assessment. Code 0815T includes assessment for one or more sites (hips, pelvis, or spine).

Clinical Example (0815T)

A 60-year-old female has been referred for a bone-density and fracture-risk analysis to determine whether to initiate hormone replacement therapy and/or an anti-osteoporotic treatment. Ultrasound-based radiofrequency echographic multi-spectrometry (REMS) is performed.

Description of Procedure (0815T)

Place the patient in a supine position. Place ultrasound probe on hips, pelvis, or spine. Adjust ultrasound depth and focus to identify targeted bone structure, and perform the echographic scan according to manufacturer instructions.

A physician interprets the report generated by the ultrasound-based REMS system, including comparison of bone density and fracture risk with standard values.

● **0816T**   Open insertion or replacement of integrated neurostimulation system for bladder dysfunction including electrode(s) (eg, array or leadless), and pulse generator or receiver, including analysis, programming, and imaging guidance, when performed, posterior tibial nerve; subcutaneous

● **0817T**   subfascial

● **0818T**   Revision or removal of integrated neurostimulation system for bladder dysfunction, including analysis, programming, and imaging, when performed, posterior tibial nerve; subcutaneous

● **0819T**   subfascial

▶(Do not report 0816T, 0817T, 0818T, 0819T in conjunction with 64555, 64566, 64575, 64590, 64596, 95970, 95971, 95972, 0588T, 0589T, 0590T)◀

▶(For percutaneous implantation or replacement of integrated neurostimulation system including electrode array and receiver for bladder dysfunction, posterior tibial nerve, use 0587T)◀

▶(For revision or removal of percutaneous integrated neurostimulation system for bladder dysfunction, posterior tibial nerve, use 0588T)◀

▶(For electronic analysis with programming of integrated or leadless neurostimulation system for bladder dysfunction, posterior tibial nerve, performed on a day subsequent to the device insertion, replacement, or revision, see 0589T, 0590T)◀

Rationale

Codes 0816T-0819T have been established to report open insertion or replacement of integrated neurostimulator services for the posterior tibial nerve (ie, bladder dysfunction) and their revisions or removals. In addition, parenthetical notes have been added following these codes to provide further instruction regarding the intended use for these codes.

Codes 0816T-0819T have been established for reporting open insertion or replacement of integrated posterior tibial nerve neurostimulator devices subcutaneously (0816T) or subfascially (0817T), as well as the revision or removal of the same (0818T, 0819T, respectively). These codes have been established to recognize the difference in work effort for surgical services for these types of integrated neurostimulators as other codes may be used for percutaneous insertions/replacements/revisions/removals of integrated neurostimulator devices of the posterior tibial nerve (eg, 0587T, 0588T). In addition, as noted in the code descriptors, programming for these services is inherently included as part of the insertion/replacement/revision procedure. This is exemplified within the parenthetical note instruction following code 0819T that directs users to report electronic analysis with programming for integrated or leadless neurostimulator systems of the bladder only when performed on a day after the device insertion, replacement, or revision (using 0589T, 0590T). Other parenthetical notes following code 0819T redirect users to the appropriate codes to report percutaneous implantation or replacement of an integrated neurostimulator system of the posterior tibial nerve (ie, for bladder dysfunction, 0587T) or to report revision or removal of the same (0588T).

An exclusionary parenthetical note has been added to restrict reporting of these new codes in conjunction with services for other types of integrated neurostimulator insertion/replacement/revision/removal/programming services.

Clinical Example (0816T)

A 65-year-old female has intractable urge urinary incontinence (UUI). Conservative remedies have been unsuccessful, and the patient has chosen to undergo an open implantation of an integrated neurostimulator system to treat UUI.

Description of Procedure (0816T)

Following positioning and preparation of the medial leg, palpate the landmarks and reference points; take precise measurements to identify the location of the posterior tibial nerve; and mark the intended location of the neurostimulation device. Under local anesthesia, make an incision and dissect the subcutaneous tissues to create the device pocket. Insert the neurostimulation device into the pocket and position it appropriately. Perform testing and program the device as appropriate. Once placement is verified, place one or more sutures, if needed, and close the incision.

Clinical Example (0817T)

A 65-year-old female has intractable UUI. Conservative remedies have been unsuccessful, and the patient has chosen to undergo an open implantation of an integrated neurostimulator system to treat UUI.

Description of Procedure (0817T)

Prepare the skin at the surgical site. Make an incision and dissect down to the subfascial plane over the posterior tibial neurovascular bundle. Place the neurostimulator over the neurovascular bundle. Use the transmitter to perform an intraoperative test of the device. Increase the stimulation intensity until the patient reports paresthesia. If results of the intraoperative test are unsatisfactory, it may be necessary to reposition the implant. Once the intraoperative test stimulation provides satisfactory results, secure the implant with sutures as needed. Close the subcutaneous tissue and skin.

Clinical Example (0818T)

A 65-year-old female has a previously placed subcutaneous posterior tibial integrated neurostimulator for the treatment of UUI that is no longer effective. She now presents for revision or removal of the device.

Description of Procedure (0818T)

Position the patient appropriately, and prepare and drape the surgical site. The physician selects, marks, prepares, and anesthetizes, and then incises the skin over the previously placed device. The subcutaneous pocket is surgically opened, and the device is revised or removed. The wound is irrigated and closed in a layered fashion, and the patient is fitted and provided with a compressive ankle support.

Clinical Example (0819T)

A 65-year-old female has a previously placed subfascial posterior tibial integrated neurostimulator for the treatment of UUI that is no longer effective. She now presents for revision or removal of the device.

Description of Procedure (0819T)

Position the patient appropriately, and prepare and drape the surgical site. The physician selects, marks, prepares, anesthetizes, and incises the skin. The physician divides the crural fascia and identifies the previously placed device, which is then revised or removed. The fascia is closed. The skin is then closed in layers.

▶Continuous In-Person Monitoring and Intervention During Psychedelic Medication Therapy◀

▶Continuous in-person monitoring and intervention (eg, psychotherapy, crisis intervention) is provided during and following supervised patient self-administration of a psychedelic medication in a therapeutic setting. Psychedelic medications induce distinctive alterations in perception that may place the patient at risk for emotional vulnerability and physiologic instability. The medications' pharmacologic risks may persist for multiple hours, and during this time, the patient may require continuous in-person monitoring and intervention by a physician or other qualified health care professional (QHP) to support the patient's physical, emotional, and psychological safety and to optimize treatment outcomes.

Code 0820T is used to report the total duration of in-person time with the patient by the physician or other QHP providing continuous monitoring, and intervention as needed, during psychedelic medication therapy. Codes 0821T, 0822T are used to report the concurrent in-person participation of a second physician or other QHP (0821T), or the concurrent in-person participation of clinical staff (0822T) based on a patient's complex presentation, that requires additional personnel in the therapy room (eg, a physician or other QHP monitoring patient needs assistance from additional clinical staff due to a crisis by the psychedelic experience that surfaces past psychological trauma). If necessary, report 0821T, 0822T, as appropriate. It is unlikely that more than two personnel need to be in the room at the same time with the patient (ie, the initial physician or other QHP and one additional physician or other QHP or clinical staff).

Psychotherapy (90832, 90833, 90834, 90836, 90837, 90838), psychotherapy for crisis (90839, 90840), neurobehavioral status examination (96116, 96121), adaptive behavior assessments (97151, 97152), adaptive behavior treatment (97153, 97154, 97155, 97156, 97157, 97158), or prolonged clinical staff services (99415, 99416) may not be reported on the same date of service.◄

● **0820T**   Continuous in-person monitoring and intervention (eg, psychotherapy, crisis intervention), as needed, during psychedelic medication therapy; first physician or other qualified health care professional, each hour

▶(Do not report 0820T in conjunction with 90832, 90833, 90834, 90836, 90837, 90838, 90839, 90840, 96116, 96121, 97151, 97152, 97153, 97154, 97155, 97156, 97157, 97158, 99415, 99416, on the same date of service)◄

✚● **0821T**   second physician or other qualified health care professional, concurrent with first physician or other qualified health care professional, each hour (List separately in addition to code for primary procedure)

✚● **0822T**   clinical staff under the direction of a physician or other qualified health care professional, concurrent with first physician or other qualified health care professional, each hour (List separately in addition to code for primary procedure)

▶(Use 0821T, 0822T in conjunction with 0820T)◄

Rationale

Three new Category III codes (0820T, 0821T, 0822T) have been established to report psychedelic drug monitoring services.

Psychedelic drug monitoring services identify physician or other QHP attendance with the patient during psychedelic medication self-administration and includes continuous in-person monitoring and intervention. The new codes focus on the personnel who may be needed to accomplish the supervision of the patient (identified within the guidelines as "physician or other QHP" and as "additional clinical staff") during psychedelic medication self-administration

with continuous in-person monitoring. Code 0820T identifies the continuous in-person monitoring and intervention during the service by the first physician or other QHP, and codes 0821T and 0822T identify the additional physician or other QHP (0821T) or clinical staff under direction of a physician or other QHP (0822T) who may be needed to accomplish the completion of the service.

To support the addition of these new codes, parenthetical notes have been added following codes 0820T and 0822T to instruct the users in the appropriate reporting for these services.

Lastly, a new heading "Continuous In-Person Monitoring and Intervention During Psychedelic Medication Therapy" and associated guidelines have been established to define psychedelic drug monitoring services and to outline the appropriate reporting of these codes.

Clinical Example (0820T)

A 38-year-old female with moderate to severe treatment-resistant depression is referred by her physician for psychedelic medication with continuous in-person monitoring and intervention.

Description of Procedure (0820T)

Prior to patient self-administration of the psychedelic medication, the physician or other QHP confirms the patient's identity and reviews pertinent clinical history and current medications. Assess the patient's current mental and emotional state, including risk factors for emotional distress and suicide, as well as protective factors. Review with the patient the goals, intentions, and any concerns regarding the psychological process that may arise during the session of psychedelic therapy.

After the patient self-administers the psychedelic medication, the physician or other QHP closely assesses the patient's mental status and emotional state at all times, introduces psychotherapeutic interventions as needed per their assessment, and maintains patient safety during the session. The physician or other QHP provides guidance and support using a range of therapeutic approaches to aid in emotional processing and resolution of psychological material as it emerges. The physician or other QHP also provides an environment conducive for self-reflection, such as eyeshades, music, and comfortable furnishings (eg, a couch or bed). The physician or other QHP supplies electrolyte-containing fluids and nourishment for the patient as needed.

At the end of the 6-hour psychedelic therapy session, the physician or other QHP re-assesses the patient's emotional state and ensures the patient is safe for discharge. A typical session will last 5 to 7 hours.

Clinical Example (0821T)

A 53-year-old male with post-traumatic stress disorder began having a complex reaction to the medication during continuous in-person monitoring and intervention for psychedelic medication. A second QHP is brought into the room to assist in the intervention. [**Note:** This is an add-on code. Only consider the additional work associated with the second physician or other QHP providing concurrent in-person monitoring and intervention.]

Description of Procedure (0821T)

Both QHPs work together to provide continuous therapeutic support, including ongoing assessment of the patient's psychological process and psychotherapeutic intervention on an intermittent and unpredictable basis. The second physician or other QHP leaves the room once the patient is stabilized, and the other physician or other QHP is comfortable with the patient's clinical state.

Clinical Example (0822T)

A 49-year-old male with treatment-resistant depression of moderate to severe degree requires the concurrent participation of clinical staff due to his complex reaction to the psychedelic medication during continuous in-person monitoring and intervention for psychedelic medication. [**Note:** This is an add-on code. Only consider the additional work associated with clinical staff providing concurrent in-person monitoring and intervention.]

Description of Procedure (0822T)

Both the physician or other QHP and clinical staff work together to provide continuous therapeutic support, including ongoing assessment of the patient's psychological process and psychotherapeutic intervention on an intermittent and unpredictable basis. The clinical staff leaves the room once the patient is stabilized, and the other physician or other QHP is comfortable with the patient's clinical state.

▶Right Atrial Leadless Pacemaker◀

▶A right atrial single-chamber leadless pacemaker includes a pulse generator with a built-in battery and electrode for implantation into the right atrium. Implantation of the atrial leadless pacemaker is performed using a catheter under fluoroscopic guidance via transvenous access.

Codes 0823T, 0824T, 0825T, 0826T only apply to single-chamber leadless pacemakers implanted in the right atrium intended for atrial pacing only and that are not part of a dual-chamber leadless system. For insertion of a right atrial single-chamber leadless pacemaker, report 0823T. For removal of a right atrial single-chamber leadless pacemaker, report 0824T. For removal and replacement of a right atrial single-chamber leadless pacemaker, report 0825T.

Leadless pacemakers are modular systems, and for clinical reasons, a dual-chamber leadless pacemaker may be implanted in stages with one pacemaker implanted into the right ventricle at the initial procedure and one pacemaker implanted into the right atrium at a subsequent session.

When a right atrial leadless pacemaker component of a dual-chamber system is modified or a right atrial leadless pacemaker is implanted to complete a dual-chamber leadless pacemaker system, see 0796T, 0799T, 0802T. For insertion of a leadless pacemaker into the right atrium when a single-chamber right ventricular leadless pacemaker already exists, in order to complete the dual-chamber system, report 0796T. If the right atrial leadless pacemaker is permanently removed when part of a dual-chamber leadless system, report 0799T. If the right atrial leadless pacemaker is removed and replaced when part of a dual-chamber leadless system, report 0802T.

Right heart catheterization (93451, 93453, 93456, 93460, 93461) may not be reported in conjunction with leadless pacemaker insertion, removal, and removal and replacement codes 33274, 33275, 0795T, 0796T, 0797T, 0798T, 0799T, 0800T, 0801T, 0802T, 0803T, 0823T, 0824T, 0825T, unless complete right heart catheterization is performed for an indication distinct from leadless pacemaker procedure.

For programming device evaluation (in person) of a right atrial single-chamber leadless pacemaker, report 0826T. Device evaluation code 93279 may not be reported in conjunction with right atrial single-chamber leadless pacemaker system codes 0823T, 0824T, 0825T.

Fluoroscopy (76000, 77002), ultrasound guidance for vascular access (76937), right ventriculography (93566), and femoral venography (75820) are included in 0823T, 0824T, 0825T, when performed.◀

● **0823T** Transcatheter insertion of permanent single-chamber leadless pacemaker, right atrial, including imaging guidance (eg, fluoroscopy, venous ultrasound, right atrial angiography and/or right ventriculography, femoral venography, cavography) and device evaluation (eg, interrogation or programming), when performed

▶(Do not report 0823T in conjunction with 33274, 0795T, 0796T, 0797T, 0802T)◀

▲ = Revised code   ● = New code   ▶◀ = Contains new or revised text   ✖ = Duplicate PLA test   ↑↓ = Category I PLA   American Medical Association   **193**

Category III 0042T-0713T

● **0824T** Transcatheter removal of permanent single-chamber leadless pacemaker, right atrial, including imaging guidance (eg, fluoroscopy, venous ultrasound, right atrial angiography and/or right ventriculography, femoral venography, cavography), when performed

▶(Do not report 0824T in conjunction with 33275, 0799T)◀

● **0825T** Transcatheter removal and replacement of permanent single-chamber leadless pacemaker, right atrial, including imaging guidance (eg, fluoroscopy, venous ultrasound, right atrial angiography and/or right ventriculography, femoral venography, cavography) and device evaluation (eg, interrogation or programming), when performed

▶(Do not report 0825T in conjunction with 33274, 0795T, 0796T, 0797T, 0802T)◀

● **0826T** Programming device evaluation (in person) with iterative adjustment of the implantable device to test the function of the device and select optimal permanent programmed values with analysis, review and report by a physician or other qualified health care professional, leadless pacemaker system in single-cardiac chamber

▶(Do not report 0826T in conjunction with 0823T, 0824T, 0825T)◀

Rationale

A new Category III subsection has been added to the code set with new guidelines, parenthetical notes, and four new codes to identify insertions, removals, removal and replacements, and programming for right atrial single-chamber leadless pacemaker systems. Guidelines and parenthetical notes have also been added and revised throughout the code set to accommodate the addition of the new codes and subsection for these procedures.

Codes 0823T-0826T are intended to identify placement, removal, revision, and programming services for right atrial, single-chamber, leadless pacemaker devices when done for right atrial, single-chamber, leadless pacemakers only. Specifically, these codes are reported for services associated with devices that are intended for leadless pacemakers that only affect function of the right atrium, ie, the device is not being placed as part of a dual-chamber device for any reason. This means that the device must be the only device that is currently implanted within the right atrium and is the only device that is intended for implantation or other services. Codes 0823T-0826T are not used: (1) if an existing right ventricular device has already been placed and the right atrial device is now being placed to complement function of the first device; or (2) if, for clinical reasons, the right atrial component of a dual-chamber system is being placed with the intent of placement of a right ventricular device at a later time. In these instances, other codes may

be reported to identify the staggered placement of the atrial component of the dual-chamber device (0796T, 0799T, 0802T) and codes 0823T-0826T should not be used to identify the service.

Common to the language included within pacemaker codes, the descriptor language within each code identifies all services that are inherently included as part of the service. As a result, services specifically identified within the code descriptor should not be separately reported when performing those services (eg, fluoroscopy, venous ultrasound).

Parenthetical notes and guidelines have been used throughout the code set to direct users to the correct code(s) to report when right atrial, leadless pacer device services are part of a component system for any reason. This includes new guidelines added within the Surgery/ Cardiovascular System/Heart and Pericardium/Pacemaker or Implantable Defibrillator subsection and the new guidelines included within the new Category III subsection for right atrial, leadless cardiac pacemaker devices. It also includes exclusionary parenthetical notes that restrict reporting of these codes in conjunction with any other single-component codes that are intended to be used either by themselves (eg, 33274) or as part of a dual-chamber system (eg, 0796T, 0799T, 0802T).

The guidelines within the Category III subsection also provide insight regarding (1) the components of these devices; (2) how these devices are placed; (3) what these codes are used to report; (4) exclusions from report services that are already included as part of the main services for these devices (such as exclusion of reporting separate catheterization [eg, 93451, 93453] and image guidance for placements, removals, or revisions [eg 76000, 77002, 76937). Instructions regarding programming device evaluation reporting have also been included.

The table within the Surgery section that provides additional insight regarding coding intent for reporting these new services also reflects the addition of the new codes to further clarify reporting intentions in a quick-to-review format.

Refer to the codebook and the Rationale for codes 0796T, 0799T, and 0802T for a full discussion of changes.

Clinical Example (0823T)

A 72-year-old male presents with persistent dizziness and shortness of breath. On work-up, the patient is diagnosed with sinus node dysfunction. A single-chamber atrial leadless pacemaker is recommended.

Category III 0042T-0713T

Description of Procedure (0823T)

In the electrophysiology laboratory, sedate the patient as clinically appropriate. Prepare the femoral region and administer local anesthesia. Depending on the leadless pacemaker system, place surface ECG electrodes and/or programming heads on the patient's chest and connect to the external pacemaker programmer. This enables transmittal of data from the implanted device to the programmer. Prior to insertion into the target chamber, load the pacemaker onto a catheter. Obtain femoral venous access using the Seldinger technique. Ultrasound guidance may be used, and femoral venography may be performed to identify the anatomy. After sequential dilation and upsizing the femoral sheath, including a small incision if needed, remove the guidewire and insert the leadless pacemaker introducer into the femoral vein. Under fluoroscopic guidance, insert the leadless pacemaker delivery catheter into the femoral vein through the introducer. Advance the delivery catheter through the IVC and then direct it into the right atrium. Contrast agent may be injected through the catheter to identify the anatomy. With the delivery catheter still attached and prior to fixation of the device, mapping may be performed to ensure accurate device placement. Electrical measurements, including intrinsic cardiac signal, can be measured and captured threshold can be performed via communication to the device from the programmer to assess device function. Then fix the leadless pacemaker to the endocardium, for example, by rotating a screw-in helix. After fixation, undock the pacemaker from the delivery system; however, it is still connected via tethers. Use the external programmer to measure pacing-capture threshold, sensing amplitude, and impedance. If values are interpreted as suboptimal, the pacemaker can be redocked, unscrewed, and repositioned within the right atrium under fluoroscopic guidance. Once appropriate parameters and adequate fixation are confirmed, release the tether and the pacemaker from the delivery catheter. Then remove the tether, delivery catheter, and sheath.

Clinical Example (0824T)

An 85-year-old female had a single-chamber atrial leadless pacemaker system placed 2 years ago. She has developed heart failure and left bundle branch block. The decision is made to remove the right atrial leadless pacemaker and place a CRT device.

Description of Procedure (0824T)

In the electrophysiology laboratory, sedate the patient as clinically appropriate. Prepare the femoral region and administer local anesthesia. Depending on the leadless pacemaker system, place surface ECG electrodes and/or programming heads on the patient's chest and connect to the external pacemaker programmer. This enables

transmittal of data from the implanted device to the programmer. Obtain femoral venous access using the Seldinger technique. Ultrasound guidance may be used, and femoral venography may be performed to identify the anatomy. After sequential dilation and upsizing the femoral sheath, including a small incision if needed, remove the guidewire and advance the retrieval catheter under fluoroscopic guidance through the IVC to the right atrium. Contrast agent may be injected through the catheter to identify the anatomy. Engage the leadless pacemaker by the retrieval catheter mechanism, for example, by snare. After confirming under fluoroscopy that the retrieval mechanism is engaged and secure, unscrew the device and remove the coupled retrieval catheter and leadless pacemaker.

Clinical Example (0825T)

An 81-year-old male had a single-chamber atrial leadless pacemaker system placed 8 years ago. Routine investigation demonstrates battery depletion associated with typical use. The decision is made to remove the existing device and replace it with a new right atrial leadless pacemaker, because the treatment has been clinically appropriate for the patient.

Description of Procedure (0825T)

In the electrophysiology laboratory, sedate the patient as clinically appropriate. Prepare the femoral region and administer local anesthesia. Depending on the leadless pacemaker system, place surface ECG electrodes and/or programming heads on the patient's chest and connect to the external pacemaker programmer. This enables transmittal of data from the implanted device to the programmer. Obtain femoral venous access using the Seldinger technique. Ultrasound guidance may be used and femoral venography may be performed to identify the anatomy. After sequential dilation and upsizing the femoral sheath, including a small incision if needed, remove the guidewire and advance the retrieval catheter under fluoroscopic guidance through the IVC to the right atrium. Contrast agent may be injected through the catheter to identify the anatomy. The leadless pacemaker is engaged by the snare integrated into the retrieval catheter, for example, by snare. After confirming under fluoroscopy that the retrieval mechanism is engaged and secure, unscrew the device and remove the coupled retrieval catheter and leadless pacemaker.

Prior to insertion into the target chamber, load the replacement pacemaker onto a catheter. Obtain femoral venous access using the Seldinger technique. Ultrasound guidance may be used and femoral venography may be performed to identify the anatomy. After sequential dilation and upsizing the femoral sheath, including a small incision if needed, remove the guidewire and insert the leadless pacemaker introducer into the femoral vein.

Under fluoroscopic guidance, insert the leadless pacemaker delivery catheter into the femoral vein through the introducer. Advance the delivery catheter through the IVC and then direct it into the right atrium. Contrast agent may be injected through the catheter to identify the anatomy. With the catheter still attached and prior to fixation of the device, mapping may be performed to ensure accurate device placement. Electrical measurements, including intrinsic cardiac signal, can be measured and captured threshold can be performed via communication to the device from the programmer to assess device function. The leadless pacemaker is then fixed to the endocardium, for example, by rotating a screw-in helix. After fixation, undock the pacemaker from the delivery system; however, it is still connected via tethers. The external programmer is used to measure pacing-capture threshold, sensing amplitude, and impedance. If values are interpreted as suboptimal, the pacemaker can be redocked, unscrewed, and repositioned within the target chamber under fluoroscopic guidance. Once appropriate parameters and adequate fixation are confirmed, release the tether and the pacemaker from the delivery catheter. Remove the tether, delivery catheter, and sheath. Close the access site with a nonabsorbable single figure-of-eight stitch or by other means.

Clinical Example (0826T)

A 65-year-old female with bradycardia had a single-chamber leadless pacemaker implanted 2 years ago. The patient contacted her internist because she had passed out. The physician has the patient come in for a symptom assessment and a programming device evaluation.

Description of Procedure (0826T)

Connect the patient to a single or multilead free-running ECG monitor. Obtain a communication link between the pacemaker and the programmer. Assess and record current rhythm. Review initial interrogation to determine if any alert conditions have occurred (eg, stored arrhythmia events, lead-function parameter out of normal range). Review alert conditions in detail. Review stored arrhythmic episodes to determine if the arrhythmia was accurately identified by the pacemaker (eg, episode identified as atrial fibrillation is not double counting far-field ventricular activity on the atrial lead).

Inhibit pacing to record the underlying rhythm. Determine pacing-capture thresholds by iteratively reducing the pacing voltage while maintaining a fixed pulse width (and/or by iteratively reducing the pulse width while maintaining a fixed voltage). Evaluate the autocapture feature (if present) to ensure appropriate function for the lead. Review alert conditions from initial interrogation in detail. Compare current

interrogation results to historical values and previous trends for battery voltage, impedance, and estimated longevity; lead sensing value; and pacing threshold and pacing impedance. Evaluate out-of-range parameters for accuracy (eg, abnormal sensing or pacing thresholds recorded by the device's autosensing and autocapture algorithms). Assess the need for reprogramming. Based on findings, adjust programmed parameters (such as pacing outputs, sensing thresholds, timing parameters, alert parameters, etc) as needed.

0827T	Code is out of numerical sequence. See 0762T-0765T
0828T	Code is out of numerical sequence. See 0762T-0765T
0829T	Code is out of numerical sequence. See 0762T-0765T
0830T	Code is out of numerical sequence. See 0762T-0765T
0831T	Code is out of numerical sequence. See 0762T-0765T
0832T	Code is out of numerical sequence. See 0762T-0765T
0833T	Code is out of numerical sequence. See 0762T-0765T
0834T	Code is out of numerical sequence. See 0762T-0765T
0835T	Code is out of numerical sequence. See 0762T-0765T
0836T	Code is out of numerical sequence. See 0762T-0765T
0837T	Code is out of numerical sequence. See 0762T-0765T
0838T	Code is out of numerical sequence. See 0762T-0765T
0839T	Code is out of numerical sequence. See 0762T-0765T
0840T	Code is out of numerical sequence. See 0762T-0765T
0841T	Code is out of numerical sequence. See 0762T-0765T
0842T	Code is out of numerical sequence. See 0762T-0765T
0843T	Code is out of numerical sequence. See 0762T-0765T
0844T	Code is out of numerical sequence. See 0762T-0765T
0845T	Code is out of numerical sequence. See 0762T-0765T
0846T	Code is out of numerical sequence. See 0762T-0765T
0847T	Code is out of numerical sequence. See 0762T-0765T
0848T	Code is out of numerical sequence. See 0762T-0765T
0849T	Code is out of numerical sequence. See 0762T-0765T
0850T	Code is out of numerical sequence. See 0762T-0765T
0851T	Code is out of numerical sequence. See 0762T-0765T
0852T	Code is out of numerical sequence. See 0762T-0765T
0853T	Code is out of numerical sequence. See 0762T-0765T
0854T	Code is out of numerical sequence. See 0762T-0765T
0855T	Code is out of numerical sequence. See 0762T-0765T
0856T	Code is out of numerical sequence. See 0762T-0765T

★ = Telemedicine   ◄ = Add-on code   ✚ = Add-on code   ✔ = FDA approval pending   # = Resequenced code   ⊘ = Modifier 51 exempt

+● 0857T Opto-acoustic imaging, breast, unilateral, including axilla when performed, real-time with image documentation, augmentative analysis and report (List separately in addition to code for primary procedure)

►(Use 0857T in conjunction with 76641, 76642)◄

Rationale

Category III code 0857T has been established to report opto-acoustic (OA) imaging for breast masses. To support the addition of the new code, a parenthetical note has been added to guide users with the appropriate reporting of this code.

Code 0857T is an add-on code; therefore, a parenthetical note following the code instructs reporting either code 76641 or 76642 for ultrasound of the breast in conjunction with it.

Clinical Example (0857T)

A 50-year-old female with a palpable lump undergoes diagnostic ultrasound that shows a solid breast mass with suspicious malignant features. The mass is further investigated with opto-acoustic (OA) imaging. [**Note:** This is an add-on code. Only consider the additional work related to the OA evaluation.]

Description of Procedure (0857T)

Following separately reported standard diagnostic breast ultrasound demonstrating a solid mass, activate laser safety protocol, including the use of protective eyewear by the patient, physician, sonographer, and staff within the room. The duplex OA probe is activated and the breast is scanned, including image documentation of abnormal tissue. Document visualized pathology. Freeze frame OA images with and without measurements and store two video sweeps. Compare and correlate the examination with previous studies. Dictate OA findings in the medical record.

►Code 0858T represents measurement of evoked cortical potentials associated with transcranial magnetic stimulation of two or more cortical areas using multiple, externally applied scalp electrode channels. Upon stimulation, the device performs automated signal processing indicating brain physiological features of connectivity, excitability, and plasticity, which may be impaired with structural and functional brain deficits. Because these physiological features may be altered in certain types of brain disease, the device's automated report of analyzed data is intended to provide clinical insight of brain function within the context of certain brain disease states.◄

● 0858T Externally applied transcranial magnetic stimulation with concomitant measurement of evoked cortical potentials with automated report

►(Do not report 0858T in conjunction with 95836, 95957, 95961, 95965, 95966)◄

Rationale

Category III code 0858T and guidelines have been established to report the measurement of evoked cortical potentials associated with transcranial magnetic stimulation of two or more cortical areas using multiple externally applied scalp electrode channels. The new guidelines provide guidance regarding what the service involves and how it is used to provide clinical insight.

Prior to the establishment of code 0858T, there were no codes available to report this service. An exclusionary parenthetical note has been added following code 0858T to preclude reporting this code with codes 95836, 95957, 95961, 95965, and 95966.

Clinical Example (0858T)

A 65-year-old male presents after complaints of cognitive decline. The physician or other QHP performs a clinical evaluation, including referral for external transcranial magnetic stimulation with concurrent measurement of evoked cortical potentials to aid in diagnosis.

Description of Procedure (0858T)

The clinical staff technician measures the patient's head to fit the correct cap size. The technician adjusts recording electrode impedances using conductive gel until electrode contact is adequate as indicated by the software. The technician records patient's brain activity for 1 minute with eyes open followed by 1 minute of recording with eyes closed. The technician locates stimulation areas: left and right primary motor cortex and left and right dorsolateral prefrontal cortex. The technician measures left and right rest motor threshold values by fixating the magnetic probe on top of the left motor cortex and stimulates in incrementing intensities until a muscle twitch is visible in right hand. The technician then performs same process for the right motor cortex and records the values in which a first muscle twitch was observed (resting motor threshold) in the appropriate software window. The technician then starts the evaluation stimulation and concomitant recording. The evaluation of each stimulated area is repeated in the exact same way and is performed for all four evaluated stimulation areas. Device software analyzes the data and produces an automated report that

Category III 0042T-0713T

quantifies the physiological evoked measures of connectivity, excitability, and plasticity with reference to validated thresholds for abnormalities.

0859T	Code is out of numerical sequence. See 0489T-0495T
0860T	Code is out of numerical sequence. See 0489T-0495T
0861T	Code is out of numerical sequence. See 0516T-0520T
0862T	Code is out of numerical sequence. See 0516T-0520T
0863T	Code is out of numerical sequence. See 0516T-0520T
● **0864T**	Low-intensity extracorporeal shock wave therapy involving corpus cavernosum, low energy

▶(Do not report 0864T in conjunction with 0101T when treating the same area)◀

Rationale

Category III code 0864T has been established to report low-energy, low-intensity extracorporeal shock wave therapy (Li-ESWT) involving the corpus cavernosum. The corpus cavernosum is in the penis and is made up of spongy tissue and blood vessels, which fill with blood to make the penis erect. Li-ESWT is used to treat disorders, such as erectile dysfunction or Peyronie's disease, a condition in which plaque develops under the skin of the penis.

There are existing CPT codes that describe ESWT. For example, code 0101T describes extracorporeal shockwave involving the musculoskeletal system. However, it should not be reported with code 0864T when treating the same area. An exclusionary parenthetical note has been added following code 0804T restricting its use with code 0101T for treatment of the same area.

Clinical Example (0864T)

A 55-year-old male presents with complaint of erectile dysfunction (ED) with the inability to achieve and maintain his penis erect throughout sexual activity, impacting intimacy for more than 2 years. He is positive for cardiovascular disease yet seeks low-intensity extracorporeal shock wave therapy to treat the ED.

Description of Procedure (0864T)

After ensuring the patient is prepared for treatment (including removal of any excessive hair from targeted areas), place a disposable cover over the applicator and apply coupling gel liberally to the applicator cover. Remove any air bubbles from the gel by working the fingers toward the edges of the disposable cover. Also apply coupling gel to the targeted areas. The penis is

manually, gently stretched for delivery of shock waves to the corpus cavernosa bilaterally along the entire shaft (avoiding the tip), the crus of the penis on each side of the penile hilum (in the direction of the prostate), and at the perineum between the scrotum and the anus (in the direction of the prostate). The shock head is coupled to the patient's penis and positioned by the physician. It is important that the applicator is held perpendicular to the treatment area and that there is good contact between the patient's skin and the shock head to ensure the most effective results. The physician instructs the technician to set the shock wave delivery rate to 3 hertz. The procedure is administered at 0.1 mJ/mm^2 (millijoule/millimeter) for the first four treatments. Energy level is not to exceed 0.13 mJ/mm^2. When applying shock waves to the perineum and crus of the penis, moderate pressure is applied to improve shock wave penetration toward the prostate.

● **0865T**	Quantitative magnetic resonance image (MRI) analysis of the brain with comparison to prior magnetic resonance (MR) study(ies), including lesion identification, characterization, and quantification, with brain volume(s) quantification and/or severity score, when performed, data preparation and transmission, interpretation and report, obtained without diagnostic MRI examination of the brain during the same session

▶(Do not report 0865T in conjunction with 70551, 70552, 70553)◀

✚● **0866T**	Quantitative magnetic resonance image (MRI) analysis of the brain with comparison to prior magnetic resonance (MR) study(ies), including lesion detection, characterization, and quantification, with brain volume(s) quantification and/or severity score, when performed, data preparation and transmission, interpretation and report, obtained with diagnostic MRI examination of the brain (List separately in addition to code for primary procedure)

▶(Use 0866T in conjunction with 70551, 70552, 70553)◀

▶(For quantitative MR for analysis of tissue composition, see 0648T, 0649T, 0697T, 0698T)◀

▶(For quantitative computed tomography tissue characterization, see 0721T, 0722T)◀

▶(For quantitative MRI analysis of the brain without comparison to prior MR study, report 0865T, 0866T with modifier 52)◀

Category III 0042T-0713T

Rationale

Two Category III codes (0865T, 0866T) have been established to report quantitative magnetic resonance image (MRI) analysis of the brain. To support the addition of the new codes, parenthetical notes have been added to guide users with the appropriate reporting of these codes.

Existing codes 0648T and 0649T describe quantitative magnetic resonance for analysis of tissue composition. Codes 0721T and 0722T describe quantitative tissue characterization using CT without (0721T) and with (0722T) concurrent CT imaging.

This new service does not analyze the composition of the tissue; instead, it provides analysis of brain lesions via software by identifying diseased areas of the brain compared over time with the use of multiple MRI images that are overlayed and analyzed. The software then quantifies the lesion volume(s), number, and locations with a comparison to prior studies, when possible, to provide results that may be analyzed by the physician to direct patient care.

Clinical Example (0865T)

A 30-year-old female presents with a 6-year history of relapsing remitting multiple sclerosis (RRMS) that has caused mild level disability (Expanded Disability Status Scale [EDSS] score 1). She is currently treated with first-line disease modifying medication for RRMS. She undergoes periodical radiological and clinical assessment to monitor clinical and subclinical disease activity.

Description of Procedure (0865T)

After acquisition of the magnetic resonance (MR) study, which has been previously interpreted (separately reported), upload the MR images manually from a local server (or potentially local picture archiving communication system [PACS]) and transfer to a secure cloud site using a gateway, which is installed on the local server of the site. Before the data leave the facility or office, encrypt all protected health information (PHI) and data using a key-based encryption for transfer. Also upload and transfer prior studies to the secure cloud site.

After processing the data, summarize the quantifications and their changes (comparing multiple time points) into an electronic quantitative report and overlay segmentations on the input images, creating the output images where the MRI scan is overlayed with the segmentations as generated by the software. A normative population graph is provided to compare the patient to age- and gender-matched normative population. Finally, the generated output undergoes an automated quality control, and once approved, the final report and output images are sent to the local server.

The physician or other QHP (typically a neurologist) reads/reviews the information provided in the quantitative MR report (in combination with the scans with overlaid segmentations), makes any corrections required, and then uses that to complete their report. A final report is generated by the physician or other QHP, including the findings of the quantitative MR image analysis, addressing any discrepancies with the original MRI if needed.

Clinical Example (0866T)

A 30-year-old female presents with a 6-year history of RRMS that has caused mild level disability (EDSS score 1). She is currently treated with first-line disease modifying medication for RRMS. She undergoes periodical radiological and clinical assessment to monitor clinical and subclinical disease activity. [**Note:** This is an add-on code. Only consider the additional work related to interpretation and report of the augmentative quantitative MR analysis of the brain.]

Description of Procedure (0866T)

After acquisition of the MR images by the technologist, upload the images either manually (by the technologist, the radiologist, or the neurologist) or automatically from the scanner/workstation or the PACS and transfer to a secure cloud site using a gateway, which is installed in the center itself. Before the data leave the hospital, encrypt all PHI and data using a key-based encryption for transfer. Also upload prior studies and transfer to the secure cloud site.

After processing the data, summarize the quantifications and their changes over time (comparing multiple time points) into an electronic pre-populated report and overlay segmentations on the input images, creating the output images where the MRI scan is overlayed with the segmentations as generated by the software. A normative population graph is provided to compare the patient to age- and gender-matched normative population. Finally, the generated output undergoes an automated quality control, and once approved, the final report and output images are sent back to the PACS. (The turnaround time is approximately 15 to 30 minutes, which allows for real-time reading of the quantitative MR report with the MR brain examination.)

The physician or other QHP (typically a radiologist) reads/reviews the information provided in the quantitative MR report (in combination with the scans with overlaid segmentations). The quantitative MR report is reviewed for technical accuracy, and adjustments are made if needed. A final report is generated by the physician or other QHP, including the findings of the MRI (separately reported) and the quantitative MR image analysis, addressing any discrepancies if needed.

▲ = Revised code   ● = New code   ▶ ◀ = Contains new or revised text   ✕ = Duplicate PLA test   ↑↓ = Category I PLA   American Medical Association   **199**

Category III 0042T-0713T

Notes

Appendix K

Summary of Additions, Deletions, and Revisions

The summary of changes shows the actual changes that have been made to the code descriptors.

New codes appear with a bullet (●) and are indicated as "Code added." Revised codes are preceded with a triangle (▲). Within revised codes, or if a code symbol has been deleted, the deleted language and code symbol appear with a ~~strikethrough~~, while new text appears <u>underlined</u>.

The ⟋ symbol is used to identify codes for vaccines that are pending FDA approval. The # symbol is used to identify codes that have been resequenced. CPT add-on codes are annotated by the ✚ symbol. The ⊘ symbol is used to identify codes that are exempt from the use of modifier 51. The ★ symbol is used to identify codes that may be used for reporting telemedicine services. The ✕ symbol is used to identify a proprietary laboratory analyses (PLA) test that has an identical descriptor as another PLA test. A PLA code that satisfies Category I code criteria and has been accepted by the CPT Editorial Panel is annotated with the ↑↓ symbol. The ◀ symbol is used to identify codes that may be used to report audio-only telemedicine services when appended by modifier 93 (**see Appendix T**).

Code
90589
90623
90683

Appendix K

Product Pending FDA Approval

▶Some vaccine and immune globulin products have been assigned a CPT Category I code in anticipation of future approval from the Food and Drug Administration (FDA). Following is a list of the vaccine and immune globulin product codes pending FDA approval status that are identified in the CPT code set with the ⟋ symbol. Upon revision of the approval status by the FDA, notation of this revision will be provided via the AMA CPT "Category I Vaccine Codes" website listing (ama-assn.org/cpt-cat-i-immunization-codes) and in subsequent publications of the CPT code set.◀

90584

90589

90623

90666

90667

90668

90671

90683

91302

91310

Rationale

The Appendix K guidelines have been revised to include the term "immune globulin" to reflect that in addition to vaccine products, immune globulin products may be assigned as CPT Category I codes pending approval from the Food and Drug Administration.

Refer to the codebook and the Rationales for Immune Globulins, Serum or Recombinant Products guidelines in the Medicine section for a full discussion of these changes.

★ = Telemedicine   ◀ = Audio-only   ✚ = Add-on code   ⟋ = FDA approval pending   # = Resequenced code   ⊘ = Modifier 51 exempt

Appendix O

Summary of Additions, Deletions, and Revisions

The summary of changes shows the actual changes that have been made to the code descriptors.

New codes appear with a bullet (●) and are indicated as "Code added." Revised codes are preceded with a triangle (▲). Within revised codes, or if a code symbol has been deleted, the deleted language and code symbol appear with a ~~strikethrough~~, while new text appears underlined.

The ⚡ symbol is used to identify codes for vaccines that are pending FDA approval. The # symbol is used to identify codes that have been resequenced. CPT add-on codes are annotated by the + symbol. The ⊘ symbol is used to identify codes that are exempt from the use of modifier 51. The ★ symbol is used to identify codes that may be used for reporting telemedicine services. The ⋈ symbol is used to identify a proprietary laboratory analyses (PLA) test that has an identical descriptor as another PLA test. A PLA code that satisfies Category I code criteria and has been accepted by the CPT Editorial Panel is annotated with the ⇅ symbol. The ◀ symbol is used to identify codes that may be used to report audio-only telemedicine services when appended by modifier 93 **(see Appendix T)**.

Proprietary Name and Clinical Laboratory or Manufacturer	Alpha-Numeric Code	Code Descriptor
Administrative Codes for Multianalyte Assays with Algorithmic Analyses (MAAA)		
~~Enhanced Liver Fibrosis™ (ELF™) Test, Siemens Healthcare Diagnostics Inc/Siemens Healthcare Laboratory LLC~~	~~0014M~~	~~Liver disease, analysis of 3 biomarkers (hyaluronic acid [HA], procollagen III amino terminal peptide [PIIINP], tissue inhibitor of metalloproteinase 1 [TIMP-1]), using immunoassays, utilizing serum, prognostic algorithm reported as a risk score and risk of liver fibrosis and liver-related clinical events within 5 years~~
	●0019M	Code added
Category I Codes for Multianalyte Assays with Algorithmic Analyses (MAAA)		
	●81517	Code added
Proprietary Laboratory Analyses (PLA)		
Oncomine™ Dx Target Test, Thermo Fisher Scientific, Thermo Fisher Scientific	▲0022U	Targeted genomic sequence analysis panel, ~~cholangiocarcinoma and~~ non-small cell lung neoplasia, DNA and RNA analysis, ~~1=~~23 genes, interrogation for sequence variants and rearrangements, reported as presence~~/~~ or absence of variants and associated therapy(ies) to consider
~~Prostate Cancer Risk Panel, Mayo Clinic, Laboratory Developed Test~~	~~0053U~~	~~Oncology (prostate cancer), FISH analysis of 4 genes (ASAP1, HDAC9, CHD1 and PTEN), needle biopsy specimen, algorithm reported as probability of higher tumor grade~~
~~PartoSure™ Test, Parsagen Diagnostics, Inc, Parsagen Diagnostics, Inc, a QIAGEN Company~~	~~0066U~~	~~Placental alpha-micro globulin-1 (PAMG-1), immunoassay with direct optical observation, cervico-vaginal fluid, each specimen~~

(Continued on page 204)

Proprietary Name and Clinical Laboratory or Manufacturer	Alpha-Numeric Code	Code Descriptor
Esophageal String Test™ (EST), ~~Cambridge Biomedical, Inc~~Children's Hospital Colorado Department of Pathology and Laboratory Medicine	▲0095U	~~Inflammation (e~~Eosinophilic esophagitis~~)~~, ~~ELISA analysis of e~~(Eotaxin-3 ¿[CCL26 ¿[C-C motif chemokine ligand 26}]}) and major basic protein ¿[PRG2 ¿[proteoglycan 2, pro eosinophil major basic protein}]), enzyme-linked immunosorbent assays (ELISA), specimen obtained by ~~swallowed nylon esophageal~~ string test device, algorithm reported as ~~predictive~~ probability ~~index for~~ of active or inactive eosinophilic esophagitis
~~CareViewRx, Newstar Medical Laboratories, LLC, Newstar Medical Laboratories, LLC~~	~~0143U~~	~~Drug assay, definitive, 120 or more drugs or metabolites, urine, quantitative liquid chromatography with tandem mass spectrometry (LC-MS/MS) using multiple reaction monitoring (MRM), with drug or metabolite description, comments including sample validation, per date of service~~
~~CareViewRx Plus, Newstar Medical Laboratories, LLC, Newstar Medical Laboratories, LLC~~	~~0144U~~	~~Drug assay, definitive, 160 or more drugs or metabolites, urine, quantitative liquid chromatography with tandem mass spectrometry (LC-MS/MS) using multiple reaction monitoring (MRM), with drug or metabolite description, comments including sample validation, per date of service~~
~~PainViewRx, Newstar Medical Laboratories, LLC, Newstar Medical Laboratories, LLC~~	~~0145U~~	~~Drug assay, definitive, 65 or more drugs or metabolites, urine, quantitative liquid chromatography with tandem mass spectrometry (LC-MS/MS) using multiple reaction monitoring (MRM), with drug or metabolite description, comments including sample validation, per date of service~~
~~PainViewRx Plus, Newstar Medical Laboratories, LLC, Newstar Medical Laboratories, LLC~~	~~0146U~~	~~Drug assay, definitive, 80 or more drugs or metabolites, urine, by quantitative liquid chromatography with tandem mass spectrometry (LC-MS/MS) using multiple reaction monitoring (MRM), with drug or metabolite description, comments including sample validation, per date of service~~
~~RiskViewRx, Newstar Medical Laboratories, LLC, Newstar Medical Laboratories, LLC~~	~~0147U~~	~~Drug assay, definitive, 85 or more drugs or metabolites, urine, quantitative liquid chromatography with tandem mass spectrometry (LC-MS/MS) using multiple reaction monitoring (MRM), with drug or metabolite description, comments including sample validation, per date of service~~
~~RiskViewRx Plus, Newstar Medical Laboratories, LLC, Newstar Medical Laboratories, LLC~~	~~0148U~~	~~Drug assay, definitive, 100 or more drugs or metabolites, urine, quantitative liquid chromatography with tandem mass spectrometry (LC-MS/MS) using multiple reaction monitoring (MRM), with drug or metabolite description, comments including sample validation, per date of service~~

★ = Telemedicine   ◀ = Audio-only   ✚ = Add-on code   ✗ = FDA approval pending   # = Resequenced code   ⊘ = Modifier 51 exempt

Proprietary Name and Clinical Laboratory or Manufacturer	Alpha-Numeric Code	Code Descriptor
~~PsychViewRx, Newstar Medical Laboratories, LLC, Newstar Medical Laboratories, LLC~~	~~0149U~~	~~Drug assay, definitive, 60 or more drugs or metabolites, urine, quantitative liquid chromatography with tandem mass spectrometry (LC-MS/MS) using multiple reaction monitoring (MRM), with drug or metabolite description, comments including sample validation, per date of service~~
~~PsychViewRx Plus, Newstar Medical Laboratories, LLC, Newstar Medical Laboratories, LLC~~	~~0150U~~	~~Drug assay, definitive, 120 or more drugs or metabolites, urine, quantitative liquid chromatography with tandem mass spectrometry (LC-MS/MS) using multiple reaction monitoring (MRM), with drug or metabolite description, comments including sample validation, per date of service~~
Versiti™ Autosomal Dominant Thrombocytopenia Panel, Versiti™ Diagnostic Laboratories, Versiti™	▲0269U	Hematology (autosomal dominant congenital thrombocytopenia), genomic sequence analysis of ~~14~~22 genes, blood, buccal swab, or amniotic fluid
Versiti™ Congenital Neutropenia Panel, Versiti™ Diagnostic Laboratories, Versiti™	▲0271U	Hematology (congenital neutropenia), genomic sequence analysis of ~~23~~24 genes, blood, buccal swab, or amniotic fluid
Versiti™ Comprehensive Bleeding Disorder Panel, Versiti™ Diagnostic Laboratories, Versiti™	▲0272U	Hematology (genetic bleeding disorders), genomic sequence analysis of ~~51~~60 genes and duplication/ deletion of *PLAU*, blood, buccal swab, or amniotic fluid, comprehensive
Versiti™ Comprehensive Platelet Disorder Panel, Versiti™ Diagnostic Laboratories, Versiti™	▲0274U	Hematology (genetic platelet disorders), genomic sequence analysis of ~~43~~62 genes and duplication/ deletion of *PLAU*, blood, buccal swab, or amniotic fluid
Versiti™ Platelet Function Disorder Panel, Versiti™ Diagnostic Laboratories, Versiti™	▲0277U	Hematology (genetic platelet function disorder), genomic sequence analysis of ~~31~~40 genes and duplication/deletion of *PLAU*, blood, buccal swab, or amniotic fluid
Versiti™ Thrombosis Panel, Versiti™ Diagnostic Laboratories, Versiti™	▲0278U	Hematology (genetic thrombosis), genomic sequence analysis of ~~12~~14 genes, blood, buccal swab, or amniotic fluid
HART CADhs®, ~~Prevencio, Inc~~Atlas Genomics, Prevencio, Inc	▲0308U	Cardiology (coronary artery disease [CAD]), analysis of 3 proteins (high sensitivity [hs] troponin, adiponectin, and kidney injury molecule-1 [KIM-1]) with 3 clinical parameters (age, sex, history of cardiac intervention), plasma, algorithm reported as a risk score for obstructive CAD
~~3D Predict™ Ovarian Doublet Panel, KIYATEC® Inc~~	~~0324U~~	~~Oncology (ovarian), spheroid cell culture, 4-drug panel (carboplatin, doxorubicin, gemcitabine, paclitaxel), tumor chemotherapy response prediction for each drug~~
~~3D Predict™ Ovarian PARP Panel, KIYATEC® Inc~~	~~0325U~~	~~Oncology (ovarian), spheroid cell culture, poly (ADP-ribose) polymerase (PARP) inhibitors (niraparib, olaparib, rucaparib, velparib), tumor response prediction for each drug~~
	●0355U	Code added

(*Continued on page 206*)

▲=Revised code   ●=New code   ►◄=Contains new or revised text   ✕=Duplicate PLA test   ↑↓=Category I PLA

American Medical Association   **205**

Appendix O

Proprietary Name and Clinical Laboratory or Manufacturer	Alpha-Numeric Code	Code Descriptor
	●0356U	Code added
~~DAWN™ IO Melanoma, InterVenn Biosciences, InterVenn Biosciences~~	~~0357U~~	~~Oncology (melanoma), artificial intelligence (AI)-enabled quantitative mass spectrometry analysis of 142 unique pairs of glycopeptide and product fragments, plasma, prognostic, and predictive algorithm reported as likely, unlikely, or uncertain benefit from immunotherapy agents~~
	●0358U	Code added
	●0359U	Code added
	●0360U	Code added
	●0361U	Code added
Thyroid GuidePx®, Protean BioDiagnostics, ~~Protean BioDiagnostics~~ Qualisure Diagnostics	▲0362U	Oncology (papillary thyroid cancer), gene-expression profiling via targeted hybrid capture–enrichment RNA sequencing of 82 content genes and 10 housekeeping genes, fine needle aspirate or formalin-fixed paraffin-_embedded (FFPE) tissue, algorithm reported as one of three molecular subtypes
	●0363U	Code added
	●0364U	Code added
	●0365U	Code added
	●0366U	Code added
	●0367U	Code added
	●0368U	Code added
	●0369U	Code added
	●0370U	Code added
	●0371U	Code added
	●0372U	Code added
	●0373U	Code added
	●0374U	Code added
	●0375U	Code added
	●0376U	Code added
	●0377U	Code added
	●0378U	Code added
	●0379U	Code added
	●0380U	Code added
	●0381U	Code added
	●0382U	Code added
	●0383U	Code added
	●0384U	Code added
	●0385U	Code added

★ = Telemedicine ◀ = Audio-only ✚ = Add-on code ✚ = FDA approval pending # = Resequenced code ⊘ = Modifier 51 exempt

Proprietary Name and Clinical Laboratory or Manufacturer	Alpha-Numeric Code	Code Descriptor
~~Envisage, Capsulomics, Inc, Capsulomics, Inc~~	~~0386U~~	~~Gastroenterology (Barrett's esophagus), P16, RUNX3, HPP1, and FBN1 methylation analysis, prognostic and predictive algorithm reported as a risk score for progression to high-grade dysplasia or esophageal cancer~~
	●0387U	Code added
	●0388U	Code added
	●0389U	Code added
	●0390U	Code added
	●0391U	Code added
	●0392U	Code added
	●0393U	Code added
	●0394U	Code added
	●0395U	Code added
	●0396U	Code added
~~Agilent Resolution ctDx FIRST, Resolution Bioscience, Inc, Resolution Bioscience, Inc~~	~~0397U~~	~~Oncology (non-small cell lung cancer), cell-free DNA from plasma, targeted sequence analysis of at least 109 genes, including sequence variants, substitutions, insertions, deletions, select rearrangements, and copy number variations~~
	●0398U	Code added
	●0399U	Code added
	●0400U	Code added
	●0401U	Code added
	●0402U	Code added
	●0403U	Code added
	●0404U	Code added
	●0405U	Code added
	●0406U	Code added
	●0407U	Code added
	●0408U	Code added
	●0409U	Code added
	●0410U	Code added
	✕●0411U	Code added
	●0412U	Code added
	●0413U	Code added
	●0414U	Code added
	●0415U	Code added
	●0416U	Code added
	●0417U	Code added
	●0418U	Code added
	●0419U	Code added

Appendix O

Multianalyte Assays with Algorithmic Analyses and Proprietary Laboratory Analyses

The following list includes three types of CPT codes:

1. Multianalyte assays with algorithmic analyses (MAAA) administrative codes
2. Category I MAAA codes
3. Proprietary laboratory analyses (PLA) codes

1. Multianalyte assays with algorithmic analyses (MAAAs) are procedures that utilize multiple results derived from assays of various types, including molecular pathology assays, fluorescent in situ hybridization assays and non-nucleic acid based assays (eg, proteins, polypeptides, lipids, carbohydrates). Algorithmic analysis using the results of these assays as well as other patient information (if used) is then performed and reported typically as a numeric score(s) or as a probability. MAAAs are typically unique to a single clinical laboratory or manufacturer. The results of individual component procedure(s) that are inputs to the MAAAs may be provided on the associated laboratory report, however these assays are not reported separately using additional codes. MAAAs, by nature, are typically unique to a single clinical laboratory or manufacturer.

The list includes a proprietary name and clinical laboratory or manufacturer in the first column, an alpha-numeric code in the second column and code descriptor in the third column. The format for the code descriptor usually includes (in order):

- Disease type (eg, oncology, autoimmune, tissue rejection),
- Chemical(s) analyzed (eg, DNA, RNA, protein, antibody),
- Number of markers (eg, number of genes, number of proteins),
- Methodology(s) (eg, microarray, real-time [RT]-PCR, in situ hybridization [ISH], enzyme linked immunosorbent assays [ELISA]),
- Number of functional domains (if indicated),
- Specimen type (eg, blood, fresh tissue, formalin-fixed paraffin-embedded),
- Algorithm result type (eg, prognostic, diagnostic),
- Report (eg, probability index, risk score).

MAAA procedures that have been assigned a Category I code are noted in the list below and additionally listed in the Category I MAAA section (81500-81599). The Category I MAAA section introductory language and associated parenthetical instruction(s) should be used to govern the appropriate use for Category I MAAA codes. If a specific MAAA procedure has not been assigned a Category I code, it is indicated as a four-digit number followed by the letter M.

When a specific MAAA procedure is not included in either the list below or in the Category I MAAA section, report the analysis using the Category I MAAA unlisted code (81599). The codes below are specific to the assays identified in Appendix O by proprietary name. In order to report an MAAA code, the analysis performed must fulfill the code descriptor **and**, if proprietary, must be the test represented by the proprietary name listed in Appendix O. When an analysis is performed that may potentially fall within a specific descriptor, however the proprietary name is not included in the list below, the MAAA unlisted code (81599) should be used.

Additions in this section may be released tri-annually (or quarterly for PLA codes) via the AMA CPT website to expedite dissemination for reporting. See the Introduction section of the CPT code set for a complete list of the dates of release and implementation.

These administrative codes encompass all analytical services required for the algorithmic analysis (eg, cell lysis, nucleic acid stabilization, extraction, digestion, amplification, hybridization and detection) in addition to the algorithmic analysis itself, when applicable. Procedures that are required prior to cell lysis (eg, microdissection, codes 88380 and 88381) should be reported separately.

The codes in this list are provided as an administrative coding set to facilitate accurate reporting of MAAA services. The minimum standard for inclusion in this list is that an analysis is generally available for patient care. The AMA has not reviewed procedures in the administrative coding set for clinical utility. The list is not a complete list of all MAAA procedures.

2. Category I MAAA codes are included below along with their proprietary names. These codes are also listed in the Pathology and Laboratory section of the CPT code set (81490-81599).

3. PLA codes created in response to the Protecting Access to Medicare Act (PAMA) of 2014 are listed along with their proprietary names. These codes are also located at the end of the Pathology and Laboratory section of the CPT code set. In some instances, the descriptor language of PLA codes may be identical, which are differentiated only by the listed propriety names.

The accuracy of a PLA code is to be maintained by the original applicant, or the current owner of the test kit or laboratory performing the proprietary test.

A new PLA code is required when:

1. Additional nucleic acid (DNA or RNA) and/or protein analysis(es) are added to the current PLA test, or

2. The name of the PLA test has changed in association with changes in test performance or test characteristics.

The addition or modification of the therapeutic applications of the test require submission of a code change application, but it may not require a new code number.

Proprietary Name and Clinical Laboratory or Manufacturer	Alpha-Numeric Code	Code Descriptor
Administrative Codes for Multianalyte Assays with Algorithmic Analyses (MAAA)		
ASH FibroSURE™, BioPredictive S.A.S	0002M	Liver disease, ten biochemical assays (ALT, A2-macroglobulin, apolipoprotein A-1, total bilirubin, GGT, haptoglobin, AST, glucose, total cholesterol and triglycerides) utilizing serum, prognostic algorithm reported as quantitative scores for fibrosis, steatosis and alcoholic steatohepatitis (ASH)
NASH FibroSURE™, BioPredictive S.A.S	0003M	Liver disease, ten biochemical assays (ALT, A2-macroglobulin, apolipoprotein A-1, total bilirubin, GGT, haptoglobin, AST, glucose, total cholesterol and triglycerides) utilizing serum, prognostic algorithm reported as quantitative scores for fibrosis, steatosis and nonalcoholic steatohepatitis (NASH)
ScoliScore™ Transgenomic	0004M	Scoliosis, DNA analysis of 53 single nucleotide polymorphisms (SNPs), using saliva, prognostic algorithm reported as a risk score
HeproDX™, GoPath Laboratories, LLC	0006M	Oncology (hepatic), mRNA expression levels of 161 genes, utilizing fresh hepatocellular carcinoma tumor tissue, with alpha-fetoprotein level, algorithm reported as a risk classifier
NETest, Wren Laboratories, LLC	0007M	Oncology (gastrointestinal neuroendocrine tumors), real-time PCR expression analysis of 51 genes, utilizing whole peripheral blood, algorithm reported as a nomogram of tumor disease index
NeoLAB™ Prostate Liquid Biopsy, NeoGenomics Laboratories	0011M	Oncology, prostate cancer, mRNA expression assay of 12 genes (10 content and 2 housekeeping), RT-PCR test utilizing blood plasma and urine, algorithms to predict high-grade prostate cancer risk

(Continued on page 210)

Proprietary Name and Clinical Laboratory or Manufacturer	Alpha-Numeric Code	Code Descriptor
Cxbladder™ Detect, Pacific Edge Diagnostics USA, Ltd	0012M	Oncology (urothelial), mRNA, gene expression profiling by real-time quantitative PCR of five genes (*MDK, HOXA13, CDC2 [CDK1], IGFBP5,* and *CXCR2*), utilizing urine, algorithm reported as a risk score for having urothelial carcinoma
Cxbladder™ Monitor, Pacific Edge Diagnostics USA, Ltd	0013M	Oncology (urothelial), mRNA, gene expression profiling by real-time quantitative PCR of five genes (*MDK, HOXA13, CDC2 [CDK1], IGFBP5,* and *CXCR2*), utilizing urine, algorithm reported as a risk score for having recurrent urothelial carcinoma
—	►(0014M has been deleted)◄ ►(For multianalyte assay with algorithmic analysis [MAAA] for liver disease using analysis of 3 biomarkers, use 81517)◄	—
Adrenal Mass Panel, 24 Hour, Urine, Mayo Clinic Laboratories (MCL), Mayo Clinic	0015M	Adrenal cortical tumor, biochemical assay of 25 steroid markers, utilizing 24-hour urine specimen and clinical parameters, prognostic algorithm reported as a clinical risk and integrated clinical steroid risk for adrenal cortical carcinoma, adenoma, or other adrenal malignancy
Decipher Bladder, Veracyte Labs SD	0016M	Oncology (bladder), mRNA, microarray gene expression profiling of 219 genes, utilizing formalin-fixed paraffin-embedded tissue, algorithm reported as molecular subtype (luminal, luminal infiltrated, basal, basal claudin-low, neuroendocrine-like)
Lymph2Cx, Mayo Clinic Arizona Molecular Diagnostics Laboratory	0017M	Oncology (diffuse large B-cell lymphoma [DLBCL]), mRNA, gene expression profiling by fluorescent probe hybridization of 20 genes, formalin-fixed paraffin-embedded tissue, algorithm reported as cell of origin (Do not report 0017M in conjunction with 0120U)
Pleximark™, Plexision, Inc	0018M	Transplantation medicine (allograft rejection, renal), measurement of donor and third-party-induced CD154+T-cytotoxic memory cells, utilizing whole peripheral blood, algorithm reported as a rejection risk score (Do not report 0018M in conjunction with 81560, 85032, 86353, 86821, 88184, 88185, 88187, 88230, 88240, 88241)
►SOMAmer®, SomaLogic◄	●0019M	►Cardiovascular disease, plasma, analysis of protein biomarkers by aptamer-based microarray and algorithm reported as 4-year likelihood of coronary event in high-risk populations◄

★ = Telemedicine   ◄ = Audio-only   ✚ = Add-on code   ✔ = FDA approval pending   # = Resequenced code   ⊘ = Modifier 51 exempt

Proprietary Name and Clinical Laboratory or Manufacturer	Alpha-Numeric Code	Code Descriptor
Category I Codes for Multianalyte Assays with Algorithmic Analyses (MAAA)		
Vectra®, ►Labcorp◄	81490	Autoimmune (rheumatoid arthritis), analysis of 12 biomarkers using immunoassays, utilizing serum, prognostic algorithm reported as a disease activity score (Do not report 81490 in conjunction with 86140)
AlloMap®, CareDx, Inc	#81595	Cardiology (heart transplant), mRNA, gene expression profiling by real-time quantitative PCR of 20 genes (11 content and 9 housekeeping), utilizing subfraction of peripheral blood, algorithm reported as a rejection risk score
Corus® CAD, CardioDx, Inc	81493	Coronary artery disease, mRNA, gene expression profiling by real-time RT-PCR of 23 genes, utilizing whole peripheral blood, algorithm reported as a risk score
PreDx Diabetes Risk Score™, Tethys Clinical Laboratory	81506	Endocrinology (type 2 diabetes), biochemical assays of seven analytes (glucose, HbA1c, insulin, hs-CRP, adiponectin, ferritin, interleukin 2-receptor alpha), utilizing serum or plasma, algorithm reporting a risk score (Do not report 81506 in conjunction with constituent components [ie, 82728, 82947, 83036, 83525, 86141], 84999 [for adopectin], and 83520 [for interleukin 2-receptor alpha])
Harmony™ Prenatal Test, Ariosa Diagnostics	81507	Fetal aneuploidy (trisomy 21, 18, and 13) DNA sequence analysis of selected regions using maternal plasma, algorithm reported as a risk score for each trisomy (Do not report 81228, 81229, 88271 when performing genomic sequencing procedures or other molecular multianalyte assays for copy number analysis)

(Continued on page 212)

Proprietary Name and Clinical Laboratory or Manufacturer	Alpha-Numeric Code	Code Descriptor
No proprietary name and clinical laboratory or manufacturer. Maternal serum screening procedures are well-established procedures and are performed by many laboratories throughout the country. The concept of prenatal screens has existed and evolved for over 10 years and is not exclusive to any one facility.	81508	Fetal congenital abnormalities, biochemical assays of two proteins (PAPP-A, hCG [any form]), utilizing maternal serum, algorithm reported as a risk score (Do not report 81508 in conjunction with 84163, 84702)
	81509	Fetal congenital abnormalities, biochemical assays of three proteins (PAPP-A, hCG [any form], DIA), utilizing maternal serum, algorithm reported as a risk score (Do not report 81509 in conjunction with 84163, 84702, 86336)
	81510	Fetal congenital abnormalities, biochemical assays of three analytes (AFP, uE3, hCG [any form]), utilizing maternal serum, algorithm reported as a risk score (Do not report 81510 in conjunction with 82105, 82677, 84702)
	81511	Fetal congenital abnormalities, biochemical assays of four analytes (AFP, uE3, hCG [any form], DIA) utilizing maternal serum, algorithm reported as a risk score (may include additional results from previous biochemical testing) (Do not report 81511 in conjunction with 82105, 82677, 84702, 86336)
	81512	Fetal congenital abnormalities, biochemical assays of five analytes (AFP, uE3, total hCG, hyperglycosylated hCG, DIA) utilizing maternal serum, algorithm reported as a risk score (Do not report 81512 in conjunction with 82105, 82677, 84702, 86336)
Aptima® BV Assay, Hologic, Inc	81513	Infectious disease, bacterial vaginosis, quantitative real-time amplification of RNA markers for Atopobium vaginae, Gardnerella vaginalis, and Lactobacillus species, utilizing vaginal-fluid specimens, algorithm reported as a positive or negative result for bacterial vaginosis
BD MAX™ Vaginal Panel, Becton Dickinson and Company	81514	Infectious disease, bacterial vaginosis and vaginitis, quantitative real-time amplification of DNA markers for Gardnerella vaginalis, Atopobium vaginae, Megasphaera type 1, Bacterial Vaginosis Associated Bacteria-2 (BVAB-2), and Lactobacillus species (L. crispatus and L. jensenii), utilizing vaginal-fluid specimens, algorithm reported as a positive or negative for high likelihood of bacterial vaginosis, includes separate detection of Trichomonas vaginalis and/or Candida species (C. albicans, C. tropicalis, C. parapsilosis, C. dubliniensis), Candida glabrata, Candida krusei, when reported (Do not report 81514 in conjunction with 87480, 87481, 87482, 87510, 87511, 87512, 87660, 87661)

Proprietary Name and Clinical Laboratory or Manufacturer	Alpha-Numeric Code	Code Descriptor
HCV FibroSURE™, FibroTest™, BioPredictive S.A.S.	#81596	Infectious disease, chronic hepatitis C virus (HCV) infection, six biochemical assays (ALT, A2-macroglobulin, apolipoprotein A-1, total bilirubin, GGT, and haptoglobin) utilizing serum, prognostic algorithm reported as scores for fibrosis and necroinflammatory activity in liver
▶Enhanced Liver Fibrosis™ (ELF™) Test, Siemens Healthcare Diagnostics Inc/Siemens Healthcare Laboratory LLC◀	●81517	▶Liver disease, analysis of 3 biomarkers (hyaluronic acid [HA], procollagen III amino terminal peptide [PIIINP], tissue inhibitor of metalloproteinase 1 [TIMP-1]), using immunoassays, utilizing serum, prognostic algorithm reported as a risk score and risk of liver fibrosis and liver-related clinical events within 5 years◀ ▶(Do not report 81517 in conjunction with 83520 for identification of biomarkers included for liver disease analysis)◀
Breast Cancer Index, Biotheranostics, Inc	81518	Oncology (breast), mRNA, gene expression profiling by real-time RT-PCR of 11 genes (7 content and 4 housekeeping), utilizing formalin-fixed paraffin-embedded tissue, algorithms reported as percentage risk for metastatic recurrence and likelihood of benefit from extended endocrine therapy
EndoPredict®, Myriad Genetic Laboratories, Inc	#81522	Oncology (breast), mRNA, gene expression profiling by RT-PCR of 12 genes (8 content and 4 housekeeping), utilizing formalin-fixed paraffin-embedded tissue, algorithm reported as recurrence risk score
Oncotype DX®, Genomic Health	81519	Oncology (breast), mRNA, gene expression profiling by real-time RT-PCR of 21 genes, utilizing formalin-fixed paraffin-embedded tissue, algorithm reported as recurrence score
Prosigna® Breast Cancer Assay, NanoString Technologies, Inc	81520	Oncology (breast), mRNA gene expression profiling by hybrid capture of 58 genes (50 content and 8 housekeeping), utilizing formalin-fixed paraffin-embedded tissue, algorithm reported as a recurrence risk score
MammaPrint®, Agendia, Inc	81521	Oncology (breast), mRNA, microarray gene expression profiling of 70 content genes and 465 housekeeping genes, utilizing fresh frozen or formalin-fixed paraffin-embedded tissue, algorithm reported as index related to risk of distant metastasis (Do not report 81521 in conjunction with 81523 for the same specimen)
MammaPrint®, Agendia, Inc	81523	Oncology (breast), mRNA, next-generation sequencing gene expression profiling of 70 content genes and 31 housekeeping genes, utilizing formalin-fixed paraffin-embedded tissue, algorithm reported as index related to risk to distant metastasis (Do not report 81523 in conjunction with 81521 for the same specimen)

(Continued on page 214)

Appendix O

Proprietary Name and Clinical Laboratory or Manufacturer	Alpha-Numeric Code	Code Descriptor
Oncotype DX® Colon Cancer Assay, Genomic Health	81525	Oncology (colon), mRNA, gene expression profiling by real-time RT-PCR of 12 genes (7 content and 5 housekeeping), utilizing formalin-fixed paraffin-embedded tissue, algorithm reported as a recurrence score
Cologuard™, Exact Sciences, Inc	81528	Oncology (colorectal) screening, quantitative real-time target and signal amplification of 10 DNA markers (*KRAS* mutations, promoter methylation of *NDRG4* and *BMP3*) and fecal hemoglobin, utilizing stool, algorithm reported as a positive or negative result (Do not report 81528 in conjunction with 81275, 82274)
DecisionDx® Melanoma, Castle Biosciences, Inc	81529	Oncology (cutaneous melanoma), mRNA, gene expression profiling by real-time RT-PCR of 31 genes (28 content and 3 housekeeping), utilizing formalin-fixed paraffin-embedded tissue, algorithm reported as recurrence risk, including likelihood of sentinel lymph node metastasis
ChemoFX®, Helomics, Corp	81535 ✚81536	Oncology (gynecologic), live tumor cell culture and chemotherapeutic response by DAPI stain and morphology, predictive algorithm reported as a drug response score; first single drug or drug combination each additional single drug or drug combination (List separately in addition to code for primary procedure) (Use 81536 in conjunction with 81535)
VeriStrat, Biodesix, Inc	81538	Oncology (lung), mass spectrometric 8-protein signature, including amyloid A, utilizing serum, prognostic and predictive algorithm reported as good versus poor overall survival
Risk of Ovarian Malignancy Algorithm (ROMA)™, Fujirebio Diagnostics	#81500	Oncology (ovarian), biochemical assays of two proteins (CA-125 and HE4), utilizing serum, with menopausal status, algorithm reported as a risk score (Do not report 81500 in conjunction with 86304, 86305)
OVA1™, Vermillion, Inc	#81503	Oncology (ovarian), biochemical assays of five proteins (CA-125, apolipoprotein A1, beta-2 microglobulin, transferrin, and pre-albumin), utilizing serum, algorithm reported as a risk score (Do not report 81503 in conjunction with 82172, 82232, 84134, 84466, 86304)
4Kscore test, OPKO Health, Inc	81539	Oncology (high-grade prostate cancer), biochemical assay of four proteins (Total PSA, Free PSA, Intact PSA, and human kallikrein-2 [hK2]), utilizing plasma or serum, prognostic algorithm reported as a probability score

Proprietary Name and Clinical Laboratory or Manufacturer	Alpha-Numeric Code	Code Descriptor
Prolaris®, Myriad Genetic Laboratories, Inc	81541	Oncology (prostate), mRNA gene expression profiling by real-time RT-PCR of 46 genes (31 content and 15 housekeeping), utilizing formalin-fixed paraffin-embedded tissue, algorithm reported as a disease-specific mortality risk score
Decipher® Prostate, Decipher® Biosciences	81542	Oncology (prostate), mRNA, microarray gene expression profiling of 22 content genes, utilizing formalin-fixed paraffin-embedded tissue, algorithm reported as metastasis risk score
ConfirmMDx® for Prostate Cancer, MDxHealth, Inc	81551	Oncology (prostate), promoter methylation profiling by real-time PCR of 3 genes (*GSTP1, APC, RASSF1*), utilizing formalin-fixed paraffin-embedded tissue, algorithm reported as a likelihood of prostate cancer detection on repeat biopsy
Afirma® Genomic Sequencing Classifier, Veracyte, Inc	#81546	Oncology (thyroid), mRNA, gene expression analysis of 10,196 genes, utilizing fine needle aspirate, algorithm reported as a categorical result (eg, benign or suspicious)
Tissue of Origin Test Kit-FFPE, Cancer Genetics, Inc	#81504	Oncology (tissue of origin), microarray gene expression profiling of > 2000 genes, utilizing formalin-fixed paraffin-embedded tissue, algorithm reported as tissue similarity scores
CancerTYPE ID, bioTheranostics, Inc	#81540	Oncology (tumor of unknown origin), mRNA, gene expression profiling by real-time RT-PCR of 92 genes (87 content and 5 housekeeping) to classify tumor into main cancer type and subtype, utilizing formalin-fixed paraffin-embedded tissue, algorithm reported as a probability of a predicted main cancer type and subtype
DecisionDx®-UM test, Castle Biosciences, Inc	81552	Oncology (uveal melanoma), mRNA, gene expression profiling by real-time RT-PCR of 15 genes (12 content and 3 housekeeping), utilizing fine needle aspirate or formalin-fixed paraffin-embedded tissue, algorithm reported as risk of metastasis
Envisia® Genomic Classifier, Veracyte, Inc	81554	Pulmonary disease (idiopathic pulmonary fibrosis [IPF]), mRNA, gene expression analysis of 190 genes, utilizing transbronchial biopsies, diagnostic algorithm reported as categorical result (eg, positive or negative for high probability of usual interstitial pneumonia [UIP])

(Continued on page 216)

Proprietary Name and Clinical Laboratory or Manufacturer	Alpha-Numeric Code	Code Descriptor
Pleximmune™, Plexision, Inc	81560	Transplantation medicine (allograft rejection, pediatric liver and small bowel), measurement of donor and third-party-induced CD154+T-cytotoxic memory cells, utilizing whole peripheral blood, algorithm reported as a rejection risk score
		(Do not report 81560 in conjunction with 85032, 86353, 86821, 88184, 88185, 88187, 88230, 88240, 88241, 0018M)
—	81599	Unlisted multianalyte assay with algorithmic analysis
		(Do not use 81599 for multianalyte assays with algorithmic analyses listed in Appendix O)
Proprietary Laboratory Analyses (PLA)		
PreciseType® HEA Test, Immucor, Inc	0001U	Red blood cell antigen typing, DNA, human erythrocyte antigen gene analysis of 35 antigens from 11 blood groups, utilizing whole blood, common RBC alleles reported
PolypDX™, Atlantic Diagnostic Laboratories, LLC, Metabolomic Technologies, Inc	0002U	Oncology (colorectal), quantitative assessment of three urine metabolites (ascorbic acid, succinic acid and carnitine) by liquid chromatography with tandem mass spectrometry (LC-MS/MS) using multiple reaction monitoring acquisition, algorithm reported as likelihood of adenomatous polyps
Overa (OVA1 Next Generation), Asprira Labs, Inc, Vermillion, Inc	0003U	Oncology (ovarian) biochemical assays of five proteins (apolipoprotein A-1, CA 125 II, follicle stimulating hormone, human epididymis protein 4, transferrin), utilizing serum, algorithm reported as a likelihood score
ExosomeDx® Prostate (IntelliScore), Exosome Diagnostics, Inc, Exosome Diagnostics, Inc	0005U	Oncology (prostate) gene expression profile by real-time RT-PCR of 3 genes (*ERG, PCA3*, and *SPDEF*), urine, algorithm reported as risk score
ToxProtect, Genotox Laboratories LTD	0007U	Drug test(s), presumptive, with definitive confirmation of positive results, any number of drug classes, urine, includes specimen verification including DNA authentication in comparison to buccal DNA, per date of service
AmHPR® H. pylori Antibiotic Resistance Panel, American Molecular Laboratories, Inc	0008U	Helicobacter pylori detection and antibiotic resistance, DNA, 16S and 23S rRNA, gyrA, pbp1, rdxA and rpoB, next generation sequencing, formalin-fixed paraffin-embedded or fresh tissue or fecal sample, predictive, reported as positive or negative for resistance to clarithromycin, fluoroquinolones, metronidazole, amoxicillin, tetracycline, and rifabutin
DEPArray™ HER2, PacificDx	0009U	Oncology (breast cancer), *ERBB2* (HER2) copy number by FISH, tumor cells from formalin-fixed paraffin-embedded tissue isolated using image-based dielectrophoresis (DEP) sorting, reported as *ERBB2* gene amplified or non-amplified
Bacterial Typing by Whole Genome Sequencing, Mayo Clinic	0010U	Infectious disease (bacterial), strain typing by whole genome sequencing, phylogenetic-based report of strain relatedness, per submitted isolate

Proprietary Name and Clinical Laboratory or Manufacturer	Alpha-Numeric Code	Code Descriptor
Cordant CORE™, Cordant Health Solutions	0011U	Prescription drug monitoring, evaluation of drugs present by LC-MS/MS, using oral fluid, reported as a comparison to an estimated steady-state range, per date of service including all drug compounds and metabolites
—	(0012U has been deleted)	—
—	(0013U has been deleted)	—
—	(0014U has been deleted)	—
BCR-ABL1 major and minor breakpoint fusion transcripts, University of Iowa, Department of Pathology, Asuragen	0016U	Oncology (hematolymphoid neoplasia), RNA, *BCR/ABL1* major and minor breakpoint fusion transcripts, quantitative PCR amplification, blood or bone marrow, report of fusion not detected or detected with quantitation
JAK2 Mutation, University of Iowa, Department of Pathology	0017U	Oncology (hematolymphoid neoplasia), *JAK2* mutation, DNA, PCR amplification of exons 12-14 and sequence analysis, blood or bone marrow, report of *JAK2* mutation not detected or detected
ThyraMIR™, Interpace Diagnostics	0018U	Oncology (thyroid), microRNA profiling by RT-PCR of 10 microRNA sequences, utilizing fine needle aspirate, algorithm reported as a positive or negative result for moderate to high risk of malignancy
OncoTarget/OncoTreat, Columbia University Department of Pathology and Cell Biology, Darwin Health	0019U	Oncology, RNA, gene expression by whole transcriptome sequencing, formalin-fixed paraffin-embedded tissue or fresh frozen tissue, predictive algorithm reported as potential targets for therapeutic agents
Apifiny®, Armune BioScience, Inc	0021U	Oncology (prostate), detection of 8 autoantibodies (ARF 6, NKX3-1, 5'-UTR-BMI1, CEP 164, 3'-UTR-Ropporin, Desmocollin, AURKAIP-1, CSNK2A2), multiplexed immunoassay and flow cytometry serum, algorithm reported as risk score
Oncomine™ Dx Target Test, Thermo Fisher Scientific, Thermo Fisher Scientific	▲0022U	▶Targeted genomic sequence analysis panel, non-small cell lung neoplasia, DNA and RNA analysis, 23 genes, interrogation for sequence variants and rearrangements, reported as presence or absence of variants and associated therapy(ies) to consider◀
LeukoStrat® CDx *FLT3* Mutation Assay, LabPMM LLC, an Invivoscribe Technologies, Inc Company, Invivoscribe Technologies, Inc	0023U	Oncology (acute myelogenous leukemia), DNA, genotyping of internal tandem duplication, p.D835, p.I836, using mononuclear cells, reported as detection or non-detection of *FLT3* mutation and indication for or against the use of midostaurin
GlycA, Laboratory Corporation of America, Laboratory Corporation of America	0024U	Glycosylated acute phase proteins (GlycA), nuclear magnetic resonance spectroscopy, quantitative
UrSure Tenofovir Quantification Test, Synergy Medical Laboratories, UrSure Inc	0025U	Tenofovir, by liquid chromatography with tandem mass spectrometry (LC-MS/MS), urine, quantitative

(Continued on page 218)

▲ = Revised code   ● = New code   ▶◀ = Contains new or revised text   ✕ = Duplicate PLA test   ↑↓ = Category I PLA   American Medical Association   **217**

Proprietary Name and Clinical Laboratory or Manufacturer	Alpha-Numeric Code	Code Descriptor
Thyroseq Genomic Classifier, CBLPath, Inc, University of Pittsburgh Medical Center	0026U	Oncology (thyroid), DNA and mRNA of 112 genes, next-generation sequencing, fine needle aspirate of thyroid nodule, algorithmic analysis reported as a categorical result ("Positive, high probability of malignancy" or "Negative, low probability of malignancy")
JAK2 Exons 12 to 15 Sequencing, Mayo Clinic, Mayo Clinic	0027U	*JAK2 (Janus kinase 2) (eg, myeloproliferative disorder) gene analysis, targeted sequence analysis exons 12-15*
Focused Pharmacogenomics Panel, Mayo Clinic, Mayo Clinic	0029U	Drug metabolism (adverse drug reactions and drug response), targeted sequence analysis (ie, *CYP1A2, CYP2C19, CYP2C9, CYP2D6, CYP3A4, CYP3A5, CYP4F2, SLCO1B1, VKORC1* and rs12777823)
Warfarin Response Genotype, Mayo Clinic, Mayo Clinic	0030U	Drug metabolism (warfarin drug response), targeted sequence analysis (ie, *CYP2C9, CYP4F2, VKORC1,* rs12777823)
Cytochrome P450 1A2 Genotype, Mayo Clinic, Mayo Clinic	0031U	*CYP1A2 (cytochrome P450 family 1, subfamily A, member 2) (eg, drug metabolism) gene analysis, common variants (ie, *1F, *1K, *6, *7)*
Catechol-O-Methyltransferase (*COMT*) Genotype, Mayo Clinic, Mayo Clinic	0032U	*COMT (catechol-O-methyltransferase) (eg, drug metabolism) gene analysis, c.472G>A (rs4680) variant*
Serotonin Receptor Genotype (*HTR2A* and *HTR2C*), Mayo Clinic, Mayo Clinic	0033U	*HTR2A (5-hydroxytryptamine receptor 2A), HTR2C (5-hydroxytryptamine receptor 2C) (eg, citalopram metabolism) gene analysis, common variants (ie, HTR2A rs7997012 [c.614-2211T>C], HTR2C rs3813929 [c.-759C>T] and rs1414334 [c.551-3008C>G])*
Thiopurine Methyltransferase (*TPMT*) and Nudix Hydrolase (*NUDT15*) Genotyping, Mayo Clinic, Mayo Clinic	0034U	*TPMT (thiopurine S-methyltransferase), NUDT15 (nudix hydroxylase 15) (eg, thiopurine metabolism) gene analysis, common variants (ie, TPMT *2, *3A, *3B, *3C, *4, *5, *6, *8, *12; NUDT15 *3, *4, *5)*
Real-time quaking-induced conversion for prion detection (RT-QuIC), National Prion Disease Pathology Surveillance Center	0035U	Neurology (prion disease), cerebrospinal fluid, detection of prion protein by quaking-induced conformational conversion, qualitative
EXaCT-1 Whole Exome Testing, Lab of Oncology-Molecular Detection, Weill Cornell Medicine-Clinical Genomics Laboratory	0036U	Exome (ie, somatic mutations), paired formalin-fixed paraffin-embedded tumor tissue and normal specimen, sequence analyses
FoundationOne CDx™ (F1CDx), Foundation Medicine, Inc, Foundation Medicine, Inc	0037U	Targeted genomic sequence analysis, solid organ neoplasm, DNA analysis of 324 genes, interrogation for sequence variants, gene copy number amplifications, gene rearrangements, microsatellite instability and tumor mutational burden
Sensieva™ Droplet 25OH Vitamin D2/D3 Microvolume LC/MS Assay, InSource Diagnostics, InSource Diagnostics	0038U	Vitamin D, 25 hydroxy D2 and D3, by LC-MS/MS, serum microsample, quantitative

Proprietary Name and Clinical Laboratory or Manufacturer	Alpha-Numeric Code	Code Descriptor
Anti-dsDNA, High Salt/Avidity, University of Washington, Department of Laboratory Medicine, Bio-Rad	0039U	Deoxyribonucleic acid (DNA) antibody, double stranded, high avidity
MRDx BCR-ABL Test, MolecularMD, MolecularMD	0040U	*BCR/ABL1 (t(9;22))* (eg, chronic myelogenous leukemia) translocation analysis, major breakpoint, quantitative
Lyme ImmunoBlot IgM, IGeneX Inc, ID-FISH Technology Inc (ASR) (Lyme ImmunoBlot IgM Strips Only)	0041U	Borrelia burgdorferi, antibody detection of 5 recombinant protein groups, by immunoblot, IgM
Lyme ImmunoBlot IgG, IGeneX Inc, ID-FISH Technology Inc (ASR) (Lyme ImmunoBlot IgG Strips Only)	0042U	Borrelia burgdorferi, antibody detection of 12 recombinant protein groups, by immunoblot, IgG
Tick-Borne Relapsing Fever (TBRF) Borrelia ImmunoBlots IgM Test, IGeneX Inc, ID-FISH Technology (Provides TBRF ImmunoBlot IgM Strips)	0043U	Tick-borne relapsing fever Borrelia group, antibody detection to 4 recombinant protein groups, by immunoblot, IgM
Tick-Borne Relapsing Fever (TBRF) Borrelia ImmunoBlots IgG Test, IGeneX Inc, ID-FISH Technology Inc (Provides TBRF ImmunoBlot IgG Strips)	0044U	Tick-borne relapsing fever Borrelia group, antibody detection to 4 recombinant protein groups, by immunoblot, IgG
The Oncotype DX® Breast DCIS Score™ Test, Genomic Health, Inc, Genomic Health, Inc	0045U	Oncology (breast ductal carcinoma in situ), mRNA, gene expression profiling by real-time RT-PCR of 12 genes (7 content and 5 housekeeping), utilizing formalin-fixed paraffin-embedded tissue, algorithm reported as recurrence score
FLT3 ITD MRD by NGS, LabPMM LLC, an Invivoscribe Technologies, Inc Company	0046U	*FLT3 (fms-related tyrosine kinase 3)* (eg, acute myeloid leukemia) internal tandem duplication (ITD) variants, quantitative
Oncotype DX Genomic Prostate Score, Genomic Health, Inc, Genomic Health, Inc	0047U	Oncology (prostate), mRNA, gene expression profiling by real-time RT-PCR of 17 genes (12 content and 5 housekeeping), utilizing formalin-fixed paraffin-embedded tissue, algorithm reported as a risk score
MSK-IMPACT (Integrated Mutation Profiling of Actionable Cancer Targets), Memorial Sloan Kettering Cancer Center	0048U	Oncology (solid organ neoplasia), DNA, targeted sequencing of protein-coding exons of 468 cancer-associated genes, including interrogation for somatic mutations and microsatellite instability, matched with normal specimens, utilizing formalin-fixed paraffin-embedded tumor tissue, report of clinically significant mutation(s)
NPM1 MRD by NGS, LabPMM LLC, an Invivoscribe Technologies, Inc Company	0049U	*NPM1 (nucleophosmin)* (eg, acute myeloid leukemia) gene analysis, quantitative
MyAML NGS Panel, LabPMM LLC, an Invivoscribe Technologies, Inc Company	0050U	Targeted genomic sequence analysis panel, acute myelogenous leukemia, DNA analysis, 194 genes, interrogation for sequence variants, copy number variants or rearrangements

(*Continued on page 220*)

▲=Revised code   ●=New code   ▶◀=Contains new or revised text   ✸=Duplicate PLA test   ↕=Category I PLA   American Medical Association   **219**

Proprietary Name and Clinical Laboratory or Manufacturer	Alpha-Numeric Code	Code Descriptor
UCompliDx, Elite Medical Laboratory Solutions, LLC, Elite Medical Laboratory Solutions, LLC (LDT)	0051U	Prescription drug monitoring, evaluation of drugs present by liquid chromatography tandem mass spectrometry (LC-MS/MS), urine or blood, 31 drug panel, reported as quantitative results, detected or not detected, per date of service
VAP Cholesterol Test, VAP Diagnostics Laboratory, Inc, VAP Diagnostics Laboratory, Inc	0052U	Lipoprotein, blood, high resolution fractionation and quantitation of lipoproteins, including all five major lipoprotein classes and subclasses of HDL, LDL, and VLDL by vertical auto profile ultracentrifugation
—	►(0053U has been deleted)◄	—
AssuranceRx Micro Serum, Firstox Laboratories, LLC, Firstox Laboratories, LLC	0054U	Prescription drug monitoring, 14 or more classes of drugs and substances, definitive tandem mass spectrometry with chromatography, capillary blood, quantitative report with therapeutic and toxic ranges, including steady-state range for the prescribed dose when detected, per date of service
myTAIHEART, TAI Diagnostics, Inc, TAI Diagnostics, Inc	0055U	Cardiology (heart transplant), cell-free DNA, PCR assay of 96 DNA target sequences (94 single nucleotide polymorphism targets and two control targets), plasma
—	(0056U has been deleted)	—
Merkel SmT Oncoprotein Antibody Titer, University of Washington, Department of Laboratory Medicine	0058U	Oncology (Merkel cell carcinoma), detection of antibodies to the Merkel cell polyoma virus oncoprotein (small T antigen), serum, quantitative
Merkel Virus VP1 Capsid Antibody, University of Washington, Department of Laboratory Medicine	0059U	Oncology (Merkel cell carcinoma), detection of antibodies to the Merkel cell polyoma virus capsid protein (VP1), serum, reported as positive or negative
Twins Zygosity PLA, Natera, Inc, Natera, Inc	0060U	Twin zygosity, genomic-targeted sequence analysis of chromosome 2, using circulating cell-free fetal DNA in maternal blood
Transcutaneous multispectral measurement of tissue oxygenation and hemoglobin using spatial frequency domain imaging (SFDI), Modulated Imaging, Inc, Modulated Imaging, Inc	0061U	Transcutaneous measurement of five biomarkers (tissue oxygenation [StO$_2$], oxyhemoglobin [ctHbO$_2$], deoxyhemoglobin [ctHbR], papillary and reticular dermal hemoglobin concentrations [ctHb1 and ctHb2]), using spatial frequency domain imaging (SFDI) and multi-spectral analysis
SLE-key® Rule Out, Veracis Inc, Veracis Inc	0062U	Autoimmune (systemic lupus erythematosus), IgG and IgM analysis of 80 biomarkers, utilizing serum, algorithm reported with a risk score
NPDX ASD ADM Panel I, Stemina Biomarker Discovery, Inc, Stemina Biomarker Discovery, Inc d/b/a NeuroPointDX	0063U	Neurology (autism), 32 amines by LC-MS/MS, using plasma, algorithm reported as metabolic signature associated with autism spectrum disorder
BioPlex 2200 Syphilis Total & RPR Assay, Bio-Rad Laboratories, Bio-Rad Laboratories	0064U	Antibody, Treponema pallidum, total and rapid plasma reagin (RPR), immunoassay, qualitative
BioPlex 2200 RPR Assay, Bio-Rad Laboratories, Bio-Rad Laboratories	0065U	Syphilis test, non-treponemal antibody, immunoassay, qualitative (RPR)

★=Telemedicine   ◀=Audio-only   ✚=Add-on code   ✗=FDA approval pending   #=Resequenced code   ⊘=Modifier 51 exempt

Appendix O

Proprietary Name and Clinical Laboratory or Manufacturer	Alpha-Numeric Code	Code Descriptor
—	▶(0066U has been deleted)◀	—
BBDRisk Dx™, Silbiotech, Inc, Silbiotech, Inc	0067U	Oncology (breast), immunohistochemistry, protein expression profiling of 4 biomarkers (matrix metalloproteinase-1 [MMP-1], carcinoembryonic antigen-related cell adhesion molecule 6 [CEACAM6], hyaluronoglucosaminidase [HYAL1], highly expressed in cancer protein [HEC1]), formalin-fixed paraffin-embedded precancerous breast tissue, algorithm reported as carcinoma risk score
MYCODART-PCR™ Dual Amplification Real Time PCR Panel for 6 Candida species, RealTime Laboratories, Inc/MycoDART, Inc, RealTime Laboratories, Inc	0068U	Candida species panel *(C. albicans, C. glabrata, C. parapsilosis, C. kruseii, C. tropicalis,* and *C. auris)*, amplified probe technique with qualitative report of the presence or absence of each species
miR-31*now*™, GoPath Laboratories, GoPath Laboratories	0069U	Oncology (colorectal), microRNA, RT-PCR expression profiling of miR-31-3p, formalin-fixed paraffin-embedded tissue, algorithm reported as an expression score
CYP2D6 Common Variants and Copy Number, Mayo Clinic, Laboratory Developed Test	0070U	*CYP2D6 (cytochrome P450, family 2, subfamily D, polypeptide 6)* (eg, drug metabolism) gene analysis, common and select rare variants (ie, *2, *3, *4, *4N, *5, *6, *7, *8, *9, *10, *11, *12, *13, *14A, *14B, *15, *17, *29, *35, *36, *41, *57, *61, *63, *68, *83, *xN)
CYP2D6 Full Gene Sequencing, Mayo Clinic, Laboratory Developed Test	✚0071U	*CYP2D6 (cytochrome P450, family 2, subfamily D, polypeptide 6)* (eg, drug metabolism) gene analysis, full gene sequence (List separately in addition to code for primary procedure) (Use 0071U in conjunction with 0070U)
CYP2D6-2D7 Hybrid Gene Targeted Sequence Analysis, Mayo Clinic, Laboratory Developed Test	✚0072U	*CYP2D6 (cytochrome P450, family 2, subfamily D, polypeptide 6)* (eg, drug metabolism) gene analysis, targeted sequence analysis (ie, *CYP2D6-2D7* hybrid gene) (List separately in addition to code for primary procedure) (Use 0072U in conjunction with 0070U)
CYP2D7-2D6 Hybrid Gene Targeted Sequence Analysis, Mayo Clinic, Laboratory Developed Test	✚0073U	*CYP2D6 (cytochrome P450, family 2, subfamily D, polypeptide 6)* (eg, drug metabolism) gene analysis, targeted sequence analysis (ie, *CYP2D7-2D6* hybrid gene) (List separately in addition to code for primary procedure) (Use 0073U in conjunction with 0070U)
CYP2D6 trans-duplication/ multiplication non-duplicated gene targeted sequence analysis, Mayo Clinic, Laboratory Developed Test	✚0074U	*CYP2D6 (cytochrome P450, family 2, subfamily D, polypeptide 6)* (eg, drug metabolism) gene analysis, targeted sequence analysis (ie, non-duplicated gene when duplication/multiplication is trans) (List separately in addition to code for primary procedure) (Use 0074U in conjunction with 0070U)

(Continued on page 222)

Proprietary Name and Clinical Laboratory or Manufacturer	Alpha-Numeric Code	Code Descriptor
CYP2D6 5' gene duplication/ multiplication targeted sequence analysis, Mayo Clinic, Laboratory Developed Test	✚0075U	*CYP2D6 (cytochrome P450, family 2, subfamily D, polypeptide 6)* (eg, drug metabolism) gene analysis, targeted sequence analysis (ie, 5' gene duplication/ multiplication) (List separately in addition to code for primary procedure) (Use 0075U in conjunction with 0070U)
CYP2D6 3' gene duplication/ multiplication targeted sequence analysis, Mayo Clinic, Laboratory Developed Test	✚0076U	*CYP2D6 (cytochrome P450, family 2, subfamily D, polypeptide 6)* (eg, drug metabolism) gene analysis, targeted sequence analysis (ie, 3' gene duplication/ multiplication) (List separately in addition to code for primary procedure) (Use 0076U in conjunction with 0070U)
M-Protein Detection and Isotyping by MALDI-TOF Mass Spectrometry, Mayo Clinic, Laboratory Developed Test	0077U	Immunoglobulin paraprotein (M-protein), qualitative, immunoprecipitation and mass spectrometry, blood or urine, including isotype
INFINITI® Neural Response Panel, PersonalizeDx Labs, AutoGenomics Inc	0078U	Pain management (opioid-use disorder) genotyping panel, 16 common variants (ie, *ABCB1, COMT, DAT1, DBH, DOR, DRD1, DRD2, DRD4, GABA, GAL, HTR2A, HTTLPR, MTHFR, MUOR, OPRK1, OPRM1)*, buccal swab or other germline tissue sample, algorithm reported as positive or negative risk of opioid-use disorder
ToxLok™, InSource Diagnostics, InSource Diagnostics	0079U	Comparative DNA analysis using multiple selected single-nucleotide polymorphisms (SNPs), urine and buccal DNA, for specimen identity verification
BDX-XL2, Biodesix®, Inc, Biodesix®, Inc	0080U	Oncology (lung), mass spectrometric analysis of galectin-3-binding protein and scavenger receptor cysteine-rich type 1 protein M130, with five clinical risk factors (age, smoking status, nodule diameter, nodule-spiculation status and nodule location), utilizing plasma, algorithm reported as a categorical probability of malignancy
NextGen Precision™ Testing, Precision Diagnostics, Precision Diagnostics LBN Precision Toxicology, LLC	0082U	Drug test(s), definitive, 90 or more drugs or substances, definitive chromatography with mass spectrometry, and presumptive, any number of drug classes, by instrument chemistry analyzer (utilizing immunoassay), urine, report of presence or absence of each drug, drug metabolite or substance with description and severity of significant interactions per date of service
Onco4D™, Animated Dynamics, Inc, Animated Dynamics, Inc	0083U	Oncology, response to chemotherapy drugs using motility contrast tomography, fresh or frozen tissue, reported as likelihood of sensitivity or resistance to drugs or drug combinations
BLOODchip® ID CORE XT™, Grifols Diagnostic Solutions Inc	0084U	Red blood cell antigen typing, DNA, genotyping of 10 blood groups with phenotype prediction of 37 red blood cell antigens

★ =Telemedicine   ◀ =Audio-only   ✚ =Add-on code   ∧ =FDA approval pending   # =Resequenced code   ⊘ =Modifier 51 exempt

Proprietary Name and Clinical Laboratory or Manufacturer	Alpha-Numeric Code	Code Descriptor
Accelerate PhenoTest™ BC kit, Accelerate Diagnostics, Inc	0086U	Infectious disease (bacterial and fungal), organism identification, blood culture, using rRNA FISH, 6 or more organism targets, reported as positive or negative with phenotypic minimum inhibitory concentration (MIC)-based antimicrobial susceptibility
Molecular Microscope® MMDx—Heart, Kashi Clinical Laboratories	0087U	Cardiology (heart transplant), mRNA gene expression profiling by microarray of 1283 genes, transplant biopsy tissue, allograft rejection and injury algorithm reported as a probability score
Molecular Microscope® MMDx—Kidney, Kashi Clinical Laboratories	0088U	Transplantation medicine (kidney allograft rejection), microarray gene expression profiling of 1494 genes, utilizing transplant biopsy tissue, algorithm reported as a probability score for rejection
Pigmented Lesion Assay (PLA), DermTech	0089U	Oncology (melanoma), gene expression profiling by RTqPCR, *PRAME* and *LINC00518*, superficial collection using adhesive patch(es)
myPath® Melanoma, Castle Biosciences, Inc	0090U	Oncology (cutaneous melanoma), mRNA gene expression profiling by RT-PCR of 23 genes (14 content and 9 housekeeping), utilizing formalin-fixed paraffin-embedded (FFPE) tissue, algorithm reported as a categorical result (ie, benign, intermediate, malignant)
FirstSight^CRC, CellMax Life	0091U	Oncology (colorectal) screening, cell enumeration of circulating tumor cells, utilizing whole blood, algorithm, for the presence of adenoma or cancer, reported as a positive or negative result
REVEAL Lung Nodule Characterization, MagArray, Inc	0092U	Oncology (lung), three protein biomarkers, immunoassay using magnetic nanosensor technology, plasma, algorithm reported as risk score for likelihood of malignancy
ComplyRX, Claro Labs	0093U	Prescription drug monitoring, evaluation of 65 common drugs by LC-MS/MS, urine, each drug reported detected or not detected
RCIGM Rapid Whole Genome Sequencing, Rady Children's Institute for Genomic Medicine (RCIGM)	0094U	Genome (eg, unexplained constitutional or heritable disorder or syndrome), rapid sequence analysis
Esophageal String Test™ (EST), ▶Children's Hospital Colorado Department of Pathology and Laboratory Medicine◀	▲0095U	▶Eosinophilic esophagitis (Eotaxin-3 *[CCL26 {C-C motif chemokine ligand 26}]* and major basic protein *[PRG2 {proteoglycan 2, pro eosinophil major basic protein}]*), enzyme-linked immunosorbent assays (ELISA), specimen obtained by esophageal string test device, algorithm reported as probability of active or inactive eosinophilic esophagitis◀
HPV, High-Risk, Male Urine, Molecular Testing Labs	0096U	Human papillomavirus (HPV), high-risk types (ie, 16, 18, 31, 33, 35, 39, 45, 51, 52, 56, 58, 59, 66, 68), male urine
—	(0097U has been deleted)	—
—	(0098U has been deleted)	—
—	(0099U has been deleted)	—

(Continued on page 224)

▲=Revised code   ●=New code   ▶◀=Contains new or revised text   ✖=Duplicate PLA test   ↿⇂=Category I PLA   American Medical Association   **223**

Proprietary Name and Clinical Laboratory or Manufacturer	Alpha-Numeric Code	Code Descriptor
—	(0100U has been deleted)	—
ColoNext®, Ambry Genetics®, Ambry Genetics®	0101U	Hereditary colon cancer disorders (eg, Lynch syndrome, *PTEN* hamartoma syndrome, Cowden syndrome, familial adenomatosis polyposis), genomic sequence analysis panel utilizing a combination of NGS, Sanger, MLPA, and array CGH, with mRNA analytics to resolve variants of unknown significance when indicated (15 genes [sequencing and deletion/duplication], *EPCAM* and *GREM1* [deletion/duplication only])
BreastNext®, Ambry Genetics®, Ambry Genetics®	0102U	Hereditary breast cancer-related disorders (eg, hereditary breast cancer, hereditary ovarian cancer, hereditary endometrial cancer), genomic sequence analysis panel utilizing a combination of NGS, Sanger, MLPA, and array CGH, with mRNA analytics to resolve variants of unknown significance when indicated (17 genes [sequencing and deletion/duplication])
OvaNext®, Ambry Genetics®, Ambry Genetics®	0103U	Hereditary ovarian cancer (eg, hereditary ovarian cancer, hereditary endometrial cancer), genomic sequence analysis panel utilizing a combination of NGS, Sanger, MLPA, and array CGH, with mRNA analytics to resolve variants of unknown significance when indicated (24 genes [sequencing and deletion/duplication], *EPCAM* [deletion/duplication only])
KidneyIntelX™, RenalytixAI, RenalytixAI	0105U	Nephrology (chronic kidney disease), multiplex electrochemiluminescent immunoassay (ECLIA) of tumor necrosis factor receptor 1A, receptor superfamily 2 *(TNFR1, TNFR2)*, and kidney injury molecule-1 (KIM-1) combined with longitudinal clinical data, including *APOL1* genotype if available, and plasma (isolated fresh or frozen), algorithm reported as probability score for rapid kidney function decline (RKFD)
13C-Spirulina Gastric Emptying Breath Test (GEBT), Cairn Diagnostics d/b/a Advanced Breath Diagnostics, LLC, Cairn Diagnostics d/b/a Advanced Breath Diagnostics, LLC	0106U	Gastric emptying, serial collection of 7 timed breath specimens, non-radioisotope carbon-13 (^{13}C) spirulina substrate, analysis of each specimen by gas isotope ratio mass spectrometry, reported as rate of $^{13}CO_2$ excretion
Singulex Clarity C. diff toxins A/B Assay, Singulex	0107U	Clostridium difficile toxin(s) antigen detection by immunoassay technique, stool, qualitative, multiple-step method
TissueCypher® Barrett's Esophagus Assay, Cernostics, Cernostics	0108U	Gastroenterology (Barrett's esophagus), whole slide–digital imaging, including morphometric analysis, computer-assisted quantitative immunolabeling of 9 protein biomarkers (p16, AMACR, p53, CD68, COX-2, CD45RO, HIF1a, HER-2, K20) and morphology, formalin-fixed paraffin-embedded tissue, algorithm reported as risk of progression to high-grade dysplasia or cancer

★ = Telemedicine   ◀ = Audio-only   ✛ = Add-on code   ✗ = FDA approval pending   # = Resequenced code   ⊘ = Modifier 51 exempt

Proprietary Name and Clinical Laboratory or Manufacturer	Alpha-Numeric Code	Code Descriptor
MYCODART Dual Amplification Real Time PCR Panel for 4 Aspergillus species, RealTime Laboratories, Inc/MycoDART, Inc	0109U	Infectious disease (Aspergillus species), real-time PCR for detection of DNA from 4 species (*A. fumigatus, A. terreus, A. niger,* and *A. flavus),* blood, lavage fluid, or tissue, qualitative reporting of presence or absence of each species
Oral OncolyticAssuranceRX, Firstox Laboratories, LLC, Firstox Laboratories, LLC	0110U	Prescription drug monitoring, one or more oral oncology drug(s) and substances, definitive tandem mass spectrometry with chromatography, serum or plasma from capillary blood or venous blood, quantitative report with steady-state range for the prescribed drug(s) when detected
Praxis™ Extended RAS Panel, Illumina, Illumina	0111U	Oncology (colon cancer), targeted *KRAS* (codons 12, 13, and 61) and *NRAS* (codons 12, 13, and 61) gene analysis, utilizing formalin-fixed paraffin-embedded tissue
MicroGenDX qPCR & NGS For Infection, MicroGenDX, MicroGenDX	0112U	Infectious agent detection and identification, targeted sequence analysis (16S and 18S rRNA genes) with drug-resistance gene
▶MyProstateScore, Lynx DX, Lynx DX◀	0113U	Oncology (prostate), measurement of *PCA3* and *TMPRSS2-ERG* in urine and PSA in serum following prostatic massage, by RNA amplification and fluorescence-based detection, algorithm reported as risk score
EsoGuard™, Lucid Diagnostics, Lucid Diagnostics	0114U	Gastroenterology (Barrett's esophagus), *VIM* and *CCNA1* methylation analysis, esophageal cells, algorithm reported as likelihood for Barrett's esophagus
ePlex Respiratory Pathogen (RP) Panel, GenMark Diagnostics, Inc, GenMark Diagnostics, Inc	0115U	Respiratory infectious agent detection by nucleic acid (DNA and RNA), 18 viral types and subtypes and 2 bacterial targets, amplified probe technique, including multiplex reverse transcription for RNA targets, each analyte reported as detected or not detected
Snapshot Oral Fluid Compliance, Ethos Laboratories	0116U	Prescription drug monitoring, enzyme immunoassay of 35 or more drugs confirmed with LC-MS/MS, oral fluid, algorithm results reported as a patient-compliance measurement with risk of drug to drug interactions for prescribed medications
Foundation PI℠, Ethos Laboratories	0117U	Pain management, analysis of 11 endogenous analytes (methylmalonic acid, xanthurenic acid, homocysteine, pyroglutamic acid, vanilmandelate, 5-hydroxyindoleacetic acid, hydroxymethylglutarate, ethylmalonate, 3-hydroxypropyl mercapturic acid (3-HPMA), quinolinic acid, kynurenic acid), LC-MS/MS, urine, algorithm reported as a pain-index score with likelihood of atypical biochemical function associated with pain
Viracor TRAC™ dd-cfDNA, Viracor Eurofins, Viracor Eurofins	0118U	Transplantation medicine, quantification of donor-derived cell-free DNA using whole genome next-generation sequencing, plasma, reported as percentage of donor-derived cell-free DNA in the total cell-free DNA

(Continued on page 226)

▲ = Revised code   ● = New code   ▶ ◀ = Contains new or revised text   ✕ = Duplicate PLA test   ⇅ = Category I PLA   American Medical Association   **225**

Proprietary Name and Clinical Laboratory or Manufacturer	Alpha-Numeric Code	Code Descriptor
MI-HEART Ceramides, Plasma, Mayo Clinic, Laboratory Developed Test	0119U	Cardiology, ceramides by liquid chromatography–tandem mass spectrometry, plasma, quantitative report with risk score for major cardiovascular events
Lymph3Cx Lymphoma Molecular Subtyping Assay, Mayo Clinic, Laboratory Developed Test	0120U	Oncology (B-cell lymphoma classification), mRNA, gene expression profiling by fluorescent probe hybridization of 58 genes (45 content and 13 housekeeping genes), formalin-fixed paraffin-embedded tissue, algorithm reported as likelihood for primary mediastinal B-cell lymphoma (PMBCL) and diffuse large B-cell lymphoma (DLBCL) with cell of origin subtyping in the latter (Do not report 0120U in conjunction with 0017M)
Flow Adhesion of Whole Blood on VCAM-1 (FAB-V), Functional Fluidics, Functional Fluidics	0121U	Sickle cell disease, microfluidic flow adhesion (VCAM-1), whole blood
Flow Adhesion of Whole Blood to P-SELECTIN (WB-PSEL), Functional Fluidics, Functional Fluidics	0122U	Sickle cell disease, microfluidic flow adhesion (P-Selectin), whole blood
Mechanical Fragility, RBC by shear stress profiling and spectral analysis, Functional Fluidics, Functional Fluidics	0123U	Mechanical fragility, RBC, shear stress and spectral analysis profiling
BRCAplus, Ambry Genetics	0129U	Hereditary breast cancer–related disorders (eg, hereditary breast cancer, hereditary ovarian cancer, hereditary endometrial cancer), genomic sequence analysis and deletion/duplication analysis panel *(ATM, BRCA1, BRCA2, CDH1, CHEK2, PALB2, PTEN,* and *TP53)*
+RNAinsight™ for ColoNext®, Ambry Genetics	+0130U	Hereditary colon cancer disorders (eg, Lynch syndrome, PTEN hamartoma syndrome, Cowden syndrome, familial adenomatosis polyposis), targeted mRNA sequence analysis panel *(APC, CDH1, CHEK2, MLH1, MSH2, MSH6, MUTYH, PMS2, PTEN,* and *TP53)* (List separately in addition to code for primary procedure) (Use 0130U in conjunction with 81435, 0101U)
+RNAinsight™ for BreastNext®, Ambry Genetics	+0131U	Hereditary breast cancer–related disorders (eg, hereditary breast cancer, hereditary ovarian cancer, hereditary endometrial cancer), targeted mRNA sequence analysis panel (13 genes) (List separately in addition to code for primary procedure) (Use 0131U in conjunction with 81162, 81432, 0102U)
+RNAinsight™ for OvaNext®, Ambry Genetics	+0132U	Hereditary ovarian cancer–related disorders (eg, hereditary breast cancer, hereditary ovarian cancer, hereditary endometrial cancer), targeted mRNA sequence analysis panel (17 genes) (List separately in addition to code for primary procedure) (Use 0132U in conjunction with 81162, 81432, 0103U)

Proprietary Name and Clinical Laboratory or Manufacturer	Alpha-Numeric Code	Code Descriptor
+RNAinsight™ for ProstateNext®, Ambry Genetics	✚0133U	Hereditary prostate cancer–related disorders, targeted mRNA sequence analysis panel (11 genes) (List separately in addition to code for primary procedure) (Use 0133U in conjunction with 81162)
+RNAinsight™ for CancerNext®, Ambry Genetics	✚0134U	Hereditary pan cancer (eg, hereditary breast and ovarian cancer, hereditary endometrial cancer, hereditary colorectal cancer), targeted mRNA sequence analysis panel (18 genes) (List separately in addition to code for primary procedure) (Use 0134U in conjunction with 81162, 81432, 81435)
+RNAinsight™ for GYNPlus®, Ambry Genetics	✚0135U	Hereditary gynecological cancer (eg, hereditary breast and ovarian cancer, hereditary endometrial cancer, hereditary colorectal cancer), targeted mRNA sequence analysis panel (12 genes) (List separately in addition to code for primary procedure) (Use 0135U in conjunction with 81162)
+RNAinsight™ for *ATM*, Ambry Genetics	✚0136U	*ATM (ataxia telangiectasia mutated)* (eg, ataxia telangiectasia) mRNA sequence analysis (List separately in addition to code for primary procedure) (Use 0136U in conjunction with 81408)
+RNAinsight™ for *PALB2*, Ambry Genetics	✚0137U	*PALB2 (partner and localizer of BRCA2)* (eg, breast and pancreatic cancer) mRNA sequence analysis (List separately in addition to code for primary procedure) (Use 0137U in conjunction with 81307)
+RNAinsight™ for *BRCA1/2*, Ambry Genetics	✚0138U	*BRCA1 (BRCA1, DNA repair associated), BRCA2 (BRCA2, DNA repair associated)* (eg, hereditary breast and ovarian cancer) mRNA sequence analysis (List separately in addition to code for primary procedure) (Use 0138U in conjunction with 81162)
—	(0139U has been deleted)	—
ePlex® BCID Fungal Pathogens Panel, GenMark Diagnostics, Inc, GenMark Diagnostics, Inc	0140U	Infectious disease (fungi), fungal pathogen identification, DNA (15 fungal targets), blood culture, amplified probe technique, each target reported as detected or not detected
ePlex® BCID Gram-Positive Panel, GenMark Diagnostics, Inc, GenMark Diagnostics, Inc	0141U	Infectious disease (bacteria and fungi), gram-positive organism identification and drug resistance element detection, DNA (20 gram-positive bacterial targets, 4 resistance genes, 1 pan gram-negative bacterial target, 1 pan Candida target), blood culture, amplified probe technique, each target reported as detected or not detected
ePlex® BCID Gram-Negative Panel, GenMark Diagnostics, Inc, GenMark Diagnostics, Inc	0142U	Infectious disease (bacteria and fungi), gram-negative bacterial identification and drug resistance element detection, DNA (21 gram-negative bacterial targets, 6 resistance genes, 1 pan gram-positive bacterial target, 1 pan Candida target), amplified probe technique, each target reported as detected or not detected

(Continued on page 228)

Proprietary Name and Clinical Laboratory or Manufacturer	Alpha-Numeric Code	Code Descriptor
—	▶(0143U has been deleted)◀	—
—	▶(0144U has been deleted)◀	—
—	▶(0145U has been deleted)◀	—
—	▶(0146U has been deleted)◀	—
—	▶(0147U has been deleted)◀	—
—	▶(0148U has been deleted)◀	—
—	▶(0149U has been deleted)◀	—
—	▶(0150U has been deleted)◀	—
—	(0151U has been deleted)	—
Karius® Test, Karius Inc, Karius Inc	0152U	Infectious disease (bacteria, fungi, parasites, and DNA viruses), microbial cell-free DNA, plasma, untargeted next-generation sequencing, report for significant positive pathogens
Insight TNBCtype™, Insight Molecular Labs	0153U	Oncology (breast), mRNA, gene expression profiling by next-generation sequencing of 101 genes, utilizing formalin-fixed paraffin-embedded tissue, algorithm reported as a triple negative breast cancer clinical subtype(s) with information on immune cell involvement
therascreen® *FGFR* RGQ RT-PCR Kit, QIAGEN, QIAGEN GmbH	0154U	Oncology (urothelial cancer), RNA, analysis by real-time RT-PCR of the *FGFR3 (fibroblast growth factor receptor 3)* gene analysis (ie, p.R248C [c.742C>T], p.S249C [c.746C>G], p.G370C [c.1108G>T], p.Y373C [c.1118A>G], FGFR3-TACC3v1, and FGFR3-TACC3v3), utilizing formalin-fixed paraffin-embedded urothelial cancer tumor tissue, reported as *FGFR* gene alteration status
therascreen *PIK3CA* RGQ PCR Kit, QIAGEN, QIAGEN GmbH	0155U	Oncology (breast cancer), DNA, *PIK3CA (phosphatidylinositol-4,5-bisphosphate 3-kinase, catalytic subunit alpha)* (eg, breast cancer) gene analysis (ie, p.C420R, p.E542K, p.E545A, p.E545D [g.1635G>T only], p.E545G, p.E545K, p.Q546E, p.Q546R, p.H1047L, p.H1047R, p.H1047Y), utilizing formalin-fixed paraffin-embedded breast tumor tissue, reported as *PIK3CA* gene mutation status
SMASH™, New York Genome Center, Marvel Genomics™	0156U	Copy number (eg, intellectual disability, dysmorphology), sequence analysis

★ = Telemedicine   ◀ = Audio-only   ✛ = Add-on code   ✚ = FDA approval pending   # = Resequenced code   ⊘ = Modifier 51 exempt

Proprietary Name and Clinical Laboratory or Manufacturer	Alpha-Numeric Code	Code Descriptor
CustomNext + RNA: *APC*, Ambry Genetics®, Ambry Genetics®	✚0157U	*APC (APC regulator of WNT signaling pathway)* (eg, familial adenomatosis polyposis [FAP]) mRNA sequence analysis (List separately in addition to code for primary procedure) (Use 0157U in conjunction with 81201)
CustomNext + RNA: *MLH1*, Ambry Genetics®, Ambry Genetics®	✚0158U	*MLH1 (mutL homolog 1)* (eg, hereditary non-polyposis colorectal cancer, Lynch syndrome) mRNA sequence analysis (List separately in addition to code for primary procedure) (Use 0158U in conjunction with 81292)
CustomNext + RNA: *MSH2*, Ambry Genetics®, Ambry Genetics®	✚0159U	*MSH2 (mutS homolog 2)* (eg, hereditary colon cancer, Lynch syndrome) mRNA sequence analysis (List separately in addition to code for primary procedure) (Use 0159U in conjunction with 81295)
CustomNext + RNA: *MSH6*, Ambry Genetics®, Ambry Genetics®	✚0160U	*MSH6 (mutS homolog 6)* (eg, hereditary colon cancer, Lynch syndrome) mRNA sequence analysis (List separately in addition to code for primary procedure) (Use 0160U in conjunction with 81298)
CustomNext + RNA: *PMS2*, Ambry Genetics®, Ambry Genetics®	✚0161U	*PMS2 (PMS1 homolog 2, mismatch repair system component)* (eg, hereditary non-polyposis colorectal cancer, Lynch syndrome) mRNA sequence analysis (List separately in addition to code for primary procedure) (Use 0161U in conjunction with 81317)
CustomNext + RNA: Lynch *(MLH1, MSH2, MSH6, PMS2)*, Ambry Genetics®, Ambry Genetics®	✚0162U	Hereditary colon cancer (Lynch syndrome), targeted mRNA sequence analysis panel *(MLH1, MSH2, MSH6, PMS2)* (List separately in addition to code for primary procedure) (Use 0162U in conjunction with 81292, 81295, 81298, 81317, 81435)
BeScreened™-CRC, Beacon Biomedical Inc, Beacon Biomedical Inc	0163U	Oncology (colorectal) screening, biochemical enzyme-linked immunosorbent assay (ELISA) of 3 plasma or serum proteins (teratocarcinoma derived growth factor-1 [TDGF-1, Cripto-1], carcinoembryonic antigen [CEA], extracellular matrix protein [ECM]), with demographic data (age, gender, CRC-screening compliance) using a proprietary algorithm and reported as likelihood of CRC or advanced adenomas
ibs-smart™, Gemelli Biotech, Gemelli Biotech	0164U	Gastroenterology (irritable bowel syndrome [IBS]), immunoassay for anti-CdtB and anti-vinculin antibodies, utilizing plasma, algorithm for elevated or not elevated qualitative results
VeriMAP™ Peanut Dx – Bead-based Epitope Assay, AllerGenis™ Clinical Laboratory, AllerGenis™ LLC	0165U	Peanut allergen-specific quantitative assessment of multiple epitopes using enzyme-linked immunosorbent assay (ELISA), blood, individual epitope results and probability of peanut allergy

(Continued on page 230)

Proprietary Name and Clinical Laboratory or Manufacturer	Alpha-Numeric Code	Code Descriptor
LiverFASt™, Fibronostics	0166U	Liver disease, 10 biochemical assays (α2-macroglobulin, haptoglobin, apolipoprotein A1, bilirubin, GGT, ALT, AST, triglycerides, cholesterol, fasting glucose) and biometric and demographic data, utilizing serum, algorithm reported as scores for fibrosis, necroinflammatory activity, and steatosis with a summary interpretation
ADEXUSDx hCG Test, NOWDiagnostics, NOWDiagnostics	0167U	Gonadotropin, chorionic (hCG), immunoassay with direct optical observation, blood
—	(0168U has been deleted)	—
NT (*NUDT15* and *TPMT*) genotyping panel, RPRD Diagnostics	0169U	*NUDT15 (nudix hydrolase 15)* and *TPMT (thiopurine S-methyltransferase)* (eg, drug metabolism) gene analysis, common variants
Clarifi™, Quadrant Biosciences, Inc, Quadrant Biosciences, Inc	0170U	Neurology (autism spectrum disorder [ASD]), RNA, next-generation sequencing, saliva, algorithmic analysis, and results reported as predictive probability of ASD diagnosis
MyMRD® NGS Panel, Laboratory for Personalized Molecular Medicine, Laboratory for Personalized Molecular Medicine	0171U	Targeted genomic sequence analysis panel, acute myeloid leukemia, myelodysplastic syndrome, and myeloproliferative neoplasms, DNA analysis, 23 genes, interrogation for sequence variants, rearrangements and minimal residual disease, reported as presence/absence
myChoice® CDx, Myriad Genetics Laboratories, Inc, Myriad Genetics Laboratories, Inc	0172U	Oncology (solid tumor as indicated by the label), somatic mutation analysis of *BRCA1 (BRCA1, DNA repair associated), BRCA2 (BRCA2, DNA repair associated)* and analysis of homologous recombination deficiency pathways, DNA, formalin-fixed paraffin-embedded tissue, algorithm quantifying tumor genomic instability score
Psych HealthPGx Panel, RPRD Diagnostics, RPRD Diagnostics	0173U	Psychiatry (ie, depression, anxiety), genomic analysis panel, includes variant analysis of 14 genes
LC-MS/MS Targeted Proteomic Assay, OncoOmicDx Laboratory, LDT	0174U	Oncology (solid tumor), mass spectrometric 30 protein targets, formalin-fixed paraffin-embedded tissue, prognostic and predictive algorithm reported as likely, unlikely, or uncertain benefit of 39 chemotherapy and targeted therapeutic oncology agents
Genomind® Professional PGx Express™ CORE, Genomind, Inc, Genomind, Inc	0175U	Psychiatry (eg, depression, anxiety), genomic analysis panel, variant analysis of 15 genes
IB*Schek*®, Commonwealth Diagnostics International, Inc, Commonwealth Diagnostics International, Inc	0176U	Cytolethal distending toxin B (CdtB) and vinculin IgG antibodies by immunoassay (ie, ELISA)
therascreen® *PIK3CA* RGQ PCR Kit, QIAGEN, QIAGEN GmbH	0177U	Oncology (breast cancer), DNA, *PIK3CA (phosphatidylinositol-4,5-bisphosphate 3-kinase catalytic subunit alpha)* gene analysis of 11 gene variants utilizing plasma, reported as *PIK3CA* gene mutation status

Appendix O

Proprietary Name and Clinical Laboratory or Manufacturer	Alpha-Numeric Code	Code Descriptor
VeriMAP™ Peanut Reactivity Threshold–Bead Based Epitope Assay, AllerGenis™ Clinical Laboratory, AllerGenis™ LLC	0178U	Peanut allergen-specific quantitative assessment of multiple epitopes using enzyme-linked immunosorbent assay (ELISA), blood, report of minimum eliciting exposure for a clinical reaction
Resolution ctDx Lung™, Resolution Bioscience, Resolution Bioscience, Inc	0179U	Oncology (non-small cell lung cancer), cell-free DNA, targeted sequence analysis of 23 genes (single nucleotide variations, insertions and deletions, fusions without prior knowledge of partner/breakpoint, copy number variations), with report of significant mutation(s)
Navigator ABO Sequencing, Grifols Immunohematology Center, Grifols Immunohematology Center	0180U	Red cell antigen (ABO blood group) genotyping (ABO), gene analysis Sanger/chain termination/conventional sequencing, *ABO (ABO, alpha 1-3-N-acetylgalactosaminyltransferase and alpha 1-3-galactosyltransferase)* gene, including subtyping, 7 exons
Navigator CO Sequencing, Grifols Immunohematology Center, Grifols Immunohematology Center	0181U	Red cell antigen (Colton blood group) genotyping (CO), gene analysis, *AQP1 (aquaporin 1 [Colton blood group])* exon 1
Navigator CROM Sequencing, Grifols Immunohematology Center, Grifols Immunohematology Center	0182U	Red cell antigen (Cromer blood group) genotyping (CROM), gene analysis, *CD55 (CD55 molecule [Cromer blood group])* exons 1-10
Navigator DI Sequencing, Grifols Immunohematology Center, Grifols Immunohematology Center	0183U	Red cell antigen (Diego blood group) genotyping (DI), gene analysis, *SLC4A1 (solute carrier family 4 member 1 [Diego blood group])* exon 19
Navigator DO Sequencing, Grifols Immunohematology Center, Grifols Immunohematology Center	0184U	Red cell antigen (Dombrock blood group) genotyping (DO), gene analysis, *ART4 (ADP-ribosyltransferase 4 [Dombrock blood group])* exon 2
Navigator FUT1 Sequencing, Grifols Immunohematology Center, Grifols Immunohematology Center	0185U	Red cell antigen (H blood group) genotyping (FUT1), gene analysis, *FUT1 (fucosyltransferase 1 [H blood group])* exon 4
Navigator FUT2 Sequencing, Grifols Immunohematology Center, Grifols Immunohematology Center	0186U	Red cell antigen (H blood group) genotyping (FUT2), gene analysis, *FUT2 (fucosyltransferase 2)* exon 2
Navigator FY Sequencing, Grifols Immunohematology Center, Grifols Immunohematology Center	0187U	Red cell antigen (Duffy blood group) genotyping (FY), gene analysis, *ACKR1 (atypical chemokine receptor 1 [Duffy blood group])* exons 1-2
Navigator GE Sequencing, Grifols Immunohematology Center, Grifols Immunohematology Center	0188U	Red cell antigen (Gerbich blood group) genotyping (GE), gene analysis, *GYPC (glycophorin C [Gerbich blood group])* exons 1-4
Navigator GYPA Sequencing, Grifols Immunohematology Center, Grifols Immunohematology Center	0189U	Red cell antigen (MNS blood group) genotyping (GYPA), gene analysis, *GYPA (glycophorin A [MNS blood group])* introns 1, 5, exon 2
Navigator GYPB Sequencing, Grifols Immunohematology Center, Grifols Immunohematology Center	0190U	Red cell antigen (MNS blood group) genotyping (GYPB), gene analysis, *GYPB (glycophorin B [MNS blood group])* introns 1, 5, pseudoexon 3
Navigator IN Sequencing, Grifols Immunohematology Center, Grifols Immunohematology Center	0191U	Red cell antigen (Indian blood group) genotyping (IN), gene analysis, *CD44 (CD44 molecule [Indian blood group])* exons 2, 3, 6

(Continued on page 232)

Proprietary Name and Clinical Laboratory or Manufacturer	Alpha-Numeric Code	Code Descriptor
Navigator JK Sequencing, Grifols Immunohematology Center, Grifols Immunohematology Center	0192U	Red cell antigen (Kidd blood group) genotyping (JK), gene analysis, *SLC14A1 (solute carrier family 14 member 1 [Kidd blood group])* gene promoter, exon 9
Navigator JR Sequencing, Grifols Immunohematology Center, Grifols Immunohematology Center	0193U	Red cell antigen (JR blood group) genotyping (JR), gene analysis, *ABCG2 (ATP binding cassette subfamily G member 2 [Junior blood group])* exons 2-26
Navigator KEL Sequencing, Grifols Immunohematology Center, Grifols Immunohematology Center	0194U	Red cell antigen (Kell blood group) genotyping (KEL), gene analysis, *KEL (Kell metallo-endopeptidase [Kell blood group])* exon 8
Navigator *KLF1* Sequencing, Grifols Immunohematology Center, Grifols Immunohematology Center	0195U	*KLF1 (Kruppel-like factor 1)*, targeted sequencing (ie, exon 13)
Navigator LU Sequencing, Grifols Immunohematology Center, Grifols Immunohematology Center	0196U	Red cell antigen (Lutheran blood group) genotyping (LU), gene analysis, *BCAM (basal cell adhesion molecule [Lutheran blood group])* exon 3
Navigator LW Sequencing, Grifols Immunohematology Center, Grifols Immunohematology Center	0197U	Red cell antigen (Landsteiner-Wiener blood group) genotyping (LW), gene analysis, *ICAM4 (intercellular adhesion molecule 4 [Landsteiner-Wiener blood group])* exon 1
Navigator RHD/CE Sequencing, Grifols Immunohematology Center, Grifols Immunohematology Center	0198U	Red cell antigen (RH blood group) genotyping (RHD and RHCE), gene analysis Sanger/chain termination/conventional sequencing, *RHD (Rh blood group D antigen) exons 1-10 and RHCE (Rh blood group CcEe antigens)* exon 5
Navigator SC Sequencing, Grifols Immunohematology Center, Grifols Immunohematology Center	0199U	Red cell antigen (Scianna blood group) genotyping (SC), gene analysis, *ERMAP (erythroblast membrane associated protein [Scianna blood group])* exons 4, 12
Navigator XK Sequencing, Grifols Immunohematology Center, Grifols Immunohematology Center	0200U	Red cell antigen (Kx blood group) genotyping (XK), gene analysis, *XK (X-linked Kx blood group)* exons 1-3
Navigator YT Sequencing, Grifols Immunohematology Center, Grifols Immunohematology Center	0201U	Red cell antigen (Yt blood group) genotyping (YT), gene analysis, *ACHE (acetylcholinesterase [Cartwright blood group])* exon 2
BioFire® Respiratory Panel 2.1 (RP2.1), BioFire® Diagnostics, BioFire® Diagnostics, LLC	✳0202U	Infectious disease (bacterial or viral respiratory tract infection), pathogen-specific nucleic acid (DNA or RNA), 22 targets including severe acute respiratory syndrome coronavirus 2 (SARS-CoV-2), qualitative RT-PCR, nasopharyngeal swab, each pathogen reported as detected or not detected (For additional PLA code with identical clinical descriptor, see 0223U. See Appendix O or the most current listing on the AMA CPT website to determine appropriate code assignment)
PredictSURE IBD™ Test, KSL Diagnostics, PredictImmune Ltd	0203U	Autoimmune (inflammatory bowel disease), mRNA, gene expression profiling by quantitative RT-PCR, 17 genes (15 target and 2 reference genes), whole blood, reported as a continuous risk score and classification of inflammatory bowel disease aggressiveness

Proprietary Name and Clinical Laboratory or Manufacturer	Alpha-Numeric Code	Code Descriptor
Afirma Xpression Atlas, Veracyte, Inc, Veracyte, Inc	0204U	Oncology (thyroid), mRNA, gene expression analysis of 593 genes (including *BRAF, RAS, RET, PAX8,* and *NTRK)* for sequence variants and rearrangements, utilizing fine needle aspirate, reported as detected or not detected
Vita Risk®, Arctic Medical Laboratories, Arctic Medical Laboratories	0205U	Ophthalmology (age-related macular degeneration), analysis of 3 gene variants (2 *CFH* gene, 1 *ARMS2* gene), using PCR and MALDI-TOF, buccal swab, reported as positive or negative for neovascular age-related macular-degeneration risk associated with zinc supplements
DISCERN™, NeuroDiagnostics, NeuroDiagnostics	0206U	Neurology (Alzheimer disease); cell aggregation using morphometric imaging and protein kinase C-epsilon (PKCe) concentration in response to amylospheroid treatment by ELISA, cultured skin fibroblasts, each reported as positive or negative for Alzheimer disease
	+0207U	quantitative imaging of phosphorylated *ERK1* and *ERK2* in response to bradykinin treatment by in situ immunofluorescence, using cultured skin fibroblasts, reported as a probability index for Alzheimer disease (List separately in addition to code for primary procedure) (Use 0207U in conjunction with 0206U)
—	(0208U has been deleted)	—
CNGnome™, PerkinElmer Genomics, PerkinElmer Genomics	0209U	Cytogenomic constitutional (genome-wide) analysis, interrogation of genomic regions for copy number, structural changes and areas of homozygosity for chromosomal abnormalities
BioPlex 2200 RPR Assay – Quantitative, Bio-Rad Laboratories, Bio-Rad Laboratories	0210U	Syphilis test, non-treponemal antibody, immunoassay, quantitative (RPR)
MI Cancer Seek™ - NGS Analysis, Caris MPI d/b/a Caris Life Sciences, Caris MPI d/b/a Caris Life Sciences	0211U	Oncology (pan-tumor), DNA and RNA by next-generation sequencing, utilizing formalin-fixed paraffin-embedded tissue, interpretative report for single nucleotide variants, copy number alterations, tumor mutational burden, and microsatellite instability, with therapy association
Genomic Unity® Whole Genome Analysis – Proband, Variantyx Inc, Variantyx Inc	0212U	Rare diseases (constitutional/heritable disorders), whole genome and mitochondrial DNA sequence analysis, including small sequence changes, deletions, duplications, short tandem repeat gene expansions, and variants in non-uniquely mappable regions, blood or saliva, identification and categorization of genetic variants, proband (Do not report 0212U in conjunction with 81425)

(Continued on page 234)

Proprietary Name and Clinical Laboratory or Manufacturer	Alpha-Numeric Code	Code Descriptor
Genomic Unity® Whole Genome Analysis – Comparator, Variantyx Inc, Variantyx Inc	0213U	Rare diseases (constitutional/heritable disorders), whole genome and mitochondrial DNA sequence analysis, including small sequence changes, deletions, duplications, short tandem repeat gene expansions, and variants in non-uniquely mappable regions, blood or saliva, identification and categorization of genetic variants, each comparator genome (eg, parent, sibling) (Do not report 0213U in conjunction with 81426)
Genomic Unity® Exome Plus Analysis – Proband, Variantyx Inc, Variantyx Inc	0214U	Rare diseases (constitutional/heritable disorders), whole exome and mitochondrial DNA sequence analysis, including small sequence changes, deletions, duplications, short tandem repeat gene expansions, and variants in non-uniquely mappable regions, blood or saliva, identification and categorization of genetic variants, proband (Do not report 0214U in conjunction with 81415)
Genomic Unity® Exome Plus Analysis – Comparator, Variantyx Inc, Variantyx Inc	0215U	Rare diseases (constitutional/heritable disorders), whole exome and mitochondrial DNA sequence analysis, including small sequence changes, deletions, duplications, short tandem repeat gene expansions, and variants in non-uniquely mappable regions, blood or saliva, identification and categorization of genetic variants, each comparator exome (eg, parent, sibling) (Do not report 0215U in conjunction with 81416)
Genomic Unity® Ataxia Repeat Expansion and Sequence Analysis, Variantyx Inc, Variantyx Inc	0216U	Neurology (inherited ataxias), genomic DNA sequence analysis of 12 common genes including small sequence changes, deletions, duplications, short tandem repeat gene expansions, and variants in non-uniquely mappable regions, blood or saliva, identification and categorization of genetic variants
Genomic Unity® Comprehensive Ataxia Repeat Expansion and Sequence Analysis, Variantyx Inc, Variantyx Inc	0217U	Neurology (inherited ataxias), genomic DNA sequence analysis of 51 genes including small sequence changes, deletions, duplications, short tandem repeat gene expansions, and variants in non-uniquely mappable regions, blood or saliva, identification and categorization of genetic variants
Genomic Unity® DMD Analysis, Variantyx Inc, Variantyx Inc	0218U	Neurology (muscular dystrophy), *DMD* gene sequence analysis, including small sequence changes, deletions, duplications, and variants in non-uniquely mappable regions, blood or saliva, identification and characterization of genetic variants
Sentosa® SQ HIV-1 Genotyping Assay, Vela Diagnostics USA, Inc, Vela Operations Singapore Pte Ltd	0219U	Infectious agent (human immunodeficiency virus), targeted viral next-generation sequence analysis (ie, protease [PR], reverse transcriptase [RT], integrase [INT]), algorithm reported as prediction of antiviral drug susceptibility
PreciseDx™ Breast Cancer Test, PreciseDx, PreciseDx	0220U	Oncology (breast cancer), image analysis with artificial intelligence assessment of 12 histologic and immunohistochemical features, reported as a recurrence score

★ =Telemedicine ◀ =Audio-only ✚ =Add-on code 𝒩 =FDA approval pending # =Resequenced code ⊘ =Modifier 51 exempt

Proprietary Name and Clinical Laboratory or Manufacturer	Alpha-Numeric Code	Code Descriptor
Navigator ABO Blood Group NGS, Grifols Immunohematology Center, Grifols Immunohematology Center	0221U	Red cell antigen (ABO blood group) genotyping (ABO), gene analysis, next-generation sequencing, *ABO (ABO, alpha 1-3-N-acetylgalactosaminyltransferase and alpha 1-3-galactosyltransferase)* gene
Navigator Rh Blood Group NGS, Grifols Immunohematology Center, Grifols Immunohematology Center	0222U	Red cell antigen (RH blood group) genotyping (RHD and RHCE), gene analysis, next-generation sequencing, RH proximal promoter, exons 1-10, portions of introns 2-3
QIAstat-Dx Respiratory SARS CoV-2 Panel, QIAGEN Sciences, QIAGEN GmbH	✕0223U	Infectious disease (bacterial or viral respiratory tract infection), pathogen-specific nucleic acid (DNA or RNA), 22 targets including severe acute respiratory syndrome coronavirus 2 (SARS-CoV-2), qualitative RT-PCR, nasopharyngeal swab, each pathogen reported as detected or not detected (For additional PLA code with identical clinical descriptor, see 0202U. See Appendix O or the most current listing on the AMA CPT website to determine appropriate code assignment)
COVID-19 Antibody Test, Mt Sinai, Mount Sinai Laboratory	0224U	Antibody, severe acute respiratory syndrome coronavirus 2 (SARS-CoV-2) (coronavirus disease [COVID-19]), includes titer(s), when performed (Do not report 0224U in conjunction with 86769)
ePlex® Respiratory Pathogen Panel 2, GenMark Dx, GenMark Diagnostics, Inc	0225U	Infectious disease (bacterial or viral respiratory tract infection) pathogen-specific DNA and RNA, 21 targets, including severe acute respiratory syndrome coronavirus 2 (SARS-CoV-2), amplified probe technique, including multiplex reverse transcription for RNA targets, each analyte reported as detected or not detected
Tru-Immune™, Ethos Laboratories, GenScript® USA Inc	0226U	Surrogate viral neutralization test (sVNT), severe acute respiratory syndrome coronavirus 2 (SARS-CoV-2) (coronavirus disease [COVID-19]), ELISA, plasma, serum
Comprehensive Screen, Aspenti Health	0227U	Drug assay, presumptive, 30 or more drugs or metabolites, urine, liquid chromatography with tandem mass spectrometry (LC-MS/MS) using multiple reaction monitoring (MRM), with drug or metabolite description, includes sample validation
PanGIA Prostate, Genetics Institute of America, Entopsis, LLC	0228U	Oncology (prostate), multianalyte molecular profile by photometric detection of macromolecules adsorbed on nanosponge array slides with machine learning, utilizing first morning voided urine, algorithm reported as likelihood of prostate cancer
Colvera®, Clinical Genomics Pathology Inc	0229U	*BCAT1 (Branched chain amino acid transaminase 1)* and *IKZF1 (IKAROS family zinc finger 1)* (eg, colorectal cancer) promoter methylation analysis

(Continued on page 236)

Proprietary Name and Clinical Laboratory or Manufacturer	Alpha-Numeric Code	Code Descriptor
Genomic Unity® AR Analysis, Variantyx Inc, Variantyx Inc	0230U	*AR (androgen receptor)* (eg, spinal and bulbar muscular atrophy, Kennedy disease, X chromosome inactivation), full sequence analysis, including small sequence changes in exonic and intronic regions, deletions, duplications, short tandem repeat (STR) expansions, mobile element insertions, and variants in non-uniquely mappable regions
Genomic Unity® CACNA1A Analysis, Variantyx Inc, Variantyx Inc	0231U	*CACNA1A (calcium voltage-gated channel subunit alpha 1A)* (eg, spinocerebellar ataxia), full gene analysis, including small sequence changes in exonic and intronic regions, deletions, duplications, short tandem repeat (STR) gene expansions, mobile element insertions, and variants in non-uniquely mappable regions
Genomic Unity® CSTB Analysis, Variantyx Inc, Variantyx Inc	0232U	*CSTB (cystatin B)* (eg, progressive myoclonic epilepsy type 1A, Unverricht-Lundborg disease), full gene analysis, including small sequence changes in exonic and intronic regions, deletions, duplications, short tandem repeat (STR) expansions, mobile element insertions, and variants in non-uniquely mappable regions
Genomic Unity® FXN Analysis, Variantyx Inc, Variantyx Inc	0233U	*FXN (frataxin)* (eg, Friedreich ataxia), gene analysis, including small sequence changes in exonic and intronic regions, deletions, duplications, short tandem repeat (STR) expansions, mobile element insertions, and variants in non-uniquely mappable regions
Genomic Unity® MECP2 Analysis, Variantyx Inc, Variantyx Inc	0234U	*MECP2 (methyl CpG binding protein 2)* (eg, Rett syndrome), full gene analysis, including small sequence changes in exonic and intronic regions, deletions, duplications, mobile element insertions, and variants in non-uniquely mappable regions
Genomic Unity® PTEN Analysis, Variantyx Inc, Variantyx Inc	0235U	*PTEN (phosphatase and tensin homolog)* (eg, Cowden syndrome, PTEN hamartoma tumor syndrome), full gene analysis, including small sequence changes in exonic and intronic regions, deletions, duplications, mobile element insertions, and variants in non-uniquely mappable regions
Genomic Unity® SMN1/2 Analysis, Variantyx Inc, Variantyx Inc	0236U	*SMN1 (survival of motor neuron 1, telomeric)* and *SMN2 (survival of motor neuron 2, centromeric)* (eg, spinal muscular atrophy) full gene analysis, including small sequence changes in exonic and intronic regions, duplications, deletions, and mobile element insertions
Genomic Unity® Cardiac Ion Channelopathies Analysis, Variantyx Inc, Variantyx Inc	0237U	Cardiac ion channelopathies (eg, Brugada syndrome, long QT syndrome, short QT syndrome, catecholaminergic polymorphic ventricular tachycardia), genomic sequence analysis panel including *ANK2, CASQ2, CAV3, KCNE1, KCNE2, KCNH2, KCNJ2, KCNQ1, RYR2,* and *SCN5A,* including small sequence changes in exonic and intronic regions, deletions, duplications, mobile element insertions, and variants in non-uniquely mappable regions

★=Telemedicine　◀=Audio-only　✚=Add-on code　✗=FDA approval pending　#=Resequenced code　⊘=Modifier 51 exempt

Proprietary Name and Clinical Laboratory or Manufacturer	Alpha-Numeric Code	Code Descriptor
Genomic Unity® Lynch Syndrome Analysis, Variantyx Inc, Variantyx Inc	0238U	Oncology (Lynch syndrome), genomic DNA sequence analysis of *MLH1, MSH2, MSH6, PMS2,* and *EPCAM,* including small sequence changes in exonic and intronic regions, deletions, duplications, mobile element insertions, and variants in non-uniquely mappable regions
FoundationOne® Liquid CDx, Foundation Medicine, Inc, Foundation Medicine, Inc	0239U	Targeted genomic sequence analysis panel, solid organ neoplasm, cell-free DNA, analysis of 311 or more genes, interrogation for sequence variants, including substitutions, insertions, deletions, select rearrangements, and copy number variations
Xpert® Xpress CoV-2/Flu/RSV plus (SARS-CoV-2 and Flu targets), Cepheid®	0240U	Infectious disease (viral respiratory tract infection), pathogen-specific RNA, 3 targets (severe acute respiratory syndrome coronavirus 2 [SARS-CoV-2], influenza A, influenza B), upper respiratory specimen, each pathogen reported as detected or not detected
Xpert® Xpress CoV-2/Flu/RSV plus (all targets), Cepheid®	0241U	Infectious disease (viral respiratory tract infection), pathogen-specific RNA, 4 targets (severe acute respiratory syndrome coronavirus 2 [SARS-CoV-2], influenza A, influenza B, respiratory syncytial virus [RSV]), upper respiratory specimen, each pathogen reported as detected or not detected
Guardant360® CDx, Guardant Health Inc, Guardant Health Inc	0242U	Targeted genomic sequence analysis panel, solid organ neoplasm, cell-free circulating DNA analysis of 55-74 genes, interrogation for sequence variants, gene copy number amplifications, and gene rearrangements
PlGF Preeclampsia Screen, PerkinElmer Genetics, PerkinElmer Genetics, Inc	0243U	Obstetrics (preeclampsia), biochemical assay of placental-growth factor, time-resolved fluorescence immunoassay, maternal serum, predictive algorithm reported as a risk score for preeclampsia
Oncotype MAP™ Pan-Cancer Tissue Test, Paradigm Diagnostics, Inc, Paradigm Diagnostics, Inc	0244U	Oncology (solid organ), DNA, comprehensive genomic profiling, 257 genes, interrogation for single-nucleotide variants, insertions/deletions, copy number alterations, gene rearrangements, tumor-mutational burden and microsatellite instability, utilizing formalin-fixed paraffin-embedded tumor tissue
ThyGeNEXT® Thyroid Oncogene Panel, Interpace Diagnostics, Interpace Diagnostics	0245U	Oncology (thyroid), mutation analysis of 10 genes and 37 RNA fusions and expression of 4 mRNA markers using next-generation sequencing, fine needle aspirate, report includes associated risk of malignancy expressed as a percentage
PrecisionBlood™, San Diego Blood Bank, San Diego Blood Bank	0246U	Red blood cell antigen typing, DNA, genotyping of at least 16 blood groups with phenotype prediction of at least 51 red blood cell antigens
PreTRM®, Sera Prognostics, Sera Prognostics, Inc®	0247U	Obstetrics (preterm birth), insulin-like growth factor–binding protein 4 (IBP4), sex hormone–binding globulin (SHBG), quantitative measurement by LC-MS/MS, utilizing maternal serum, combined with clinical data, reported as predictive-risk stratification for spontaneous preterm birth

(Continued on page 238)

Proprietary Name and Clinical Laboratory or Manufacturer	Alpha-Numeric Code	Code Descriptor
3D Predict Glioma, KIYATEC®, Inc	0248U	Oncology (brain), spheroid cell culture in a 3D microenvironment, 12 drug panel, tumor-response prediction for each drug
Theralink® Reverse Phase Protein Array (RPPA), Theralink® Technologies, Inc, Theralink® Technologies, Inc	0249U	Oncology (breast), semiquantitative analysis of 32 phosphoproteins and protein analytes, includes laser capture microdissection, with algorithmic analysis and interpretative report
PGDx elio™ tissue complete, Personal Genome Diagnostics, Inc, Personal Genome Diagnostics, Inc	0250U	Oncology (solid organ neoplasm), targeted genomic sequence DNA analysis of 505 genes, interrogation for somatic alterations (SNVs [single nucleotide variant], small insertions and deletions, one amplification, and four translocations), microsatellite instability and tumor-mutation burden
Intrinsic Hepcidin IDx™ Test, IntrinsicDx, Intrinsic LifeSciences™ LLC	0251U	Hepcidin-25, enzyme-linked immunosorbent assay (ELISA), serum or plasma
POC (Products of Conception), Igenomix®, Igenomix® USA	0252U	Fetal aneuploidy short tandem–repeat comparative analysis, fetal DNA from products of conception, reported as normal (euploidy), monosomy, trisomy, or partial deletion/duplication, mosaicism, and segmental aneuploidy
ERA® (Endometrial Receptivity Analysis), Igenomix®, Igenomix® USA	0253U	Reproductive medicine (endometrial receptivity analysis), RNA gene expression profile, 238 genes by next-generation sequencing, endometrial tissue, predictive algorithm reported as endometrial window of implantation (eg, pre-receptive, receptive, post-receptive)
SMART PGT-A (Pre-implantation Genetic Testing - Aneuploidy), Igenomix®, Igenomix® USA	0254U	Reproductive medicine (preimplantation genetic assessment), analysis of 24 chromosomes using embryonic DNA genomic sequence analysis for aneuploidy, and a mitochondrial DNA score in euploid embryos, results reported as normal (euploidy), monosomy, trisomy, or partial deletion/duplication, mosaicism, and segmental aneuploidy, per embryo tested
Cap-Score™ Test, Androvia LifeSciences, Avantor Clinical Services (previously known as Therapak)	0255U	Andrology (infertility), sperm-capacitation assessment of ganglioside GM1 distribution patterns, fluorescence microscopy, fresh or frozen specimen, reported as percentage of capacitated sperm and probability of generating a pregnancy score
Trimethylamine (TMA) and TMA N-Oxide, Children's Hospital Colorado Laboratory	0256U	Trimethylamine/trimethylamine N-oxide (TMA/TMAO) profile, tandem mass spectrometry (MS/MS), urine, with algorithmic analysis and interpretive report
Very-Long Chain Acyl-CoA Dehydrogenase (VLCAD) Enzyme Activity, Children's Hospital Colorado Laboratory	0257U	Very long chain acyl-coenzyme A (CoA) dehydrogenase (VLCAD), leukocyte enzyme activity, whole blood

★ = Telemedicine   ◀ = Audio-only   ✦ = Add-on code   ✗ = FDA approval pending   # = Resequenced code   ⊘ = Modifier 51 exempt

Proprietary Name and Clinical Laboratory or Manufacturer	Alpha-Numeric Code	Code Descriptor
Mind.Px, Mindera, Mindera Corporation	0258U	Autoimmune (psoriasis), mRNA, next-generation sequencing, gene expression profiling of 50-100 genes, skin-surface collection using adhesive patch, algorithm reported as likelihood of response to psoriasis biologics
GFR by NMR, Labtech™ Diagnostics	0259U	Nephrology (chronic kidney disease), nuclear magnetic resonance spectroscopy measurement of myo-inositol, valine, and creatinine, algorithmically combined with cystatin C (by immunoassay) and demographic data to determine estimated glomerular filtration rate (GFR), serum, quantitative
Augusta Optical Genome Mapping, Georgia Esoteric and Molecular (GEM) Laboratory, LLC, Bionano Genomics Inc	✕0260U	Rare diseases (constitutional/heritable disorders), identification of copy number variations, inversions, insertions, translocations, and other structural variants by optical genome mapping (For additional PLA code with identical clinical descriptor, see 0264U. See Appendix O or the most current listing on the AMA CPT website to determine appropriate code assignment)
Immunoscore®, HalioDx, HalioDx	0261U	Oncology (colorectal cancer), image analysis with artificial intelligence assessment of 4 histologic and immunohistochemical features (CD3 and CD8 within tumor-stroma border and tumor core), tissue, reported as immune response and recurrence-risk score
OncoSignal 7 Pathway Signal, Protean BioDiagnostics, Philips Electronics Nederland BV	0262U	Oncology (solid tumor), gene expression profiling by real-time RT-PCR of 7 gene pathways (ER, AR, PI3K, MAPK, HH, TGFB, Notch), formalin-fixed paraffin-embedded (FFPE), algorithm reported as gene pathway activity score
NPDX ASD and Central Carbon Energy Metabolism, Stemina Biomarker Discovery, Inc, Stemina Biomarker Discovery, Inc	0263U	Neurology (autism spectrum disorder [ASD]), quantitative measurements of 16 central carbon metabolites (ie, α-ketoglutarate, alanine, lactate, phenylalanine, pyruvate, succinate, carnitine, citrate, fumarate, hypoxanthine, inosine, malate, S-sulfocysteine, taurine, urate, and xanthine), liquid chromatography tandem mass spectrometry (LC-MS/MS), plasma, algorithmic analysis with result reported as negative or positive (with metabolic subtypes of ASD)
Praxis Optical Genome Mapping, Praxis Genomics LLC	✕0264U	Rare diseases (constitutional/heritable disorders), identification of copy number variations, inversions, insertions, translocations, and other structural variants by optical genome mapping (For additional PLA code with identical clinical descriptor, see 0260U. See Appendix O or the most current listing on the AMA CPT website to determine appropriate code assignment)

(Continued on page 240)

Proprietary Name and Clinical Laboratory or Manufacturer	Alpha-Numeric Code	Code Descriptor
Praxis Whole Genome Sequencing, Praxis Genomics LLC	0265U	Rare constitutional and other heritable disorders, whole genome and mitochondrial DNA sequence analysis, blood, frozen and formalin-fixed paraffin-embedded (FFPE) tissue, saliva, buccal swabs or cell lines, identification of single nucleotide and copy number variants
Praxis Transcriptome, Praxis Genomics LLC	0266U	Unexplained constitutional or other heritable disorders or syndromes, tissue-specific gene expression by whole-transcriptome and next-generation sequencing, blood, formalin-fixed paraffin-embedded (FFPE) tissue or fresh frozen tissue, reported as presence or absence of splicing or expression changes
Praxis Combined Whole Genome Sequencing and Optical Genome Mapping, Praxis Genomics LLC	0267U	Rare constitutional and other heritable disorders, identification of copy number variations, inversions, insertions, translocations, and other structural variants by optical genome mapping and whole genome sequencing
Versiti™ aHUS Genetic Evaluation, Versiti™ Diagnostic Laboratories, Versiti™	0268U	Hematology (atypical hemolytic uremic syndrome [aHUS]), genomic sequence analysis of 15 genes, blood, buccal swab, or amniotic fluid
Versiti™ Autosomal Dominant Thrombocytopenia Panel, Versiti™ Diagnostic Laboratories, Versiti™	▲0269U	►Hematology (autosomal dominant congenital thrombocytopenia), genomic sequence analysis of 22 genes, blood, buccal swab, or amniotic fluid◄
Versiti™ Coagulation Disorder Panel, Versiti™ Diagnostic Laboratories, Versiti™	0270U	Hematology (congenital coagulation disorders), genomic sequence analysis of 20 genes, blood, buccal swab, or amniotic fluid
Versiti™ Congenital Neutropenia Panel, Versiti™ Diagnostic Laboratories, Versiti™	▲0271U	►Hematology (congenital neutropenia), genomic sequence analysis of 24 genes, blood, buccal swab, or amniotic fluid◄
Versiti™ Comprehensive Bleeding Disorder Panel, Versiti™ Diagnostic Laboratories, Versiti™	▲0272U	►Hematology (genetic bleeding disorders), genomic sequence analysis of 60 genes and duplication/deletion of *PLAU*, blood, buccal swab, or amniotic fluid, comprehensive◄
Versiti™ Fibrinolytic Disorder Panel, Versiti™ Diagnostic Laboratories, Versiti™	0273U	Hematology (genetic hyperfibrinolysis, delayed bleeding), analysis of 9 genes (*F13A1, F13B, FGA, FGB, FGG, SERPINA1, SERPINE1, SERPINF2* by next-generation sequencing, and *PLAU* by array comparative genomic hybridization), blood, buccal swab, or amniotic fluid
Versiti™ Comprehensive Platelet Disorder Panel, Versiti™ Diagnostic Laboratories, Versiti™	▲0274U	►Hematology (genetic platelet disorders), genomic sequence analysis of 62 genes and duplication/deletion of *PLAU*, blood, buccal swab, or amniotic fluid◄
Versiti™ Heparin-Induced Thrombocytopenia Evaluation – PEA, Versiti™ Diagnostic Laboratories, Versiti™	0275U	Hematology (heparin-induced thrombocytopenia), platelet antibody reactivity by flow cytometry, serum
Versiti™ Inherited Thrombocytopenia Panel, Versiti™ Diagnostic Laboratories, Versiti™	0276U	Hematology (inherited thrombocytopenia), genomic sequence analysis of 42 genes , blood, buccal swab, or amniotic fluid

★ =Telemedicine   ◀ =Audio-only   ✚ =Add-on code   ✎ =FDA approval pending   # =Resequenced code   ⊘ =Modifier 51 exempt

Proprietary Name and Clinical Laboratory or Manufacturer	Alpha-Numeric Code	Code Descriptor
Versiti™ Platelet Function Disorder Panel, Versiti™ Diagnostic Laboratories, Versiti™	▲0277U	▶Hematology (genetic platelet function disorder), genomic sequence analysis of 40 genes and duplication/deletion of *PLAU*, blood, buccal swab, or amniotic fluid◀
Versiti™ Thrombosis Panel, Versiti™ Diagnostic Laboratories, Versiti™	▲0278U	▶Hematology (genetic thrombosis), genomic sequence analysis of 14 genes, blood, buccal swab, or amniotic fluid◀
Versiti™ VWF Collagen III Binding, Versiti™ Diagnostic Laboratories, Versiti™	0279U	Hematology (von Willebrand disease [VWD]), von Willebrand factor (VWF) and collagen III binding by enzyme-linked immunosorbent assays (ELISA), plasma, report of collagen III binding
Versiti™ VWF Collagen IV Binding, Versiti™ Diagnostic Laboratories, Versiti™	0280U	Hematology (von Willebrand disease [VWD]), von Willebrand factor (VWF) and collagen IV binding by enzyme-linked immunosorbent assays (ELISA), plasma, report of collagen IV binding
Versiti™ VWF Propeptide Antigen, Versiti™ Diagnostic Laboratories, Versiti™	0281U	Hematology (von Willebrand disease [VWD]), von Willebrand propeptide, enzyme-linked immunosorbent assays (ELISA), plasma, diagnostic report of von Willebrand factor (VWF) propeptide antigen level
Versiti™ Red Cell Genotyping Panel, Versiti™ Diagnostic Laboratories, Versiti™	0282U	Red blood cell antigen typing, DNA, genotyping of 12 blood group system genes to predict 44 red blood cell antigen phenotypes
Versiti™ VWD Type 2B Evaluation, Versiti™ Diagnostic Laboratories, Versiti™	0283U	von Willebrand factor (VWF), type 2B, platelet-binding evaluation, radioimmunoassay, plasma
Versiti™ VWD Type 2N Binding, Versiti™ Diagnostic Laboratories, Versiti™	0284U	von Willebrand factor (VWF), type 2N, factor VIII and VWF binding evaluation, enzyme-linked immunosorbent assays (ELISA), plasma
RadTox™ cfDNA test, DiaCarta Clinical Lab, DiaCarta Inc	0285U	Oncology, response to radiation, cell-free DNA, quantitative branched chain DNA amplification, plasma, reported as a radiation toxicity score
CNT (*CEP72, TPMT* and *NUDT15*) genotyping panel, RPRD Diagnostics	0286U	*CEP72 (centrosomal protein, 72-KDa), NUDT15 (nudix hydrolase 15)* and *TPMT (thiopurine S-methyltransferase)* (eg, drug metabolism) gene analysis, common variants
ThyroSeq® CRC, CBLPath, Inc, University of Pittsburgh Medical Center	0287U	Oncology (thyroid), DNA and mRNA, next-generation sequencing analysis of 112 genes, fine needle aspirate or formalin-fixed paraffin-embedded (FFPE) tissue, algorithmic prediction of cancer recurrence, reported as a categorical risk result (low, intermediate, high)
DetermaRx™, Oncocyte Corporation	0288U	Oncology (lung), mRNA, quantitative PCR analysis of 11 genes *(BAG1, BRCA1, CDC6, CDK2AP1, ERBB3, FUT3, IL11, LCK, RND3, SH3BGR, WNT3A)* and 3 reference genes *(ESD, TBP, YAP1)*, formalin-fixed paraffin-embedded (FFPE) tumor tissue, algorithmic interpretation reported as a recurrence risk score

(Continued on page 242)

Proprietary Name and Clinical Laboratory or Manufacturer	Alpha-Numeric Code	Code Descriptor
MindX Blood Test™ - Memory/ Alzheimer's, MindX Sciences™ Laboratory, MindX Sciences™ Inc	0289U	Neurology (Alzheimer disease), mRNA, gene expression profiling by RNA sequencing of 24 genes, whole blood, algorithm reported as predictive risk score
MindX Blood Test™ - Pain, MindX Sciences™ Laboratory, MindX Sciences™ Inc	0290U	Pain management, mRNA, gene expression profiling by RNA sequencing of 36 genes, whole blood, algorithm reported as predictive risk score
MindX Blood Test™ - Mood, MindX Sciences™ Laboratory, MindX Sciences™ Inc	0291U	Psychiatry (mood disorders), mRNA, gene expression profiling by RNA sequencing of 144 genes, whole blood, algorithm reported as predictive risk score
MindX Blood Test™ - Stress, MindX Sciences™ Laboratory, MindX Sciences™ Inc	0292U	Psychiatry (stress disorders), mRNA, gene expression profiling by RNA sequencing of 72 genes, whole blood, algorithm reported as predictive risk score
MindX Blood Test™ - Suicidality, MindX Sciences™ Laboratory, MindX Sciences™ Inc	0293U	Psychiatry (suicidal ideation), mRNA, gene expression profiling by RNA sequencing of 54 genes, whole blood, algorithm reported as predictive risk score
MindX Blood Test™ - Longevity, MindX Sciences™ Laboratory, MindX Sciences™ Inc	0294U	Longevity and mortality risk, mRNA, gene expression profiling by RNA sequencing of 18 genes, whole blood, algorithm reported as predictive risk score
DCISionRT®, PreludeDx™, Prelude Corporation	0295U	Oncology (breast ductal carcinoma in situ), protein expression profiling by immunohistochemistry of 7 proteins (COX2, FOXA1, HER2, Ki-67, p16, PR, SIAH2), with 4 clinicopathologic factors (size, age, margin status, palpability), utilizing formalin-fixed paraffin-embedded (FFPE) tissue, algorithm reported as a recurrence risk score
mRNA CancerDetect™, Viome Life Sciences, Inc, Viome Life Sciences, Inc	0296U	Oncology (oral and/or oropharyngeal cancer), gene expression profiling by RNA sequencing of at least 20 molecular features (eg, human and/or microbial mRNA), saliva, algorithm reported as positive or negative for signature associated with malignancy
Praxis Somatic Whole Genome Sequencing, Praxis Genomics LLC	0297U	Oncology (pan tumor), whole genome sequencing of paired malignant and normal DNA specimens, fresh or formalin-fixed paraffin-embedded (FFPE) tissue, blood or bone marrow, comparative sequence analyses and variant identification
Praxis Somatic Transcriptome, Praxis Genomics LLC	0298U	Oncology (pan tumor), whole transcriptome sequencing of paired malignant and normal RNA specimens, fresh or formalin-fixed paraffin-embedded (FFPE) tissue, blood or bone marrow, comparative sequence analyses and expression level and chimeric transcript identification
Praxis Somatic Optical Genome Mapping, Praxis Genomics LLC	0299U	Oncology (pan tumor), whole genome optical genome mapping of paired malignant and normal DNA specimens, fresh frozen tissue, blood, or bone marrow, comparative structural variant identification

★=Telemedicine   ◀=Audio-only   ✚=Add-on code   ✵=FDA approval pending   #=Resequenced code   ⊘=Modifier 51 exempt

Proprietary Name and Clinical Laboratory or Manufacturer	Alpha-Numeric Code	Code Descriptor
Praxis Somatic Combined Whole Genome Sequencing and Optical Genome Mapping, Praxis Genomics LLC	0300U	Oncology (pan tumor), whole genome sequencing and optical genome mapping of paired malignant and normal DNA specimens, fresh tissue, blood, or bone marrow, comparative sequence analyses and variant identification
Bartonella ddPCR, Galaxy Diagnostics Inc	0301U	Infectious agent detection by nucleic acid (DNA or RNA), Bartonella henselae and Bartonella quintana, droplet digital PCR (ddPCR);
Bartonella Digital ePCR™, Galaxy Diagnostics Inc	0302U	following liquid enrichment
Hypoxic BioChip Adhesion, BioChip Labs™, BioChip Labs™	0303U	Hematology, red blood cell (RBC) adhesion to endothelial/subendothelial adhesion molecules, functional assessment, whole blood, with algorithmic analysis and result reported as an RBC adhesion index; hypoxic
Normoxic BioChip Adhesion, BioChip Labs™, BioChip Labs™	0304U	normoxic
Ektacytometry, BioChip Labs™, BioChip Labs™	0305U	Hematology, red blood cell (RBC) functionality and deformity as a function of shear stress, whole blood, reported as a maximum elongation index
Invitae PCM Tissue Profiling and MRD Baseline Assay, Invitae Corporation, Invitae Corporation	0306U	Oncology (minimal residual disease [MRD]), next-generation targeted sequencing analysis, cell-free DNA, initial (baseline) assessment to determine a patient-specific panel for future comparisons to evaluate for MRD (Do not report 0306U in conjunction with 0307U)
Invitae PCM MRD Monitoring, Invitae Corporation, Invitae Corporation	0307U	Oncology (minimal residual disease [MRD]), next-generation targeted sequencing analysis of a patient-specific panel, cell-free DNA, subsequent assessment with comparison to previously analyzed patient specimens to evaluate for MRD (Do not report 0307U in conjunction with 0306U)
HART CADhs®, ▶Atlas Genomics, Prevencio, Inc◀	▲0308U	▶Cardiology (coronary artery disease [CAD]), analysis of 3 proteins (high sensitivity [hs] troponin, adiponectin, and kidney injury molecule-1 [KIM-1]) with 3 clinical parameters (age, sex, history of cardiac intervention), plasma, algorithm reported as a risk score for obstructive CAD◀
HART CVE®, ▶Atlas Genomics, Prevencio, Inc◀	0309U	Cardiology (cardiovascular disease), analysis of 4 proteins (NT-proBNP, osteopontin, tissue inhibitor of metalloproteinase-1 [TIMP-1], and kidney injury molecule-1 [KIM-1]), plasma, algorithm reported as a risk score for major adverse cardiac event
HART KD®, ▶Atlas Genomics, Prevencio, Inc◀	0310U	Pediatrics (vasculitis, Kawasaki disease [KD]), analysis of 3 biomarkers (NT-proBNP, C-reactive protein, and T-uptake), plasma, algorithm reported as a risk score for KD

(Continued on page 244)

Proprietary Name and Clinical Laboratory or Manufacturer	Alpha-Numeric Code	Code Descriptor
Accelerate PhenoTest® BC kit, AST configuration, Accelerate Diagnostics, Inc, Accelerate Diagnostics, Inc	0311U	Infectious disease (bacterial), quantitative antimicrobial susceptibility reported as phenotypic minimum inhibitory concentration (MIC)–based antimicrobial susceptibility for each organism identified (Do not report 0311U in conjunction with 87076, 87077, 0086U)
Avise® Lupus, Exagen Inc, Exagen Inc	0312U	Autoimmune diseases (eg, systemic lupus erythematosus [SLE]), analysis of 8 IgG autoantibodies and 2 cell-bound complement activation products using enzyme-linked immunosorbent immunoassay (ELISA), flow cytometry and indirect immunofluorescence, serum, or plasma and whole blood, individual components reported along with an algorithmic SLE-likelihood assessment
PancreaSeq® Genomic Classifier, Molecular and Genomic Pathology Laboratory, University of Pittsburgh Medical Center	0313U	Oncology (pancreas), DNA and mRNA next-generation sequencing analysis of 74 genes and analysis of CEA (CEACAM5) gene expression, pancreatic cyst fluid, algorithm reported as a categorical result (ie, negative, low probability of neoplasia or positive, high probability of neoplasia)
DecisionDx® DiffDx™- Melanoma, Castle Biosciences, Inc, Castle Biosciences, Inc	0314U	Oncology (cutaneous melanoma), mRNA gene expression profiling by RT-PCR of 35 genes (32 content and 3 housekeeping), utilizing formalin-fixed paraffin-embedded (FFPE) tissue, algorithm reported as a categorical result (ie, benign, intermediate, malignant)
DecisionDx®-SCC, Castle Biosciences, Inc, Castle Biosciences, Inc	0315U	Oncology (cutaneous squamous cell carcinoma), mRNA gene expression profiling by RT-PCR of 40 genes (34 content and 6 housekeeping), utilizing formalin-fixed paraffin-embedded (FFPE) tissue, algorithm reported as a categorical risk result (ie, Class 1, Class 2A, Class 2B)
Lyme Borrelia Nanotrap® Urine Antigen Test, Galaxy Diagnostics Inc	0316U	Borrelia burgdorferi (Lyme disease), OspA protein evaluation, urine
LungLB®, LungLife AI®, LungLife AI®	0317U	Oncology (lung cancer), four-probe FISH (3q29, 3p22.1, 10q22.3, 10cen) assay, whole blood, predictive algorithm-generated evaluation reported as decreased or increased risk for lung cancer
EpiSign Complete, Greenwood Genetic Center	0318U	Pediatrics (congenital epigenetic disorders), whole genome methylation analysis by microarray for 50 or more genes, blood
Clarava™, Verici Dx, Verici Dx, Inc	0319U	Nephrology (renal transplant), RNA expression by select transcriptome sequencing, using pretransplant peripheral blood, algorithm reported as a risk score for early acute rejection
Tuteva™, Verici Dx, Verici Dx, Inc	0320U	Nephrology (renal transplant), RNA expression by select transcriptome sequencing, using posttransplant peripheral blood, algorithm reported as a risk score for acute cellular rejection

★ = Telemedicine   ◀ = Audio-only   ✦ = Add-on code   ✇ = FDA approval pending   # = Resequenced code   ⊘ = Modifier 51 exempt

Proprietary Name and Clinical Laboratory or Manufacturer	Alpha-Numeric Code	Code Descriptor
Bridge Urinary Tract Infection Detection and Resistance Test, Bridge Diagnostics	0321U	Infectious agent detection by nucleic acid (DNA or RNA), genitourinary pathogens, identification of 20 bacterial and fungal organisms and identification of 16 associated antibiotic-resistance genes, multiplex amplified probe technique
NPDX ASD Test Panel III, Stemina Biomarker Discovery d/b/a NeuroPointDX, Stemina Biomarker Discovery d/b/a NeuroPointDX	0322U	Neurology (autism spectrum disorder [ASD]), quantitative measurements of 14 acyl carnitines and microbiome-derived metabolites, liquid chromatography with tandem mass spectrometry (LC-MS/MS), plasma, results reported as negative or positive for risk of metabolic subtypes associated with ASD
Johns Hopkins Metagenomic Next-Generation Sequencing Assay for Infectious Disease Diagnostics, Johns Hopkins Medical Microbiology Laboratory	0323U	Infectious agent detection by nucleic acid (DNA and RNA), central nervous system pathogen, metagenomic next-generation sequencing, cerebrospinal fluid (CSF), identification of pathogenic bacteria, viruses, parasites, or fungi
—	▶(0324U has been deleted)◀	—
—	▶(0325U has been deleted)◀	—
Guardant360®, Guardant Health, Inc, Guardant Health, Inc	0326U	Targeted genomic sequence analysis panel, solid organ neoplasm, cell-free circulating DNA analysis of 83 or more genes, interrogation for sequence variants, gene copy number amplifications, gene rearrangements, microsatellite instability and tumor mutational burden
Vasistera™, Natera, Inc, Natera, Inc	0327U	Fetal aneuploidy (trisomy 13, 18, and 21), DNA sequence analysis of selected regions using maternal plasma, algorithm reported as a risk score for each trisomy, includes sex reporting, if performed
CareView360, Newstar Medical Laboratories, LLC, Newstar Medical Laboratories, LLC	0328U	Drug assay, definitive, 120 or more drugs and metabolites, urine, quantitative liquid chromatography with tandem mass spectrometry (LC-MS/MS), includes specimen validity and algorithmic analysis describing drug or metabolite and presence or absence of risks for a significant patient-adverse event, per date of service
Oncomap™ ExTra, Exact Sciences, Inc, Genomic Health Inc	0329U	Oncology (neoplasia), exome and transcriptome sequence analysis for sequence variants, gene copy number amplifications and deletions, gene rearrangements, microsatellite instability and tumor mutational burden utilizing DNA and RNA from tumor with DNA from normal blood or saliva for subtraction, report of clinically significant mutation(s) with therapy associations
Bridge Women's Health Infectious Disease Detection Test, Bridge Diagnostics, Thermo Fisher and Hologic Test Kit on Panther Instrument	0330U	Infectious agent detection by nucleic acid (DNA or RNA), vaginal pathogen panel, identification of 27 organisms, amplified probe technique, vaginal swab

(Continued on page 246)

Proprietary Name and Clinical Laboratory or Manufacturer	Alpha-Numeric Code	Code Descriptor
Augusta Hematology Optical Genome Mapping, Georgia Esoteric and Molecular Labs, Augusta University, Bionano	0331U	Oncology (hematolymphoid neoplasia), optical genome mapping for copy number alterations and gene rearrangements utilizing DNA from blood or bone marrow, report of clinically significant alterations
EpiSwitch® CiRT (Checkpoint-inhibitor Response Test), Next Bio-Research Services, LLC, Oxford BioDynamics, PLC	0332U	Oncology (pan-tumor), genetic profiling of 8 DNA-regulatory (epigenetic) markers by quantitative polymerase chain reaction (qPCR), whole blood, reported as a high or low probability of responding to immune checkpoint–inhibitor therapy
HelioLiver™ Test, Fulgent Genetics, LLC, Helio Health, Inc	0333U	Oncology (liver), surveillance for hepatocellular carcinoma (HCC) in high-risk patients, analysis of methylation patterns on circulating cell-free DNA (cfDNA) plus measurement of serum of AFP/AFP-L3 and oncoprotein des-gamma-carboxy-prothrombin (DCP), algorithm reported as normal or abnormal result
Guardant360 TissueNext™, Guardant Health, Inc, Guardant Health, Inc	0334U	Oncology (solid organ), targeted genomic sequence analysis, formalin-fixed paraffin-embedded (FFPE) tumor tissue, DNA analysis, 84 or more genes, interrogation for sequence variants, gene copy number amplifications, gene rearrangements, microsatellite instability and tumor mutational burden
IriSight™ Prenatal Analysis – Proband, Variantyx, Inc, Variantyx, Inc	0335U	Rare diseases (constitutional/heritable disorders), whole genome sequence analysis, including small sequence changes, copy number variants, deletions, duplications, mobile element insertions, uniparental disomy (UPD), inversions, aneuploidy, mitochondrial genome sequence analysis with heteroplasmy and large deletions, short tandem repeat (STR) gene expansions, fetal sample, identification and categorization of genetic variants (Do not report 0335U in conjunction with 81425, 0212U)
IriSight™ Prenatal Analysis – Comparator, Variantyx, Inc, Variantyx, Inc	0336U	Rare diseases (constitutional/heritable disorders), whole genome sequence analysis, including small sequence changes, copy number variants, deletions, duplications, mobile element insertions, uniparental disomy (UPD), inversions, aneuploidy, mitochondrial genome sequence analysis with heteroplasmy and large deletions, short tandem repeat (STR) gene expansions, blood or saliva, identification and categorization of genetic variants, each comparator genome (eg, parent) (Do not report 0336U in conjunction with 81426, 0213U)

★ = Telemedicine   ◀ = Audio-only   ✚ = Add-on code   ✗ = FDA approval pending   # = Resequenced code   ⊘ = Modifier 51 exempt

Proprietary Name and Clinical Laboratory or Manufacturer	Alpha-Numeric Code	Code Descriptor
CELLSEARCH® Circulating Multiple Myeloma Cell (CMMC) Test, Menarini Silicon Biosystems, Inc, Menarini Silicon Biosystems, Inc	0337U	Oncology (plasma cell disorders and myeloma), circulating plasma cell immunologic selection, identification, morphological characterization, and enumeration of plasma cells based on differential CD138, CD38, CD19, and CD45 protein biomarker expression, peripheral blood
CELLSEARCH® HER2 Circulating Tumor Cell (CTC-HER2) Test, Menarini Silicon Biosystems, Inc, Menarini Silicon Biosystems, Inc	0338U	Oncology (solid tumor), circulating tumor cell selection, identification, morphological characterization, detection and enumeration based on differential EpCAM, cytokeratins 8, 18, and 19, and CD45 protein biomarkers, and quantification of HER2 protein biomarker–expressing cells, peripheral blood
SelectMDx® for Prostate Cancer, MDxHealth®, Inc, MDxHealth®, Inc	0339U	Oncology (prostate), mRNA expression profiling of *HOXC6* and *DLX1*, reverse transcription polymerase chain reaction (RT-PCR), first-void urine following digital rectal examination, algorithm reported as probability of high-grade cancer
Signatera™, Natera, Inc, Natera, Inc	0340U	Oncology (pan-cancer), analysis of minimal residual disease (MRD) from plasma, with assays personalized to each patient based on prior next-generation sequencing of the patient's tumor and germline DNA, reported as absence or presence of MRD, with disease-burden correlation, if appropriate
Single Cell Prenatal Diagnosis (SCPD) Test, Luna Genetics, Inc, Luna Genetics, Inc	0341U	Fetal aneuploidy DNA sequencing comparative analysis, fetal DNA from products of conception, reported as normal (euploidy), monosomy, trisomy, or partial deletion/duplication, mosaicism, and segmental aneuploid
IMMray® PanCan-d, Immunovia, Inc, Immunovia, Inc	0342U	Oncology (pancreatic cancer), multiplex immunoassay of C5, C4, cystatin C, factor B, osteoprotegerin (OPG), gelsolin, IGFBP3, CA125 and multiplex electrochemiluminescent immunoassay (ECLIA) for CA19-9, serum, diagnostic algorithm reported qualitatively as positive, negative, or borderline
miR Sentinel™ Prostate Cancer Test, miR Scientific, LLC, miR Scientific, LLC	0343U	Oncology (prostate), exosome-based analysis of 442 small noncoding RNAs (sncRNAs) by quantitative reverse transcription polymerase chain reaction (RT-qPCR), urine, reported as molecular evidence of no-, low-, intermediate- or high-risk of prostate cancer
OWLiver®, CIMA Sciences, LLC	0344U	Hepatology (nonalcoholic fatty liver disease [NAFLD]), semiquantitative evaluation of 28 lipid markers by liquid chromatography with tandem mass spectrometry (LC-MS/MS), serum, reported as at-risk for nonalcoholic steatohepatitis (NASH) or not NASH

(*Continued on page 248*)

Proprietary Name and Clinical Laboratory or Manufacturer	Alpha-Numeric Code	Code Descriptor
GeneSight® Psychotropic, Assurex Health, Inc, Myriad Genetics, Inc	✳0345U	Psychiatry (eg, depression, anxiety, attention deficit hyperactivity disorder [ADHD]), genomic analysis panel, variant analysis of 15 genes, including deletion/duplication analysis of *CYP2D6* ▶(For additional PLA code with identical clinical descriptor, see 0411U. See Appendix O to determine appropriate code assignment)◀
QUEST AD-Detect™, Beta-Amyloid 42/40 Ratio, Plasma, Quest Diagnostics	0346U	Beta amyloid, Aß40 and Aß42 by liquid chromatography with tandem mass spectrometry (LC-MS/MS), ratio, plasma
RightMed® PGx16 Test, OneOme®, OneOme®, LLC	0347U	Drug metabolism or processing (multiple conditions), whole blood or buccal specimen, DNA analysis, 16 gene report, with variant analysis and reported phenotypes
RightMed® Comprehensive Test Exclude F2 and F5, OneOme®, OneOme®, LLC	0348U	Drug metabolism or processing (multiple conditions), whole blood or buccal specimen, DNA analysis, 25 gene report, with variant analysis and reported phenotypes
RightMed® Comprehensive Test, OneOme®, OneOme®, LLC	0349U	Drug metabolism or processing (multiple conditions), whole blood or buccal specimen, DNA analysis, 27 gene report, with variant analysis, including reported phenotypes and impacted gene-drug interactions
RightMed® Gene Report, OneOme®, OneOme®, LLC	0350U	Drug metabolism or processing (multiple conditions), whole blood or buccal specimen, DNA analysis, 27 gene report, with variant analysis and reported phenotypes
MeMed BV®, MeMed Diagnostics, Ltd, MeMed Diagnostics, Ltd	0351U	Infectious disease (bacterial or viral), biochemical assays, tumor necrosis factor-related apoptosis-inducing ligand (TRAIL), interferon gamma-induced protein-10 (IP-10), and C-reactive protein, serum, algorithm reported as likelihood of bacterial infection
Xpert® Xpress MVP, Cepheid®	0352U	Infectious disease (bacterial vaginosis and vaginitis), multiplex amplified probe technique, for detection of bacterial vaginosis–associated bacteria (BVAB-2, Atopobium vaginae, and Megasphera type 1), algorithm reported as detected or not detected and separate detection of Candida species (C. albicans, C. tropicalis, C. parapsilosis, C. dubliniensis), Candida glabrata/Candida krusei, and trichomonas vaginalis, vaginal-fluid specimen, each result reported as detected or not detected
Xpert® CT/NG, Cepheid®	0353U	Infectious agent detection by nucleic acid (DNA), Chlamydia trachomatis and Neisseria gonorrhoeae, multiplex amplified probe technique, urine, vaginal, pharyngeal, or rectal, each pathogen reported as detected or not detected
PreTect HPV-Proofer' 7, GenePace Laboratories, LLC, PreTech	0354U	Human papilloma virus (HPV), high-risk types (ie, 16, 18, 31, 33, 45, 52 and 58) qualitative mRNA expression of E6/E7 by quantitative polymerase chain reaction (qPCR)

Appendix O

Proprietary Name and Clinical Laboratory or Manufacturer	Alpha-Numeric Code	Code Descriptor
▶Apolipoprotein L1 *(APOL1)* Renal Risk Variant Genotyping, Quest Diagnostics®, Quest Diagnostics®◀	●0355U	▶*APOL1 (apolipoprotein L1)* (eg, chronic kidney disease), risk variants (G1, G2)◀
▶NavDx®, Naveris, Inc, Naveris, Inc◀	●0356U	▶Oncology (oropharyngeal), evaluation of 17 DNA biomarkers using droplet digital PCR (ddPCR), cell-free DNA, algorithm reported as a prognostic risk score for cancer recurrence◀
—	▶(0357U has been deleted)◀	—
▶Lumipulse® G ß-Amyloid Ratio (1-42/1-40) Test, Fujirebio Diagnostics, Inc, Fujirebio Diagnostics, Inc◀	●0358U	▶Neurology (mild cognitive impairment), analysis of ß-amyloid 1-42 and 1-40, chemiluminescence enzyme immunoassay, cerebral spinal fluid, reported as positive, likely positive, or negative◀
▶IsoPSA®, Cleveland Diagnostics, Inc, Cleveland Diagnostics, Inc◀	●0359U	▶Oncology (prostate cancer), analysis of all prostate-specific antigen (PSA) structural isoforms by phase separation and immunoassay, plasma, algorithm reports risk of cancer◀
▶Nodify CDT®, Biodesix, Inc, Biodesix, Inc◀	●0360U	▶Oncology (lung), enzyme-linked immunosorbent assay (ELISA) of 7 autoantibodies (p53, NY-ESO-1, CAGE, GBU4-5, SOX2, MAGE A4, and HuD), plasma, algorithm reported as a categorical result for risk of malignancy◀
▶Neurofilament Light Chain (NfL), Mayo Clinic, Mayo Clinic◀	●0361U	▶Neurofilament light chain, digital immunoassay, plasma, quantitative◀
▶Thyroid GuidePx®, Protean BioDiagnostics, Qualisure Diagnostics◀	▲0362U	▶Oncology (papillary thyroid cancer), gene-expression profiling via targeted hybrid capture–enrichment RNA sequencing of 82 content genes and 10 housekeeping genes, fine needle aspirate or formalin-fixed paraffin-embedded (FFPE) tissue, algorithm reported as one of three molecular subtypes◀
▶Cxbladder™ Triage, Pacific Edge Diagnostics USA, Ltd, Pacific Edge Diagnostics USA, Ltd◀	●0363U	▶Oncology (urothelial), mRNA, gene-expression profiling by real-time quantitative PCR of 5 genes *(MDK, HOXA13, CDC2 [CDK1], IGFBP5,* and *CXCR2),* utilizing urine, algorithm incorporates age, sex, smoking history, and macrohematuria frequency, reported as a risk score for having urothelial carcinoma◀
▶clonoSEQ® Assay, Adaptive Biotechnologies◀	●0364U	▶Oncology (hematolymphoid neoplasm), genomic sequence analysis using multiplex (PCR) and next-generation sequencing with algorithm, quantification of dominant clonal sequence(s), reported as presence or absence of minimal residual disease (MRD) with quantitation of disease burden, when appropriate◀
▶Oncuria® Detect, DiaCarta Clinical Lab, DiaCarta, Inc◀	●0365U	▶Oncology (bladder), analysis of 10 protein biomarkers (A1AT, ANG, APOE, CA9, IL8, MMP9, MMP10, PAI1, SDC1, and VEGFA) by immunoassays, urine, algorithm reported as a probability of bladder cancer◀

(Continued on page 250)

Proprietary Name and Clinical Laboratory or Manufacturer	Alpha-Numeric Code	Code Descriptor
▶Oncuria® Monitor, DiaCarta Clinical Lab, DiaCarta, Inc◀	●0366U	▶Oncology (bladder), analysis of 10 protein biomarkers (A1AT, ANG, APOE, CA9, IL8, MMP9, MMP10, PAI1, SDC1, and VEGFA) by immunoassays, urine, algorithm reported as a probability of recurrent bladder cancer◀
▶Oncuria® Predict, DiaCarta Clinical Lab, DiaCarta, Inc◀	●0367U	▶Oncology (bladder), analysis of 10 protein biomarkers (A1AT, ANG, APOE, CA9, IL8, MMP9, MMP10, PAI1, SDC1, and VEGFA) by immunoassays, urine, diagnostic algorithm reported as a risk score for probability of rapid recurrence of recurrent or persistent cancer following transurethral resection◀
▶ColoScape™ Colorectal Cancer Detection, DiaCarta Clinical Lab, DiaCarta, Inc◀	●0368U	▶Oncology (colorectal cancer), evaluation for mutations of *APC, BRAF, CTNNB1, KRAS, NRAS, PIK3CA, SMAD4,* and *TP53,* and methylation markers (MYO1G, KCNQ5, C9ORF50, FLI1, CLIP4, ZNF132, and TWIST1), multiplex quantitative polymerase chain reaction (qPCR), circulating cell-free DNA (cfDNA), plasma, report of risk score for advanced adenoma or colorectal cancer◀
▶GI assay (Gastrointestinal Pathogen with ABR), Lab Genomics LLC, Thermo Fisher Scientific◀	●0369U	▶Infectious agent detection by nucleic acid (DNA and RNA), gastrointestinal pathogens, 31 bacterial, viral, and parasitic organisms and identification of 21 associated antibiotic-resistance genes, multiplex amplified probe technique◀
▶Lesion Infection (Wound), Lab Genomics LLC, Thermo Fisher Scientific◀	●0370U	▶Infectious agent detection by nucleic acid (DNA and RNA), surgical wound pathogens, 34 microorganisms and identification of 21 associated antibiotic-resistance genes, multiplex amplified probe technique, wound swab◀
▶Qlear UTI, Lifescan Labs of Illinois, Thermo Fisher Scientific◀	●0371U	▶Infectious agent detection by nucleic acid (DNA or RNA), genitourinary pathogen, semiquantitative identification, DNA from 16 bacterial organisms and 1 fungal organism, multiplex amplified probe technique via quantitative polymerase chain reaction (qPCR), urine◀
▶Qlear UTI - Reflex ABR, Lifescan Labs of Illinois, Thermo Fisher Scientific◀	●0372U	▶Infectious disease (genitourinary pathogens), antibiotic-resistance gene detection, multiplex amplified probe technique, urine, reported as an antimicrobial stewardship risk score◀
▶Respiratory Pathogen with ABR (RPX), Lab Genomics LLC, Thermo Fisher Scientific◀	●0373U	▶Infectious agent detection by nucleic acid (DNA and RNA), respiratory tract infection, 17 bacteria, 8 fungus, 13 virus, and 16 antibiotic-resistance genes, multiplex amplified probe technique, upper or lower respiratory specimen◀
▶Urogenital Pathogen with Rx Panel (UPX), Lab Genomics LLC, Thermo Fisher Scientific◀	●0374U	▶Infectious agent detection by nucleic acid (DNA or RNA), genitourinary pathogens, identification of 21 bacterial and fungal organisms and identification of 21 associated antibiotic-resistance genes, multiplex amplified probe technique, urine◀

★ = Telemedicine ◀ = Audio-only ✚ = Add-on code ✎ = FDA approval pending # = Resequenced code ⊘ = Modifier 51 exempt

Proprietary Name and Clinical Laboratory or Manufacturer	Alpha-Numeric Code	Code Descriptor
▶OvaWatch^{SM}, Aspira Women's Health^{SM}, Aspira Labs, Inc◀	●0375U	▶Oncology (ovarian), biochemical assays of 7 proteins (follicle stimulating hormone, human epididymis protein 4, apolipoprotein A-1, transferrin, beta-2 macroglobulin, prealbumin [ie, transthyretin], and cancer antigen 125), algorithm reported as ovarian cancer risk score◀
▶ArteraAI Prostate Test, Artera Inc®, Artera Inc®◀	●0376U	▶Oncology (prostate cancer), image analysis of at least 128 histologic features and clinical factors, prognostic algorithm determining the risk of distant metastases, and prostate cancer-specific mortality, includes predictive algorithm to androgen deprivation-therapy response, if appropriate◀
▶Liposcale®, CIMA Sciences, LLC◀	●0377U	▶Cardiovascular disease, quantification of advanced serum or plasma lipoprotein profile, by nuclear magnetic resonance (NMR) spectrometry with report of a lipoprotein profile (including 23 variables)◀
▶UCGSL *RFC1* Repeat Expansion Test, University of Chicago Genetic Services Laboratories◀	●0378U	▶*RFC1 (replication factor C subunit 1),* repeat expansion variant analysis by traditional and repeat-primed PCR, blood, saliva, or buccal swab◀
▶Solid Tumor Expanded Panel, Quest Diagnostics®, Quest Diagnostics®◀	●0379U	▶Targeted genomic sequence analysis panel, solid organ neoplasm, DNA (523 genes) and RNA (55 genes) by next-generation sequencing, interrogation for sequence variants, gene copy number amplifications, gene rearrangements, microsatellite instability, and tumor mutational burden◀
▶PersonalisedRX, Lab Genomics LLC, Agena Bioscience, Inc◀	●0380U	▶Drug metabolism (adverse drug reactions and drug response), targeted sequence analysis, 20 gene variants and *CYP2D6* deletion or duplication analysis with reported genotype and phenotype◀
▶Branched-Chain Amino Acids, Self-Collect, Blood Spot, Mayo Clinic, Laboratory Developed Test◀	●0381U	▶Maple syrup urine disease monitoring by patient-collected blood card sample, quantitative measurement of allo-isoleucine, leucine, isoleucine, and valine, liquid chromatography with tandem mass spectrometry (LC-MS/MS)◀
▶Phenylalanine and Tyrosine, Self-Collect, Blood Spot, Mayo Clinic, Laboratory Developed Test◀	●0382U	▶Hyperphenylalaninemia monitoring by patient-collected blood card sample, quantitative measurement of phenylalanine and tyrosine, liquid chromatography with tandem mass spectrometry (LC-MS/MS)◀
▶Tyrosinemia Follow-Up Panel, Self-Collect, Blood Spot, Mayo Clinic, Laboratory Developed Test◀	●0383U	▶Tyrosinemia type I monitoring by patient-collected blood card sample, quantitative measurement of tyrosine, phenylalanine, methionine, succinylacetone, nitisinone, liquid chromatography with tandem mass spectrometry (LC-MS/MS)◀

(*Continued on page 252*)

Appendix O

Proprietary Name and Clinical Laboratory or Manufacturer	Alpha-Numeric Code	Code Descriptor
►NaviDKD™ Predictive Diagnostic Screening for Kidney Health, Journey Biosciences, Inc, Journey Biosciences, Inc◄	●0384U	►Nephrology (chronic kidney disease), carboxymethyllysine, methylglyoxal hydroimidazolone, and carboxyethyl lysine by liquid chromatography with tandem mass spectrometry (LC-MS/MS) and HbA1c and estimated glomerular filtration rate (GFR), with risk score reported for predictive progression to high-stage kidney disease◄
►PromarkerD, Sonic Reference Laboratory, Proteomics International Pty Ltd◄	●0385U	►Nephrology (chronic kidney disease), apolipoprotein A4 (ApoA4), CD5 antigen-like (CD5L), and insulin-like growth factor binding protein 3 (IGFBP3) by enzyme-linked immunoassay (ELISA), plasma, algorithm combining results with HDL, estimated glomerular filtration rate (GFR) and clinical data reported as a risk score for developing diabetic kidney disease◄
—	►(0386U has been deleted)◄	—
►AMBLor® melanoma prognostic test, Avero® Diagnostics◄	●0387U	►Oncology (melanoma), autophagy and beclin 1 regulator 1 (AMBRA1) and loricrin (AMLo) by immunohistochemistry, formalin-fixed paraffin-embedded (FFPE) tissue, report for risk of progression◄ ►(Do not report 0387U in conjunction with 88341, 88342)◄
►InVisionFirst®-Lung Liquid Biopsy, Inivata, Inc, Inivata, Inc◄	●0388U	►Oncology (non-small cell lung cancer), next-generation sequencing with identification of single nucleotide variants, copy number variants, insertions and deletions, and structural variants in 37 cancer-related genes, plasma, with report for alteration detection◄
►KawasakiDx, OncoOmicsDx Laboratory, mProbe◄	●0389U	►Pediatric febrile illness (Kawasaki disease [KD]), interferon alpha-inducible protein 27 (IFI27) and mast cell-expressed membrane protein 1 (MCEMP1), RNA, using quantitative reverse transcription polymerase chain reaction (RT-qPCR), blood, reported as a risk score for KD◄
►PEPredictDx, OncoOmicsDx Laboratory, mProbe◄	●0390U	►Obstetrics (preeclampsia), kinase insert domain receptor (KDR), Endoglin (ENG), and retinol-binding protein 4 (RBP4), by immunoassay, serum, algorithm reported as a risk score◄
►Strata Select™, Strata Oncology, Inc, Strata Oncology, Inc◄	●0391U	►Oncology (solid tumor), DNA and RNA by next-generation sequencing, utilizing formalin-fixed paraffin-embedded (FFPE) tissue, 437 genes, interpretive report for single nucleotide variants, splice-site variants, insertions/deletions, copy number alterations, gene fusions, tumor mutational burden, and microsatellite instability, with algorithm quantifying immunotherapy response score◄

★=Telemedicine ◄=Audio-only ✦=Add-on code ✚=FDA approval pending #=Resequenced code ⊘=Modifier 51 exempt

Proprietary Name and Clinical Laboratory or Manufacturer	Alpha-Numeric Code	Code Descriptor
▶Medication Management Neuropsychiatric Panel, RCA Laboratory Services LLC d/b/a GENETWORx, GENETWORx◀	●0392U	▶Drug metabolism (depression, anxiety, attention deficit hyperactivity disorder [ADHD]), gene-drug interactions, variant analysis of 16 genes, including deletion/duplication analysis of *CYP2D6*, reported as impact of gene-drug interaction for each drug◀
▶SYNTap® Biomarker Test, Amprion Clinical Laboratory, Amprion Clinical Laboratory◀	●0393U	▶Neurology (eg, Parkinson disease, dementia with Lewy bodies), cerebrospinal fluid (CSF), detection of misfolded α-synuclein protein by seed amplification assay, qualitative◀
▶PFAS Testing & PFASure™, National Medical Services, NMS Labs, Inc◀	●0394U	▶Perfluoroalkyl substances (PFAS) (eg, perfluorooctanoic acid, perfluorooctane sulfonic acid), 16 PFAS compounds by liquid chromatography with tandem mass spectrometry (LC-MS/MS), plasma or serum, quantitative◀
▶OncobiotaLUNG, Micronoma™, Micronoma™◀	●0395U	▶Oncology (lung), multi-omics (microbial DNA by shotgun next-generation sequencing and carcinoembryonic antigen and osteopontin by immunoassay), plasma, algorithm reported as malignancy risk for lung nodules in early-stage disease◀
▶Spectrum PGT-M, Natera, Inc, Natera, Inc◀	●0396U	▶Obstetrics (pre-implantation genetic testing), evaluation of 300000 DNA single-nucleotide-polymorphisms (SNPs) by microarray, embryonic tissue, algorithm reported as a probability for single gene germline conditions◀
—	▶(0397U has been deleted)◀	—
▶ESOPREDICT® Barrett's Esophagus Risk Classifier Assay, Capsulomics, Inc d/b/a Previse◀	●0398U	▶Gastroenterology (Barrett's esophagus), *P16, RUNX3, HPP1*, and *FBN1* DNA methylation analysis using PCR, formalin-fixed paraffin-embedded (FFPE) tissue, algorithm reported as risk score for progression to high-grade dysplasia or cancer◀
▶FRAT® (Folate Receptor Antibody Test), Religen Inc, Religen Inc◀	●0399U	▶Neurology (cerebral folate deficiency), serum, detection of anti-human folate receptor IgG-binding antibody and blocking autoantibodies by enzyme-linked immunoassay (ELISA), qualitative, and blocking autoantibodies, using a functional blocking assay for IgG or IgM, quantitative, reported as positive or not detected◀
▶Genesys Carrier Panel, Genesys Diagnostics, Inc◀	●0400U	▶Obstetrics (expanded carrier screening), 145 genes by next-generation sequencing, fragment analysis and multiplex ligation-dependent probe amplification, DNA, reported as carrier positive or negative◀
▶CARDIO inCode-Score (CIC-SCORE), GENinCode U.S. Inc, GENinCode U.S. Inc◀	●0401U	▶Cardiology (coronary heart disease [CHD]), 9 genes (12 variants), targeted variant genotyping, blood, saliva, or buccal swab, algorithm reported as a genetic risk score for a coronary event◀

(Continued on page 254)

▲ = Revised code   ● = New code   ▶ ◀ = Contains new or revised text   ✕ = Duplicate PLA test   ↑↓ = Category I PLA

Proprietary Name and Clinical Laboratory or Manufacturer	Alpha-Numeric Code	Code Descriptor
▶Abbott Alinity™ m STI Assay, Abbott Molecular, Inc◀	●0402U	▶Infectious agent (sexually transmitted infection), Chlamydia trachomatis, Neisseria gonorrhoeae, Trichomonas vaginalis, Mycoplasma genitalium, multiplex amplified probe technique, vaginal, endocervical, or male urine, each pathogen reported as detected or not detected◀
▶MyProstateScore 2.0, LynxDX, LynxDX◀	●0403U	▶Oncology (prostate), mRNA, gene expression profiling of 18 genes, first-catch post-digital rectal examination urine (or processed first-catch urine), algorithm reported as percentage of likelihood of detecting clinically significant prostate cancer◀
▶DiviTum®TKa, Biovica Inc, Biovica International AB◀	●0404U	▶Oncology (breast), semiquantitative measurement of thymidine kinase activity by immunoassay, serum, results reported as risk of disease progression◀
▶BTG Early Detection of Pancreatic Cancer, Breakthrough Genomics, Breakthrough Genomics◀	●0405U	▶Oncology (pancreatic), 59 methylation haplotype block markers, next-generation sequencing, plasma, reported as cancer signal detected or not detected◀
▶CyPath® Lung, Precision Pathology Services, bioAffinity Technologies, Inc◀	●0406U	▶Oncology (lung), flow cytometry, sputum, 5 markers (meso-tetra [4-carboxyphenyl] porphyrin [TCPP], CD206, CD66b, CD3, CD19), algorithm reported as likelihood of lung cancer◀
▶IntelxDKD™, Renalytix Inc, Renalytix Inc, NYC, NY◀	●0407U	▶Nephrology (diabetic chronic kidney disease [CKD]), multiplex electrochemiluminescent immunoassay (ECLIA) of soluble tumor necrosis factor receptor 1 (sTNFR1), soluble tumor necrosis receptor 2 (sTNFR2), and kidney injury molecule 1 (KIM-1) combined with clinical data, plasma, algorithm reported as risk for progressive decline in kidney function◀
▶Omnia™ SARS-CoV-2 Antigen Test, Qorvo Biotechnologies, Qorvo Biotechnologies◀	●0408U	▶Infectious agent antigen detection by bulk acoustic wave biosensor immunoassay, severe acute respiratory syndrome coronavirus 2 (SARS-CoV-2) (coronavirus disease [COVID-19])◀
▶LiquidHALLMARK®, Lucence Health, Inc◀	●0409U	▶Oncology (solid tumor), DNA (80 genes) and RNA (36 genes), by next-generation sequencing from plasma, including single nucleotide variants, insertions/deletions, copy number alterations, microsatellite instability, and fusions, report showing identified mutations with clinical actionability◀
▶Avantect™ Pancreatic Cancer Test, ClearNote™ Health, ClearNote™ Health◀	●0410U	▶Oncology (pancreatic), DNA, whole genome sequencing with 5-hydroxymethylcytosine enrichment, whole blood or plasma, algorithm reported as cancer detected or not detected◀

★ = Telemedicine   ◀ = Audio-only   ✚ = Add-on code   ✗ = FDA approval pending   # = Resequenced code   ⊘ = Modifier 51 exempt

Proprietary Name and Clinical Laboratory or Manufacturer	Alpha-Numeric Code	Code Descriptor
▶IDgenetix®, Castle Biosciences, Inc, Castle Biosciences, Inc◀	✖●0411U	▶Psychiatry (eg, depression, anxiety, attention deficit hyperactivity disorder [ADHD]), genomic analysis panel, variant analysis of 15 genes, including deletion/duplication analysis of *CYP2D6*◀
		▶(For additional PLA code with identical clinical descriptor, see 0345U. See Appendix O to determine appropriate code assignment)◀
▶PrecivityAD® blood test, C2N Diagnostics LLC, C2N Diagnostics LLC◀	●0412U	▶Beta amyloid, Aß42/40 ratio, immunoprecipitation with quantitation by liquid chromatography with tandem mass spectrometry (LC-MS/MS) and qualitative ApoE isoform-specific proteotyping, plasma combined with age, algorithm reported as presence or absence of brain amyloid pathology◀
▶DH Optical Genome Mapping/ Digital Karyotyping Assay, The Clinical Genomics and Advanced Technology (CGAT) Laboratory at Dartmouth Health, Bionano Genomics◀	●0413U	▶Oncology (hematolymphoid neoplasm), optical genome mapping for copy number alterations, aneuploidy, and balanced/complex structural rearrangements, DNA from blood or bone marrow, report of clinically significant alterations◀
▶LungOI, Imagene◀	●0414U	▶Oncology (lung), augmentative algorithmic analysis of digitized whole slide imaging for 8 genes *(ALK, BRAF, EGFR, ERBB2, MET, NTRK1-3, RET, ROS1)*, and *KRAS* G12C and PD-L1, if performed, formalin-fixed paraffin-embedded (FFPE) tissue, reported as positive or negative for each biomarker◀
▶SmartHealth Vascular Dx™, Morningstar Laboratories, LLC, SmartHealth DX◀	●0415U	▶Cardiovascular disease (acute coronary syndrome [ACS]), IL-16, FAS, FASLigand, HGF, CTACK, EOTAXIN, and MCP-3 by immunoassay combined with age, sex, family history, and personal history of diabetes, blood, algorithm reported as a 5-year (deleted risk) score for ACS◀
▶GENETWORx UTI with ABR, RCA Laboratory Services LLC d/b/a GENETWORx, GENETWORx◀	●0416U	▶Infectious agent detection by nucleic acid (DNA), genitourinary pathogens, identification of 20 bacterial and fungal organisms, including identification of 20 associated antibiotic-resistance genes, if performed, multiplex amplified probe technique, urine◀
▶Genomic Unity® Comprehensive Mitochondrial Disorders Analysis, Variantyx Inc, Variantyx Inc◀	●0417U	▶Rare diseases (constitutional/heritable disorders), whole mitochondrial genome sequence with heteroplasmy detection and deletion analysis, nuclear-encoded mitochondrial gene analysis of 335 nuclear genes, including sequence changes, deletions, insertions, and copy number variants analysis, blood or saliva, identification and categorization of mitochondrial disorder–associated genetic variants◀
▶PreciseDx Breast Biopsy Test, PreciseDx, PreciseDx, Inc NYC, NY◀	●0418U	▶Oncology (breast), augmentative algorithmic analysis of digitized whole slide imaging of 8 histologic and immunohistochemical features, reported as a recurrence score◀

(*Continued on page 256*)

Proprietary Name and Clinical Laboratory or Manufacturer	Alpha-Numeric Code	Code Descriptor
▶Tempus nP, Tempus Labs, Inc, Tempus Labs, Inc◀	●0419U	▶Neuropsychiatry (eg, depression, anxiety), genomic sequence analysis panel, variant analysis of 13 genes, saliva or buccal swab, report of each gene phenotype◀

Rationale

Numerous changes have occurred throughout Appendix O. Administrative Multianalyte Assays with Algorithmic Analyses (MAAA) code 0014M has been deleted and code 81517 has been established to report liver disease analysis of three biomarkers for the risk assessment of liver disease progression and other liver-related events in patients with advanced fibrosis due to nonalcoholic steatohepatitis.

Refer to the codebook and the Rationale for code 81517 for a full discussion of this change.

New administrative MAAA code 0019M has been established to report a residual cardiovascular risk MAAA for risk-prediction of cardiovascular (CV) events or death in at-risk patients.

Code 0019M is an administrative MAAA procedure in which protein analytes are processed from a blood sample to compute relationships between individual proteins and protein-network patterns. An algorithm-generated risk score based on the analysis of 27 of these proteins generates a risk score that predicts and stratifies risk of CV events or death for patients who belong to an elevated-risk group. These may include patients with prior CV event history, patients aged 65 years or older with no prior CV, and individuals diagnosed with type 2 diabetes, with chronic kidney disease, or experiencing non-acute chest pain. Stratifying a patient's CV risk helps decision making for additional cardio-protective therapies.

Appendix O has also been updated by replacing the name of "Vectra® DA, Crescendo Bioscience, Inc" to its new name of "Vectra® (Labcorp)" for code 81490.

In addition, a total of 61 new proprietary laboratory analyses (PLA) codes have been established for the CPT 2024 code set. PLA test codes are released and posted online at https://www.ama-assn.org/practice-management/cpt/cpt-pla-codes on a quarterly basis (fall, winter, spring, and summer). New codes are effective the quarter following their publication online. Other changes include the deletion of 15 codes (0053U, 0066U, 0143U-0150U, 0324U, 0325U, 0357U, 0386U, 0397U); the revision of 10 codes (0022U, 0095U, 0269U, 0271U, 0272U, 0274U, 0277U, 0278U, 0308U, 0362U); the revision of three test names (0308U-0310U); and the revision of the test name, laboratory name, and manufacturer name for code 0113U.

Clinical Example (0019M)

A 57-year-old female presents with type 2 diabetes and chronic kidney disease. A blood sample is collected and sent for a residual cardiovascular risk (RCVR) multianalyte assay with algorithm analysis.

Description of Procedure (0019M)

Run an assay and measure 27 analytes in the RCVR test with an output of relative fluorescent units (RFUs) as raw data. The RFU data are normalized and the RCVR algorithm is applied to calculate the risk score for the likelihood of a cardiovascular event in the next 4 years. A report is generated and sent to the ordering provider.

★ = Telemedicine ◀ = Audio-only ✛ = Add-on code ✐ = FDA approval pending # = Resequenced code ⊘ = Modifier 51 exempt

Appendix P

▶CPT Codes That May Be Used for Synchronous Real-Time Interactive Audio-Video Telemedicine Services◀

▶This listing is a summary of CPT codes that are typically rendered in person but may be used for reporting synchronous (real-time) interactive audio-video telemedicine services when appended by modifier 95. Procedures on this list involve electronic communication using interactive telecommunications equipment that includes, at a minimum, audio and video. The codes listed below are identified in CPT 2024 with the ★ symbol.◀

90785	90970	96164	99212
90791	92227	96165	99213
90792	92228	96167	99214
90832	92507	96168	99215
90833	92508	96170	99231
90834	92521	96171	99232
90836	92522	97110	99233
90837	92523	97112	99242
90838	92524	97116	99243
90839	92526	97161	99244
90840	92601	97162	99245
90845	92602	97165	99252
90846	92603	97166	99253
90847	92604	97530	99254
90863	93228	97535	99255
90951	93229	97750	99307
90952	93268	97755	99308
90954	93270	97760	99309
90955	93271	97761	99310
90957	93272	97802	99406
90958	96040	97803	99407
90960	96105	97804	99408
90961	96116	98960	99409
90963	96121	98961	99417
90964	96125	98962	99418
90965	96156	99202	99495
90966	96158	99203	99496
90967	96159	99204	99497
90968	96160	99205	99498
90969	96161	99211	

Rationale

In accordance with the addition of the new criteria for Appendixes P and T, the title for Appendix P has been revised by adding "Real-Time Interactive Audio-Video." The introduction also has been revised to indicate that these services are typically rendered in person and to include the new verbiage that has been added to the title.

Refer to the codebook and the Rationale for the Introduction for a full discussion of these changes.

Notes

Appendix Q

Severe Acute Respiratory Syndrome Coronavirus 2 (SARS-CoV-2) (coronavirus disease [COVID-19]) Vaccines

▶This table links the individual severe acute respiratory syndrome coronavirus 2 (SARS-CoV-2) (coronavirus disease [COVID-19]) vaccine product codes (91300-91317) to their associated immunization administration codes (0001A, 0002A, 0003A, 0004A, 0011A, 0012A, 0013A, 0021A, 0022A, 0031A, 0034A, 0041A, 0042A, 0044A, 0051A, 0052A, 0053A, 0054A, 0064A, 0071A, 0072A, 0073A, 0074A, 0081A, 0082A, 0083A, 0091A, 0092A, 0093A, 0094A, 0104A, 0111A, 0112A, 0113A, 0121A, 0124A, 0134A, 0141A, 0142A, 0144A, 0151A, 0154A, 0164A, 0171A, 0172A, 0173A, 0174A), patient age, manufacturer name, vaccine name(s), 10- and 11-digit National Drug Code (NDC) Labeler Product ID, and interval between doses. These codes are also located in the **Medicine** section of the CPT code set.

Additional introductory and instructional information for codes 0001A, 0002A, 0003A, 0004A, 0011A, 0012A, 0013A, 0021A, 0022A, 0031A, 0034A, 0041A, 0042A, 0044A, 0051A, 0052A, 0053A, 0054A, 0064A, 0071A, 0072A, 0073A, 0074A, 0081A, 0082A, 0083A, 0091A, 0092A, 0093A, 0094A, 0104A, 0111A, 0112A, 0113A, 0121A, 0124A, 0134A, 0141A, 0142A, 0144A, 0151A, 0154A, 0164A, 0171A, 0172A, 0173A, 0174A and 91300-91317 can be found in the **Immunization Administration for Vaccines/Toxoids** and **Vaccines, Toxoids** guidelines in the **Medicine** section of the CPT code set.◀

Appendix Q

Vaccine Code	Vaccine Administration Code(s)	Patient Age	Vaccine Manufacturer	Vaccine Name(s)	NDC 10/NDC 11 Labeler Product ID (Vial)	Dosing Interval
#91300 Severe acute respiratory syndrome coronavirus 2 (SARS-CoV-2) (coronavirus disease [COVID-19]) vaccine, mRNA-LNP, spike protein, preservative free, 30 mcg/0.3 mL dosage, diluent reconstituted, for intramuscular use	0001A (1st Dose) 0002A (2nd Dose) 0003A (3rd Dose) 0004A (Booster)	12 years and older	Pfizer, Inc	Pfizer-BioNTech COVID-19 Vaccine/Comirnaty	59267-1000-1 59267-1000-01	▲All Dosing: Refer to FDA/ CDC Guidance▼
#91305 Severe acute respiratory syndrome coronavirus 2 (SARS-CoV-2) (coronavirus disease [COVID-19]) vaccine, mRNA-LNP, spike protein, preservative free, 30 mcg/0.3 mL dosage, tris-sucrose formulation, for intramuscular use	#0051A (1st Dose) #0052A (2nd Dose) #0053A (3rd Dose) #0054A (Booster)	12 years and older	Pfizer, Inc	Pfizer-BioNTech COVID-19 Vaccine	59267-1025-1 59267-1025-01 00069-2025-1 00069-2025-01	▲All Dosing: Refer to FDA/ CDC Guidance▼
#●91312 Severe acute respiratory syndrome coronavirus 2 (SARS-CoV-2) (coronavirus disease [COVID-19]) vaccine, mRNA-LNP, bivalent spike protein, preservative free, 30 mcg/0.3 mL dosage, tris-sucrose formulation, for intramuscular use	#●0121A (1st Dose) #▲0124A (Additional Dose)	▲12 years and older▼	▲Pfizer, Inc▼	▲Pfizer-BioNTech COVID-19 Bivalent▼	▲59267-0304-1 59267-0304-01 59267-1404-1 59267-1404-01▼	▲All Dosing: Refer to FDA/ CDC Guidance▼
#91307 Severe acute respiratory syndrome coronavirus 2 (SARS-CoV-2) (coronavirus disease [COVID-19]) vaccine, mRNA-LNP, spike protein, preservative free, 10 mcg/0.2 mL dosage, diluent reconstituted, tris-sucrose formulation, for intramuscular use	#0071A (1st Dose) #0072A (2nd Dose) #0073A (3rd Dose) #0074A (Booster)	5 years through 11 years	Pfizer, Inc	Pfizer-BioNTech COVID-19 Vaccine	59267-1055-1 59267-1055-01	▲All Dosing: Refer to FDA/ CDC Guidance▼
#●91315 Severe acute respiratory syndrome coronavirus 2 (SARS-CoV-2) (coronavirus disease [COVID-19]) vaccine, mRNA-LNP, bivalent spike protein, preservative free, 10 mcg/0.2 mL dosage, diluent reconstituted, tris-sucrose formulation, for intramuscular use	#●0151A (1st Dose) #▲0154A (Additional Dose)	▲5 years through 11 years▼	▲Pfizer, Inc▼	▲Pfizer-BioNTech COVID-19 Bivalent▼	▲59267-0565-1 59267-0565-01▼	▲All Dosing: Refer to FDA/ CDC Guidance▼

★=Telemedicine ◀=Audio-only ✚=Add-on code ✗=FDA approval pending #=Resequenced code ⊘=Modifier 51 exempt

Vaccine Code	Vaccine Administration Code(s)	Patient Age	Vaccine Manufacturer	Vaccine Name(s)	NDC 10/NDC 11 Labeler Product ID (Vial)	Dosing Interval
#91308 Severe acute respiratory syndrome coronavirus 2 (SARS-CoV-2) (coronavirus disease [COVID-19]) vaccine, mRNA-LNP, spike protein, preservative free, 3 mcg/0.2 mL dosage, diluent reconstituted, tris-sucrose formulation, for intramuscular use	#0081A (1st Dose) #0082A (2nd Dose) #0083A (3rd Dose)	6 months through 4 years	Pfizer, Inc	Pfizer-BioNTech COVID-19 Vaccine	59267-0078-1 59267-0078-01 59267-0078-4 59267-0078-04	▲All Dosing: Refer to FDA/ CDC Guidance ▼
#●91317 Severe acute respiratory syndrome coronavirus 2 (SARS-CoV-2) (coronavirus disease [COVID-19]) vaccine, mRNA-LNP, bivalent spike protein, preservative free, 3 mcg/0.2 mL dosage, diluent reconstituted, tris-sucrose formulation, for intramuscular use	#●0171A (1st Dose) #●0172A (2nd Dose) #▲0173A (3rd Dose) #▲0174A (Additional Dose)	▲6 months through 4 years ▼	▲Pfizer, Inc ▼	▲Pfizer-BioNTech COVID-19 Bivalent ▼	▲59267-0609-1 59267-0609-01 ▼	▲All Dosing: Refer to FDA/ CDC Guidance ▼
#91301 Severe acute respiratory syndrome coronavirus 2 (SARS-CoV-2) (coronavirus disease [COVID-19]) vaccine, mRNA-LNP, spike protein, preservative free, 100 mcg/0.5 mL dosage, for intramuscular use	0011A (1st Dose) 0012A (2nd Dose) 0013A (3rd Dose)	12 years and older	Moderna, Inc	▲Moderna COVID-19 Vaccine/ spikevax ▼	▲80777-273-10 80777-0273-10 80777-100-11 80777-0100-11 ▼	▲All Dosing: Refer to FDA/ CDC Guidance ▼
#91306 Severe acute respiratory syndrome coronavirus 2 (SARS-CoV-2) (coronavirus disease [COVID-19]) vaccine, mRNA-LNP, spike protein, preservative free, 50 mcg/0.25 mL dosage, for intramuscular use	#0064A (Booster)	18 years and older	Moderna, Inc	Moderna COVID-19 Vaccine	80777-273-10 80777-0273-10	▲All Dosing: Refer to FDA/ CDC Guidance ▼
#●91313 Severe acute respiratory syndrome coronavirus 2 (SARS-CoV-2) (coronavirus disease [COVID-19]) vaccine, mRNA-LNP, spike protein, bivalent, preservative free, 50 mcg/0.5 mL dosage, for intramuscular use	#▲0134A (Additional Dose)	▲12 years and older ▼	▲Moderna, Inc ▼	▲Moderna COVID-19 Vaccine, Bivalent ▼	▲80777-282-05 80777-0282-05 ▼	▲Additional Dose: Refer to FDA/CDC Guidance ▼
#●91314 Severe acute respiratory syndrome coronavirus 2 (SARS-CoV-2) (coronavirus disease [COVID-19]) vaccine, mRNA-LNP, spike protein, bivalent, preservative free, 25 mcg/0.25 mL dosage, for intramuscular use	#●0141A (1st Dose) #●0142A (2nd Dose) #▲0144A (Additional Dose)	▲6 months through 11 years ▼	▲Moderna, Inc ▼	▲Moderna COVID-19 Vaccine, Bivalent ▼	▲80777-282-05 80777-0282-05 ▼	▲All Dosing: Refer to FDA/ CDC Guidance ▼

▲ = Revised code   ● = New code   ▶◀ = Contains new or revised text   ✕ = Duplicate PLA test   ↕ = Category I PLA

Vaccine Code	Vaccine Administration Code(s)	Patient Age	Vaccine Manufacturer	Vaccine Name(s)	NDC 10/NDC 11 Labeler Product ID (Vial)	Dosing Interval
#91311 Severe acute respiratory syndrome coronavirus 2 (SARS-CoV-2) (coronavirus disease [COVID-19]) vaccine, mRNA-LNP, spike protein, preservative free, 25 mcg/0.25 mL dosage, for intramuscular use	0111A (1st Dose) 0112A (2nd Dose) ●0113A (3rd Dose)	6 months through 5 years	Moderna, Inc	Moderna COVID-19 Vaccine	80777-279-05 80777-0279-05	▲All Dosing: Refer to FDA/CDC Guidance▼
#●91316 Severe acute respiratory syndrome coronavirus 2 (SARS-CoV-2) (coronavirus disease [COVID-19]) vaccine, mRNA-LNP, spike protein, bivalent, preservative free, 10 mcg/0.2 mL dosage, for intramuscular use	▲0164A (Additional Dose)	▲6 months through 5 years▼	▲Moderna, Inc▼	▲Moderna COVID-19 Vaccine, Bivalent▼	▲80777-283-02 80777-0283-02▼	▲Additional Dose: Refer to FDA/CDC Guidance▼
#91309 Severe acute respiratory syndrome coronavirus 2 (SARS-CoV-2) (coronavirus disease [COVID-19]) vaccine, mRNA-LNP, spike protein, preservative free, 50 mcg/0.5 mL dosage, for intramuscular use	#●0091A (1st Dose) #●0092A (2nd Dose) #●0093A (3rd Dose) #▲0094A (Booster)	▲6 years through 11 years▼	▲Moderna, Inc▼	▲Moderna COVID-19 Vaccine▼	▲80777-275-05 80777-0275-05▼	▲All Dosing: Refer to FDA/CDC Guidance▼
		18 years and older	Moderna, Inc	Moderna COVID-19 Vaccine	80777-275-05 80777-0275-05	Booster: Refer to FDA/CDC Guidance
#⚡91302 Severe acute respiratory syndrome coronavirus 2 (SARS-CoV-2) (coronavirus disease [COVID-19]) vaccine, DNA, spike protein, chimpanzee adenovirus Oxford 1 (ChAdOx1) vector, preservative free, 5×10^{10} viral particles/0.5 mL dosage, for intramuscular use	0021A (1st Dose) 0022A (2nd Dose)	18 years and older	AstraZeneca, Plc	AstraZeneca COVID-19 Vaccine	0310-1222-10 00310-1222-10	28 Days
#91303 Severe acute respiratory syndrome coronavirus 2 (SARS-CoV-2) (coronavirus disease [COVID-19]) vaccine, DNA, spike protein, adenovirus type 26 (Ad26) vector, preservative free, 5×10^{10} viral particles/0.5 mL dosage, for intramuscular use	0031A (Single Dose) 0034A (Booster)	18 years and older	Janssen	Janssen COVID-19 Vaccine	59676-580-05 59676-0580-05	▲All Dosing: Refer to FDA/CDC Guidance▼

★ = Telemedicine   ◀ = Audio-only   ✚ = Add-on code   ⚡ = FDA approval pending   # = Resequenced code   ⊘ = Modifier 51 exempt

Appendix Q

Vaccine Code	Vaccine Administration Code(s)	Patient Age	Vaccine Manufacturer	Vaccine Name(s)	NDC 10/NDC 11 Labeler Product ID (Vial)	Dosing Interval
#91304 Severe acute respiratory syndrome coronavirus 2 (SARS-CoV-2) (coronavirus disease [COVID-19]) vaccine, recombinant spike protein nanoparticle, saponin-based adjuvant, preservative free, 5 mcg/0.5 mL dosage, for intramuscular use	0041A (1st Dose) 0042A (2nd Dose)	▲12 years and older▼	Novavax, Inc	Novavax COVID-19 Vaccine	80631-100-01 80631-1000-01	21 Days
	●0044A (Booster)	▲18 years and older▼	▲Novavax, Inc▼	▲Novavax COVID-19 Vaccine▼	▲80631-100-01 80631-1000-01 ▼	▲Booster: Refer to FDA/CDC Guidance ▼
#✔91310 Severe acute respiratory syndrome coronavirus 2 (SARS-CoV-2) (coronavirus disease [COVID-19]) vaccine, monovalent, preservative free, 5 mcg/0.5 mL dosage, adjuvant AS03 emulsion, for intramuscular use	0104A (Booster)	18 years and older	Sanofi Pasteur	Sanofi Pasteur COVID-19 Vaccine, (Adjuvanted For Booster Immunization)	49281-618-20 49281-0618-20	Booster: Refer to FDA/CDC Guidance

Abbreviations: CDC indicates Centers for Disease Control and Prevention and FDA indicates Food and Drug Administration

Rationale

It is important to note that subsequent to the printing of the CPT codebook, the CPT Editorial Panel approved five new COVID-19 vaccine product codes and one administration code in August 2023. These new COVID-19 codes replaced all previously approved, specific COVID-19 product and administration codes, with the exception of vaccine product code 91304. In addition, Appendix Q has been deleted from the CPT code set effective November 1, 2023. To view the most current CPT codes to report for COVID-19 administration and products, refer to the AMA CPT public website at ama-assn.org/cpt-cat-i-immunization-codes. Because the decision to delete these codes took place after the *CPT 2024* codebook has been finalized, these deleted codes and Appendix Q are included in the *CPT 2024* codebook and *CPT Changes 2024*. Therefore, the following rationale only discusses the content that have been included in the *CPT 2024* codebook, which was finalized before the August 2023 revisions.

In accordance with the additions and revisions of codes for reporting severe acute respiratory syndrome coronavirus 2 (SARS-CoV-2) (coronavirus disease [COVID-19]) vaccine products and their administration, Appendix Q has been updated.

For the CPT 2024 code set, six new codes for COVID-19 vaccine products (91312-91317), as well as 18 COVID-19 vaccine administration codes (0044A, 0091A-0093A, 0113A, 0121A, 0124A, 0134A, 0141A, 0142A, 0144A, 0151A, 0154A, 0164A, 0171A-0174A) have been added to the table in Appendix Q.

Refer to the codebook and the Rationale for COVID-19 product administration for a full discussion of these changes.

★ = Telemedicine   ◀ = Audio-only   ✚ = Add-on code   ✗ = FDA approval pending   # = Resequenced code   ⊘ = Modifier 51 exempt

Appendix S

Artificial Intelligence Taxonomy for Medical Services and Procedures

This taxonomy provides guidance for classifying various artificial intelligence (AI) applications (eg, expert systems, machine learning, algorithm-based services) for medical services and procedures into one of these three categories: assistive, augmentative, and autonomous. AI as applied to health care may differ from AI in other public and private sectors (eg, banking, energy, transportation). Note that there is no single product, procedure, or service for which the term "AI" is sufficient or necessary to describe its intended clinical use or utility; therefore, the term "AI" is not defined in the code set. In addition, the term "AI" is not intended to encompass or constrain the full scope of innovations that are characterized as "work done by machines." Classification of AI medical services and procedures as assistive, augmentative, and autonomous is based on the clinical procedure or service provided to the patient and the work performed by the machine on behalf of the physician or other qualified health care professional (QHP).

Assistive: The work performed by the machine for the physician or other QHP is assistive when the machine **detects** clinically relevant data without analysis or generated conclusions. Requires physician or other QHP interpretation and report.

▶**Augmentative:** The work performed by the machine for the physician or other QHP is augmentative when the machine **analyzes** and/or **quantifies** data to yield clinically meaningful output. Requires physician or other QHP interpretation and report.

Autonomous: The work performed by the machine for the physician or other QHP is autonomous when the machine automatically **interprets** data and independently generates clinically meaningful conclusions without concurrent physician or other QHP involvement. Autonomous medical services and procedures include interrogating and analyzing data. The work of the algorithm may or may not include acquisition, preparation, and/or transmission of data. The clinically meaningful conclusion may be a characterization of data (eg, likelihood of pathophysiology) to be used to establish a diagnosis or to implement a therapeutic intervention. There are three levels of autonomous AI medical services and procedures with varying physician or other QHP professional involvement:

Level I. The autonomous AI draws conclusions and offers diagnosis and/or management options, which are contestable and require physician or other QHP action to implement.

Level II. The autonomous AI draws conclusions and initiates diagnosis and/or management options with alert/opportunity for override, which may require physician or other QHP action to implement.

Level III. The autonomous AI draws conclusions and initiates management, which requires physician or other QHP initiative to contest.◀

▶Service Components	AI Category: Assistive	AI Category: Augmentative	AI Category: Autonomous
Primary objective	Detects clinically relevant data	Analyzes and/or quantifies data to yield clinically meaningful output	Interprets data and independently generates clinically meaningful conclusions
Provides independent diagnosis and/or management decision	No	No	Yes
Analyzes data	No	Yes	Yes
Requires physician or other QHP interpretation and report	Yes	Yes	No
Examples in CPT code set	Algorithmic electrocardiogram risk-based assessment for cardiac dysfunction (0764T, 0765T)	Noninvasive estimate of coronary fractional flow reserve (FFR) (75580)	Retinal imaging (92229)◀

Rationale

Appendix S has been revised to include new examples of assistive and augmentative services that were recently included in the CPT code set. In addition, the guidelines have been revised.

The terminology and definitions used to describe artificial intelligence (AI) taxonomy for medical services and procedures have been applied by the CPT Editorial Panel. As a result, there are more codes included in the code set that can be used as examples than those originally listed in Appendix S in CPT 2023 as assistive and augmentative. Those new examples better illustrate the work performed by AI on behalf of physicians or other qualified health care professionals (QHPs).

The guidelines have been revised to clarify the intent of the augmentative and Level III definitions. In the augmentative definition, the word "way" has been replaced with "output" to better focus on the results of AI and its effects on the work of physicians or other QHPs rather than the algorithmic process.

Revisions to Appendix S include removing "Computer-aided detection (CAD) imaging (77048, 77049, 77065-77067, 0042T, 0174T, 0175T)" from the "AI Category: Assistive" column and adding "Algorithmic electrocardiogram risk-based assessment for cardiac dysfunction (0764T, 0765T)." In addition, in the "AI Category: Augmentative" column, "Continuous glucose monitoring (CGM) (95251), external processing of imaging data sets" has been removed, and "Noninvasive estimate of coronary fractional flow reserve (FFR) (75580)" has been added.

★ = Telemedicine   ◀ = Audio-only   ✚ = Add-on code   ✔ = FDA approval pending   # = Resequenced code   ⃠ = Modifier 51 exempt

Appendix T

CPT Codes That May Be Used for Synchronous Real-Time Interactive Audio-Only Telemedicine Services

▶This listing is a summary of CPT codes that are typically rendered in person but may be used for reporting audio-only services when appended with modifier 93. Procedures on this list involve electronic communication using interactive telecommunications equipment that includes, at a minimum, audio. The codes listed below are identified in CPT 2024 with the ◀ symbol.◀

Rationale

In accordance with the new criteria added for Appendixes P and T, the introduction for Appendix T has been revised to indicate that these services are typically provided in person.

Refer to the codebook and the Rationale for the Introduction for a full discussion of these changes.

90785	92508	96165
90791	92521	96167
90792	92522	96168
90832	92523	96170
90833	92524	96171
90834	96040	97802
90836	96110	97803
90837	96116	97804
90838	96121	99406
90839	96156	99407
90840	96158	99408
90845	96159	99409
90846	96160	99497
90847	96161	99498
92507	96164	

Notes

Indexes

Instructions for the Use of the Changes Indexes

The Changes Indexes are not a substitute for the main text of *CPT Changes 2024* or the main text of the CPT codebook. The changes indexes consist of two types of content—coding changes and modifiers—all of which are intended to assist users in searching and locating information quickly within *CPT Changes 2024*.

Index of Coding Changes

The Index of Coding Changes list new, revised, and deleted codes, and/or some codes that may be affected by revised and/or new guidelines and parenthetical notes. This index enables users to quickly search and locate the codes within a page(s), in addition to discerning the status of a code (new, revised, deleted, or textually changed) because the status of each new, revised, or deleted code is noted in parentheses next to the code number:

0014M (deleted) 81, 203, 210, 256
27278 (new) 23, 29, 30, 174, 187

Index of Modifiers

The Index of Modifiers does not list all modifiers unless they are new, revised, or deleted, and/or if the modifier may be affected by revised and/or new codes, guidelines, and parenthetical notes. A limited Index of Modifiers, ie, limited to only those modifiers that appear in the Rationales and new or revised guidelines and/or parenthetical notes, is provided to help users quickly locate these modifiers and to know where in the book these modifiers are listed or mentioned.

50, Bilateral Procedure 4, 29, 42
51, Multiple Procedures 122

Index of Coding Changes

Codes in this index are in numerical order, with the four-digit alphanumeric codes first:

Category III changes (a four-digit code followed by the letter "T"); changes to administrative codes for multianalyte assays with algorithmic analyses (MAAA) (a four-digit code followed by the letter "M"); and changes to proprietary laboratory analysis (PLA) codes (a four-digit code followed by the letter "U"). Five-digit CPT codes follow.

0001A 21, 113, 114, 122, 123, 141, 259
0002A 21, 113, 114, 122, 123, 141, 259
0003A 21, 113, 114, 122, 123, 141, 259
0004A 21, 113, 114, 122, 123, 141, 259
0011A 21, 113, 115, 122-124, 141, 259
0012A 21, 113, 115, 122-124, 141, 259
0013A 21, 113, 115, 122, 124, 141, 259
0014M (deleted) 81, 203, 210, 256
0019M (new) 203, 210, 256
0021A 21, 113, 122, 141, 259
0022A 21, 113, 122, 141, 259
0022U (revised) 58, 94, 98, 203, 217, 256
0031A 21, 113, 122, 141, 259
0034A 21, 113, 122, 141, 259
0041A 21, 113, 122, 124, 141, 259
0042A 21, 113, 122, 124, 141, 259
0042T 266
0044A (new) 21, 110, 113, 116-118, 122, 124, 141, 259, 263, 264
0051A 21, 113, 115, 122, 123, 141, 259
0052A 21, 113, 115, 122, 123, 141, 259
0053A 21, 113, 115, 122, 123, 141, 259
0053U (deleted) 58, 94, 98, 203, 220, 256
0054A 21, 113, 115, 122, 123, 141, 259
0064A 21, 113, 115, 122, 124, 141, 259
0066U (deleted) 59, 94, 98, 203, 221, 256
0071A 21, 113, 115, 122, 123, 141, 259
0072A 21, 113, 115, 122, 123, 259
0073A 21, 113, 115, 122, 123, 141, 259
0074A 21, 113, 115, 122, 123, 141, 259
0081A 113, 115, 122, 123, 141, 259
0081A-0083A 21
0082A 113, 115, 122, 123, 141, 259
0083A 113, 115, 122, 123, 141, 259
0091A (new) 21, 110, 113, 116-118, 122-124, 141, 259, 262, 264
0092A (new) 21, 110, 113, 116-118, 122-124, 141, 259, 262, 264
0093A (new) 21, 110, 113, 116-118, 122-124, 141, 259, 262, 264
0094A (revised) 21, 110, 113, 116, 118, 119, 122-124, 141, 259

0095U (revised) 59, 94, 98, 204, 223, 256
0101T 198
0104A 21, 113, 122, 141, 259
0111A 21, 113, 116, 122-124, 141, 259
0112A 21, 113, 116, 122-124, 141, 259
0113A (new) 21, 110, 113, 116-119, 122-124, 141, 259, 262, 264
0113U 98, 256
0121A 21, 260
0121A (new) 21, 109, 113, 115-117, 119, 122, 123, 141, 259, 264
0124A 21, 260
0124A (revised) 21, 109, 113, 115-117, 119, 122, 123, 141, 259, 264
0134A 21
0134A (revised) 21, 109, 113, 116, 117, 119,
                                122-124, 141, 259, 261, 264
0141A 21
0141A (new) 21, 109, 113, 116, 117, 119,
                           120, 122-124, 141, 259, 261, 264
0142A 21
0142A (new) 21, 109, 113, 116, 117, 120,
                           122-124, 141, 259, 261, 264
0143U (deleted) 59, 94, 98, 204, 228, 256
0144A 21
0144A (revised) 21, 110, 113, 116, 117, 120,
                           122-124, 141, 259, 261, 264
0144U (deleted) 59, 94, 98, 204, 228, 256
0145U (deleted) 59, 94, 98, 204, 228, 256
0146U (deleted) 59, 94, 98, 204, 228, 256
0147U (deleted) 59, 94, 98, 204, 228, 256
0148U (deleted) 59, 94, 98, 204, 228, 256
0149U (deleted) 59, 95, 98, 205, 228, 256
0150U (deleted) 59, 95, 98, 205, 228, 256
0151A (new) 21, 109, 113, 115-117, 120,
                           122, 123, 141, 259, 260, 264
0154A (revised) 21, 109, 113, 115-117, 120,
                           122, 123, 141, 259, 260, 264
0164A (revised) 21, 110, 113, 116, 117, 120-124, 141, 259, 262, 264
0171A (new) 21, 109, 113, 115-117, 121-123, 141, 259, 261, 264
0172A (new) 21, 109, 113, 115-117, 121-123, 141, 259, 261, 264

0173A (revised).....21, 109, 113, 115-117, 121-123, 141, 259, 261, 264
0174A (revised).....21, 109, 113, 115-117, 121-124, 141, 259, 261, 264
0174T 266
0175T 266
0269U (revised) 59, 95, 98, 205, 240, 256
0271U (revised)........................59, 95, 98, 99, 205, 240, 256
0272U (revised)........................59, 95, 98, 99, 205, 240, 256
0274U (revised) 59, 95, 98, 99, 205, 240, 256
0277U (revised)........................59, 95, 98, 99, 205, 241, 256
0278T 156
0278U (revised)........................59, 95, 98, 99, 205, 241, 256
0308U (revised) 59, 95, 98, 205, 243, 256
0309U 256
0310U 256
0324U (deleted) 60, 95, 98, 205, 245, 256
0325U (deleted) 60, 95, 98, 205, 245, 256
0345T 140
0345U 97
0355U (new) 60, 95, 205, 249
0356U (new) 60, 95, 99, 206, 249
0357U (deleted) 60, 95, 98, 206, 249, 256
0358U (new) 60, 95, 99, 100, 206, 249
0359U (new) 60, 95, 100, 206, 249
0360U (new) 60, 95, 100, 206, 249
0361U (new)...............................60, 95, 100, 206, 249
0362U (revised) 60, 95, 98, 100, 206, 249, 256
0363U (new) 60, 95, 100, 206, 249
0364U (new) 60, 95, 100, 206, 249
0365U (new) 60, 95, 101, 206, 249
0366U (new) 60, 95, 101, 206, 250
0367U (new) 60, 95, 101, 206, 250
0368U (new) 60, 95, 101, 206, 250
0369U (new) 60, 96, 101, 206, 250
0370U (new)...............................60, 96, 101, 206, 250
0371U (new) 60, 96, 101, 206, 250
0372U (new)...............................60, 96, 102, 206, 250
0373U (new)...............................60, 96, 102, 206, 250
0374U (new)...............................60, 96, 102, 206, 250
0375U (new) 60, 96, 102, 206, 251
0376U (new)...............................60, 96, 102, 206, 251
0377U (new) 60, 96, 102, 206, 251
0378U (new)...............................60, 96, 102, 206, 251
0379U (new) 60, 96, 103, 206, 251
0380U (new) 60, 96, 103, 206, 251
0381U (new)...............................60, 96, 103, 206, 251
0382U (new) 61, 96, 103, 206, 251
0383U (new) 61, 96, 103, 206, 251

0384U (new) 61, 96, 103, 206, 252
0385U (new) 61, 96, 103, 104, 206, 252
0386U (deleted)........................61, 96, 98, 207, 252, 256
0387U (new) 61, 96, 104, 207, 252
0388U (new) 61, 96, 104, 207, 252
0389U (new) 61, 96, 104, 207, 252
0390U (new) 61, 96, 104, 207, 252
0391U (new) 61, 97, 104, 207, 252
0392U (new) 61, 97, 104, 207, 253
0393U (new) 61, 97, 105, 207, 253
0394U (new) 61, 97, 105, 207, 253
0395U (new) 61, 97, 105, 207, 253
0396U (new) 61, 97, 105, 207, 253
0397U (deleted) 61, 97, 98, 207, 253, 256
0398U (new) 61, 97, 105, 207, 253
0399U (new) 61, 97, 105, 207, 253
0400U (new) 61, 97, 105, 207, 253
0401U (new) 61, 97, 105, 106, 207, 253
0402U (new) 61, 97, 106, 207, 254
0403U (new) 61, 97, 106, 207, 254
0404T (deleted) 41, 151, 156
0404U (new) 61, 97, 106, 207, 254
0405U (new) 61, 97, 106, 207, 254
0406U (new) 61, 97, 106, 207, 254
0407U (new) 61, 97, 106, 207, 254
0408U (new) 61, 97, 106, 107, 207, 254
0409U (new) 61, 97, 107, 207, 254
0410U (new) 61, 97, 107, 207, 254
0411U (new) 61, 95, 97, 107, 207, 248, 255
0412U (new) 61, 97, 107, 207, 255
0413U (new) 61, 98, 107, 207, 255
0414U (new) 62, 98, 107, 207, 255
0415U (new) 62, 98, 108, 207, 255
0416U (new) 62, 98, 108, 207, 255
0417U (new) 62, 98, 108, 207, 255
0418U (new) 62, 98, 108, 207, 255
0419U (new) 62, 98, 108, 207, 256
0424T (deleted)...........................36, 134, 151, 156
0425T (deleted)...........................36, 134, 151, 156
0426T (deleted)...........................36, 134, 151, 156
0427T (deleted)...........................36, 134, 151, 156
0428T (deleted)...........................36, 134, 151, 156
0429T (deleted)...........................36, 134, 151, 156
0430T (deleted)...........................36, 134, 151, 156
0431T (deleted)...........................36, 134, 151, 156
0432T (deleted) 36, 134, 151, 156
0433T (deleted) 36, 134, 151, 156

★ = Telemedicine   ◀ = Audio-only   ✚ = Add-on code   ✗ = FDA approval pending   # = Resequenced code   ⦸ = Modifier 51 exempt

0434T (deleted)	36, 134, 151, 156
0435T (deleted)	36, 134, 151, 156
0436T (deleted)	36, 134, 151, 156
0465T (deleted)	48, 151, 156
0483T	140
0484T	140
0499T (deleted)	40, 152, 158, 163
0501T (deleted)	52, 152, 158, 159, 165
0502T (deleted)	52, 152, 158, 159, 165
0503T (deleted)	52, 152, 158, 159, 165
0504T (deleted)	52, 152, 158, 159, 165
0508T (deleted)	152, 159
0515T	56, 159, 160
0516T	53, 56, 159-161
0517T (revised)	53, 56, 152, 159-161
0518T (revised)	53, 56, 152, 159-161
0519T (revised)	53, 56, 152, 159-161
0520T (revised)	53, 56, 152, 159, 160, 162
0523T	159
0533T (deleted)	152, 162
0534T (deleted)	152, 162
0535T (deleted)	152, 162
0536T (revised)	152, 162
0543T	140
0544T	140
0545T	140
0552T	144, 162, 163
0587T (revised)	46, 47, 152, 163, 174, 190, 191
0588T (revised)	46, 47, 152, 163, 174, 190, 191
0589T (revised)	47, 153, 163, 174, 190, 191
0590T (revised)	47, 153, 163, 174, 190, 191
0619T	163
0623T	165
0624T	165
0625T	165
0626T	159, 165
0632T	176, 177
0640T (revised)	151, 156, 157
0641T (deleted)	152, 157
0642T (deleted)	152, 157
0648T	198, 199
0649T	198, 199
0656T (revised)	25-27, 32, 153, 164
0657T (revised)	25-27, 32, 153, 164
0697T	198
0698T	198
0710T	165
0711T	165
0712T	165
0713T	165
0715T (deleted)	132, 153, 165
0721T	198, 199
0722T	198, 199
0751T-0763T	166
0764T	265, 266
0765T	265, 266
0766T (revised)	45, 47, 128, 141, 144, 154, 156, 172, 173
0767T (revised)	45, 47, 128, 144, 154, 156, 172, 173
0768T (deleted)	47, 128, 141, 144, 154, 156, 172, 173
0769T (deleted)	47, 128, 141, 144, 154, 156, 172, 173
0771T	199
0775T (deleted)	29, 154, 174
0784T (new)	44, 46, 47, 154, 174
0785T (new)	44, 46, 47, 154, 174, 175
0786T (new)	44, 47, 154, 174, 175
0787T (new)	44, 46, 47, 154, 174, 175
0788T (new)	47, 154, 163, 174, 175
0789T (new)	47, 154, 174, 175
0790T (new)	25-27, 32, 153, 164, 165, 175
0791T (new)	145, 154, 175, 176
0792T (new)	154, 176
0793T (new)	154, 164, 176, 177
0794T (new)	154, 177, 178
0795T (new)	33-35, 53, 135, 140, 154, 160, 178-180, 193, 194
0796T (new)	33, 34, 53, 135, 140, 154, 160, 178-181, 193, 194
0797T (new)	33-35, 53, 135, 140, 154, 160, 178-181, 193, 194
0798T (new)	33, 35, 53, 140, 154, 160, 178-181, 182, 193
0799T (new)	33, 35, 53, 140, 154, 160, 178-180, 182, 193, 194
0800T (new)	33, 35, 53, 140, 154, 160, 178-180, 182, 193
0801T (new)	33, 35, 53, 135, 140, 155, 160, 178-180, 182, 193
0802T (new)	33, 35, 53, 135, 140, 155, 160, 178-180, 183, 193, 194
0803T (new)	33, 35, 53, 135, 140, 155, 160, 178-180, 183, 193
0804T (new)	33, 35, 155, 178, 179, 184, 198
0805T (new)	155, 184, 185
0806T (new)	155, 184, 185, 186
0807T (new)	155, 186, 187
0808T (new)	155, 186, 187
0809T	29
0809T (deleted)	29, 30, 155, 187
0810T (new)	155, 188
0811T (new)	22, 39, 40, 155, 188, 189
0812T (new)	22, 39, 40, 155, 188, 189
0813T (new)	155, 189
0814T (new)	29, 155, 189

Indexes

Indexes

0815T (new) 155, 190

0816T (new) 46, 155, 163, 174, 190, 191

0817T (new) 46, 155, 163, 174, 190, 191

0818T (new) 46, 155, 163, 174, 190, 191

0819T (new) 46, 155, 163, 174, 190, 191

0820T (new) 155, 191, 192

0821T (new) 155, 191, 192, 193

0822T (new) 155, 191, 192, 193

0823T (new) 33-35, 53, 135, 140, 155,
160, 179, 180, 193, 194, 195

0824T (new) 33, 35, 53, 135, 140, 155,
160, 179, 180, 193, 194, 195

0825T (new) 33, 35, 53, 135, 140, 155,
160, 179, 180, 193, 194, 195

0826T (new) 33, 35, 155, 179, 193, 194, 196

0827T (new) 88, 153, 166, 168, 196

0828T (new) 88, 153, 166, 168, 196

0829T (new) 88, 153, 166, 168, 196

0830T (new) 88, 153, 166, 168, 196

0831T (new) 88, 153, 166, 168, 169, 196

0832T (new) 88, 153, 166, 169, 196

0833T (new) 89, 153, 166, 169, 196

0834T (new) 89, 153, 166, 169, 196

0835T (new) 89, 153, 166, 169, 196

0836T (new) 89, 153, 166, 169, 196

0837T (new) 89, 153, 166, 169, 196

0838T (new) 90, 91, 153, 166, 167, 169, 196

0839T (new) 91, 153, 166, 167, 170, 196

0840T (new) 91, 153, 166, 167, 170, 196

0841T (new) 91, 153, 166, 167, 170, 196

0842T (new) 91, 153, 166, 167, 170, 196

0843T (new) 91, 153, 166, 167, 170, 196

0844T (new) 91, 92, 153, 166, 167, 170, 196

0845T (new) 92, 153, 166, 167, 170, 171, 196

0846T (new) 92, 153, 166, 167, 171, 196

0847T (new) 92, 153, 166, 167, 171, 196

0848T (new) 92, 154, 166, 167, 171, 196

0849T (new) 92, 93, 154, 166, 167, 171, 196

0850T (new) 93, 154, 166, 167, 171, 196

0851T (new) 93, 154, 166, 167, 171, 196

0852T (new) 93, 154, 166, 167, 171, 196

0853T (new) 93, 154, 166, 167, 172, 196

0854T (new) 83, 154, 166, 167, 172, 196

0855T (new) 83, 154, 166, 167, 172, 196

0856T (new) 92, 154, 166-168, 172, 196

0857T (new) 155, 197

0858T (new) 155, 197

0859T (new) 152, 156, 157, 158, 198

0860T (new) 152, 157, 158, 198

0861T (new) 53, 56, 152, 159, 160, 162, 198

0862T (new) 53, 54, 56, 152, 159, 160, 162, 198

0863T (new) 53, 56, 152, 159, 160, 162, 198

0864T (new) 155, 198

0865T (new) 155, 198, 199

0866T (new) 155, 198, 199

11400-11446 2

11600-11646 2

22800 .... 25, 27

22802 .... 25, 27

22804 .... 25, 27

22808 .... 25, 27

22810 .... 25, 27

22812 .... 25, 27

22818 .... 25, 27

22819 .... 25, 27

22836 (new) 23, 25-27, 32, 164

22837 (new) 23, 25-27, 28, 32, 164

22838 (new) 23, 25-27, 28, 32, 164

22845 26

22846 26

22847 26

22849 26

22855 26

26992 189

27235 29

27278 (new) 23, 29, 30, 174, 187

27279 ....29, 174, 187

27299 29

28292 (revised) 23, 30, 31

28295 (revised) 23, 30, 31

28296 (revised) 23, 30

28297 (revised) 23, 30, 31

28298 (revised) 23, 30

28299 (revised) 23, 30

28740 .... 30, 31

29999 3

30117 31

30118 31

31231 31

31242 (new) 23, 31

31243 (new) 23, 31, 32

32601 .... 26, 32

33206 34

33207 34

33208 34

★ = Telemedicine   ◀ = Audio-only   ✚ = Add-on code   ✒ = FDA approval pending   # = Resequenced code   ⊘ = Modifier 51 exempt

33210	185
33211	185
33212	34
33213	34
33214	34
33216	34
33217	34
33221	34
33224	34
33225	34, 35
33227	34
33228	34, 35
33229	34, 35
33230	34
33231	34
33233	34
33234	34
33235	34
33240	34
33241	34, 35
33244	34
33249	34
33262	34
33263	34, 35
33264	34, 35
33270	34, 35
33271	34
33272	34, 35
33274	33-35, 53, 135, 140, 178-180, 193, 194
33275	33, 35, 53, 140, 179, 180, 193
33276 (new)	23, 35-37, 39, 132, 134, 156
33277 (new)	23, 35-37, 39, 133, 134, 156
33278 (new)	23, 36, 37, 39, 133, 134
33279 (new)	23, 36, 37, 39, 133, 156
33280 (new)	23, 36, 38, 39, 133, 134, 156
33281 (new)	23, 36, 38, 39, 133, 134, 156
33287 (new)	24, 36, 38, 39, 134, 156
33288 (new)	24, 36, 38, 39, 134, 156
33340	140
33361	140
33362	140
33363	140
33364	140
33365	140
33366	140
33368	185
33369	185

33418	140
33477	140
33724	180
33741	140
33745	140
33957	53
33958	53
33959	53
33962	53
33963	53
33964	53
33967	185
33970	185
33973	185
33990	185
33991	185
33992	185
33993	185
33995	185
33997	185
33999	36
36475	3, 56
36479	56
36568	53
36569	53
36572	53
36573	53
36584	53
36836	53
36837	53
37191	53
37192	53
37193	53
37760	53, 56
37761	53, 56
37799	3
38100	142
38101	142
38102	142
38120	142
39599	3
42820	2
42825	2
42830	2
43197	189
43198	189
43235	189

Indexes

43241	189
43247	189
43281	3
43290	189
43291	189
43611	142
43620	142
43621	142
43622	142
43631	142
43632	142
43633	142
43634	142
43647	163, 174
43648	39, 163, 174
43881	163, 174
43882	39, 163, 174
43999	39
44010	142
44015	142
44110	142
44111	142
44120	142
44121	142
44125	142
44130	142
44139	142
44140	142
44141	142
44143	142
44144	142
44145	142
44146	142
44147	142
44150	142
44151	142
44155	142
44156	142
44157	142
44158	142
44160	142
44202	142
44203	142
44204	142
44207	142
44213	142
44227	142

46948	56
47001	142
47100	142
47370	56
47371	56
47380	56
47381	56
47382	56
48140	142
48145	142
48152	142
48155	142
49000	142
49010	142
49203	142
49204	142
49205	142
49320	41, 142
51610	40
51736	39, 40, 188
51741	39, 40, 188
52000	40, 163
52281	40
52283	40
52284 (new)	24, 40, 158, 163
52441	163
52442	163
52450	163
52500	163
52601	163
52630	163
52640	163
52647	163
52648	163
52649	163
53850	163
53852	163
53854	163
58200	142
58210	142
58353	41
58356	41
58541-58546	41
58548	41
58550	41
58552-58554	41
58561	41

Indexes

58570-58573	41
58575	142
58580 (new)	24, 41, 156
58661	42
58674	41
58940	142
58943	142
58950	142
58951	142
58952	142
58953	142
58954	142
58956	142
58957	142
58958	142
58960	142
61850-61888	163, 174
61885	42, 43
61886	42, 43
61888	42, 43
61889 (new)	24, 42, 43
61891 (new)	24, 42, 43
61892 (new)	24, 42, 43, 44
63650	44, 163, 174
63655	44, 163, 174
63661	44, 163, 174
63662	44, 163, 174
63663	44, 163, 174
63664	44, 163, 174
63685	163
63685 (revised)	24, 44-46, 163, 174
63688	163
63688 (revised)	24, 44-46, 163, 174
64553	163
64553-64595	163, 174
64555	45-47, 163, 190
64561	45, 46
64566	47, 163, 190
64575	163, 190
64585	47
64590 (revised)	24, 39, 45-47, 163, 174, 190
64595 (revised)	24, 39, 45-48, 163, 174
64596 (new)	24, 39, 45-48, 163, 174, 190
64597 (new)	24, 39, 45-48, 163
64598 (new)	24, 39, 45-48, 163, 174
64999	46, 47
67036	188
67039	188
67040	188
67041	188
67042	188
67043	188
67516 (new)	24, 48, 49, 156
69729	49
70551	198
70552	198
70553	198
71250	186
71260	186
71270	186
71271	186
74450	40
74710 (deleted)	51, 52
75574	52
75580 (new)	51, 52, 158, 159, 165, 265, 266
75746	176, 177
75820	178, 179, 193
75825	137, 139, 140
75827	137, 139, 140
76000	40, 53, 178, 179, 186, 193, 194
76376	159
76377	159
76641	197
76642	197
76830	41
76872	163
76937	53, 178, 179, 193, 194
76940	41
76942	53
76984 (new)	51, 54, 56
76987 (new)	51, 54-56
76988 (new)	51, 54-56
76989 (new)	54-56
76998	41, 54, 56
76999	159
77002	178, 179, 189, 193, 194
77048	266
77049	266
77065	266
77066	266
77067	266
77605	143
78579	186, 187
78582	186, 187

Indexes

78598	186, 187
81000	63
81001	63
81002	63
81003	63
81005	63
81007	63
81015	63
81020	63
81025	63
81050	63
81099	63
81171 (revised)	57, 63
81172 (revised)	57, 63
81243 (revised)	57, 63
81244 (revised)	57, 63, 64
81403 (revised)	57, 64–65, 76
81404 (revised)	57, 65–68, 76
81405 (revised)	57, 68–71, 76, 78
81406 (revised)	57, 71–75, 76, 78
81407 (revised)	58, 75–76
81445 (revised)	58, 76-79
81449 (revised)	58, 76-79
81450 (revised)	58, 76-79
81451 (revised)	58, 76-80
81455 (revised)	58, 76-80
81456 (revised)	58, 76-80
81457 (new)	58, 76-80
81458 (new)	58, 76-80
81459 (new)	58, 76-80
81462 (new)	58, 76-79, 81
81463 (new)	58, 76-79, 81
81464 (new)	58, 76-79, 81
81479	76
81490	256
81517 (new)	58, 81-83, 203, 210, 213, 256
82009-84830	63, 82-84, 86
82166 (new)	58, 82, 83
83519	84
83520	81, 83, 213
84999	82
85002-85810	83
85060	83, 167, 168
85097	83, 167, 168
85999	83
86008	84
86015-86835	83, 84, 86
86041 (new)	58, 84, 85
86042 (new)	58, 84, 85
86043 (new)	58, 84, 85
86255	84
86256	84
86304	85
86366 (new)	58, 84, 85
86692	85-87
86849	84
86850-86985	83, 86
86999	86
87003-87912	86
87380	85, 87
87523 (new)	58, 85-87
87593 (new)	58, 87
87999	86
88000-88045	87
88099	87
88104	166
88104-88189	87
88106	88, 166
88108	88, 166, 168
88112	88, 166, 168
88141	88, 166, 168
88160	88, 166, 168
88161	89, 166
88162	89, 166, 168
88172	89, 166, 168
88173	89, 166, 168
88177	89, 166, 168
88199	87
88230-88291	90
88299	90
88300-88309	90
88300-88388	90
88311-88365	90
88311-88388	90
88321	90, 91, 166-168
88323	91, 167, 168
88325	91, 167, 168
88331	91, 167, 168
88332	91, 167, 168
88333	91, 167, 168
88334	91, 92, 167, 168
88341	96
88342	96
88346	92, 167, 168

★ = Telemedicine   ◀ = Audio-only   ✛ = Add-on code   𝒩 = FDA approval pending   # = Resequenced code   ⊘ = Modifier 51 exempt

88348 ....92, 167, 168
88350 ....92, 167, 168
88363 ....92, 167, 168
88364 ....92, 93, 167, 168
88365 ....90, 92, 167, 168
88366 ....93, 167, 168
88367 90
88368 ....90, 93, 167, 168
88369 ....93, 167, 168
88377 ....93, 167, 168
88399 90
88720 94
88738 94
88740 94
88741 94
88749 94
89049-89230 94
89240 94
89250-89356 94
89398 94
90281-90399 ....114, 122
90380 (new) 109, 112, 113, 126
90381 (new) 109, 112, 113, 126
90460 ....21, 113, 114, 121, 122, 125-127, 141
90461 ....21, 113, 114, 121, 122, 125-127, 141
90471 ....21, 113, 114, 121, 122, 125-127, 141
90472 ....21, 113, 114, 121, 122, 125-127, 141
90473 ....21, 113, 114, 121, 122, 125-127
90474 ....21, 113, 114, 121, 122, 125-127
90476-90759 ....21, 113, 114, 121, 122
90589 (new) 110, 125, 126, 201, 202
90611 (new) 110, 126, 127
90622 (new) 110, 126, 127
90623 (new) 110, 126, 127, 201, 202
90679 (new) 110, 126
90683 (new) 110, 126, 201, 202
90832 192
90833 192
90834 192
90836 192
90837 192
90838 192
90839 192
90840 192
90867 128
91300 ....21, 113-115, 121-123, 259
91301 ....21, 113-116, 121-123, 259

91304 ....21, 113-117, 121, 122, 124, 259, 264
91305 ....21, 113-115, 121-123, 259
91306 ....21, 113-116, 121-123, 259
91307 ....21, 113-115, 121-123, 259
91308 ....21, 113-115, 121-123, 259
91309 ....21, 113, 115, 116, 118, 121, 122, 124, 259
91311 ....21, 113-116, 118, 121, 122, 124, 259
91312 (new) 21, 110, 114, 115, 117, 118,
                                                    122-124, 128, 259, 260, 264
91313 (new) 21, 110, 115-118, 121-124, 128, 259, 261
91314 (new) 21, 110, 115-118, 121, 122, 124, 125, 128, 259, 261
91315 (new) 21, 110, 114, 115, 117, 118,
                                                    121-124, 125, 128, 259, 260
91316 (new) 21, 110, 115-118, 121, 124, 125, 128, 259, 262
91317 (new) 21, 110, 113-115, 117, 118,
                                              121-124, 125, 128, 259, 261, 264
92229 (new) 265
92511 31
92601 ....129, 130
92602 ....129, 130
92603 ....129, 130
92604 ....129, 130
92622 (new) 49, 128-130
92623 (new) 49, 110, 128-130
92626 128-130
92627 ....129, 130
92630 ....128, 129
92633 ....128, 129
92920 ....131, 132
92920-92944 130
92924 ....131, 132
92928 ....131, 132
92933 ....131, 132
92937 ....131, 132
92941 ....131, 132
92943 ....131, 132
92972 (new) 110, 130-133, 165
92973 132
92974 132
92975 ....131, 132
92978 132
92979 132
92986 140
92987 140
92990 140
92997 140
93150 (new) 36, 110, 133, 134, 141, 156
93151 (new) 36, 110, 133, 134, 156

93152 (new) 36, 110, 133, 134, 140, 141, 156
93153 (new) 36, 110, 133, 134, 135, 141, 156
93279 .... 33, 178, 193
93286 33
93288 33
93294 33
93296 33
93451 .... 33, 140, 178, 179, 184, 185, 193, 194
93452 .... 140, 184
93453 .... 33, 140, 178, 179, 184, 185, 193, 194
93454 .... 140, 184
93455 .... 140, 184
93456 .... 33, 140, 178, 179, 184, 185, 193
93457 .... 33, 140, 178, 179, 184, 185
93458 .... 140, 184
93459 .... 140, 184
93460 .... 33, 140, 178, 179, 184, 185, 193
93461 .... 33, 140, 178, 179, 184, 185, 193
93503 .... 176, 177, 185
93505 140
93563 .... 137, 140, 184
93564 .... 137, 140, 184
93565 .... 137, 140
93566 .... 135, 137, 140, 178, 179, 185, 193
93567 .... 137, 140
93568 .... 137, 140, 176, 177
93569 .... 137, 140
93571 .... 132, 159
93572 .... 132, 159
93573 .... 137, 140
93574 .... 137, 140
93575 .... 137, 140
93580 140
93581 140
93582 140
93583 140
93584 (new) 110, 136-140
93585 (new) 111, 136-140
93586 (new) 111, 136-140, 160
93587 (new) 111, 136-140
93588 (new) 111, 136-140
93590 140
93591 140
93593 .... 33, 136, 138, 140, 178, 179, 184, 185
93594 .... 33, 138, 140, 178, 179, 184, 185
93595 .... 140, 184
93596 .... 33, 136, 138, 140, 178, 179, 184, 185

93597 .... 33, 138, 140, 178, 179, 184, 185
93598 .... 139, 184
93620 140
93653 140
93654 140
93662 .... 140, 185
95251 266
95782 133
95783 .... 133, 141
95808 133
95810 133
95811 133
95836 197
95885 141
95886 141
95887 141
95905 141
95907 141
95908 141
95909 141
95910 141
95911 141
95912 141
95913 141
95957 197
95961 197
95965 197
95966 197
95970 .... 44, 45, 163, 174, 190
95971 .... 44, 45, 163, 174, 190
95972 .... 44, 45, 163, 174, 190
95976 .... 163, 174
95977 .... 163, 174
95980 39
95981 39
95982 39
95983 .... 163, 174
95984 .... 163, 174
95999 162
96116 192
96121 192
96360 4
96361 4
96365 114
96365-96372 113
96365-96375 122
96366 114

96367	114
96368	114
96369	114
96370	114
96371	114
96372	114, 126, 142
96374	114
96374-96375	113
96446 (revised)	111, 142, 143
96547 (new)	56, 111, 142, 143
96548 (new)	56, 111, 142, 143
96920 (revised)	111, 143
96921 (revised)	111, 143
96922 (revised)	111, 143
97014	144
97026	144
97032	144
97037 (new)	111, 144, 162, 163
97116	145, 175, 176
97151	192
97152	192
97153	192
97154	192
97155	192
97156	192
97157	192
97158	192
97550 (new)	111, 145, 146
97551 (new)	111, 145, 146
97552 (new)	111, 145-147
99188	176
99202 (revised)	5, 14, 15, 21, 22, 257
99203 (revised)	4, 5, 14, 15, 21, 22, 257
99204 (revised)	4, 5, 14, 15, 21, 22, 257
99205 (revised)	4, 5, 14, 15, 20-22, 257
99212 (revised)	4, 5, 14, 15, 21, 22, 257
99213 (revised)	4, 5, 14, 15, 21, 22, 257
99214 (revised)	4, 6, 14, 15, 21, 22, 257
99215 (revised)	4, 6, 14, 15, 20-22, 257
99221	15, 17, 18
99222	15, 17, 18
99223	15, 17, 18, 20
99231	15, 16
99232	15, 16
99233	15, 16, 20
99234	8, 17, 18
99235	8, 17, 18
99236	8, 17, 18, 20
99238	17, 18
99239	17, 18
99242-99245	22
99245	20
99255	20
99306	6, 20
99306 (revised)	18-21
99308 (revised)	6, 19, 257
99310	20
99345	20
99350	20
99358	20
99359	20
99381-99397	22
99383-99387	22
99393-99397	22
99415	192
99416	192
99417	13, 20, 21
99418	13, 20, 21
99453	22, 188
99454	22, 188
99459 (new)	6, 22
99483	20

Indexes

Index of Modifiers

The modifiers in this Index of Modifiers is limited to only the modifiers that appear in the Rationales and in the new or revised guidelines and/or parenthetical notes.

Modifier, Descriptor   Page Numbers

50, Bilateral Procedures 4, 29, 42

51, Multiple Procedures 122

52, Reduced Services 3–4, 31, 32, 198

59, Distinct Procedural Service 3, 4, 185

62, Two Surgeons 25, 26, 27

80, Assistant Surgeon 4

93, Synchronous Telemedicine Service Rendered Via Telephone or Other Real-Time Interactive Audio-Only Telecommunications System 2, 4, 267

95, Synchronous Telemedicine Service Rendered Via a Real-Time Interactive Audio and Video Telecommunications System 2, 4, 257

NOTES

NOTES

NOTES

NOTES